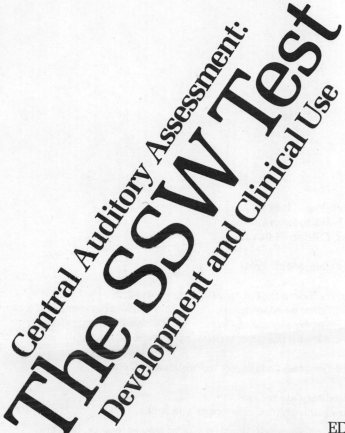

Central Auditory Assessment:
The SSW Test
Development and Clinical Use

EDITORS

DENNIS ARNST
V.A. Medical Center, San Francisco

JACK KATZ
State University of New York, Buffalo

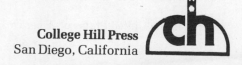

College Hill Press
San Diego, California

College-Hill Press, Inc.
4580-E Alvarado Canyon Road
San Diego, California 92120

Library of Congress Cataloging in Publication Data

Central auditory assessment.
    Includes bibliographic references and index.
    1. Staggered Spondaic Word Test—Addresses, essays, lectures.
    2. Auditory pathways—Diseases –Diagnosis—Addresses, essays,
lectures.
I. Arnst, Dennis
II. Katz, Jack
[DNLM: 1. Hearing tests. 2. Auditory diseases, Central—Complications.
WV 272 C3967]
RF294.5.S72C46   617.8'86075   81-17987

ISBN 0-933014-66-X   AACR2

Printed in the United States of America.

Dedication

To those researchers who made this book possible and to those who may be inspired to ask more questions.

Preface

In the 1950s Bocca and Calearo stressed the importance of specialized speech materials in identifying central auditory problems. They firmly pointed out that the pure tone played an ever-decreasing role in locating disorders higher in the auditory pathway. Since then the Staggered Spondaic Word (SSW) Test has emerged and has been used to evaluate auditory function from the cochlea to the cortex. It was based on a dichotic listening task involving partially overlapped, two-syllable words.

Since its inception in the early 1960s, the SSW Test has been shown to be sensitive to dysfunction at all levels of the central auditory nervous system. Although it began as a test for temporal lobe disorders, various clinical studies have shown it to be useful in identification of VIIIth nerve, brainstem, and cortical problems outside the temporal lobe as well.

The test has traveled the past 20 years with only minor modification. Its application has been expanded by the quantitative and qualitative evaluation of patient performance. In fact, coupled with other tests, its ability to detect central auditory disorders has been enhanced and expanded with age.

Two challenges have accompanied the SSW Test during its adolescence: (1) widespread and often difficult to locate literature, and (2) the need to study the test carefully, since results for specific problems do not emerge in mutually exclusive categories. The purpose of this book is directed toward the first problem in an attempt to help the reader solve the second. But, as with any effort to study or evaluate the many interconnections of the central nervous system, practice and experience remain to be elusive sisters not captured between the covers of any text.

The material in this book is divided into seven areas, each designed to contain information relevant for an in-depth understanding of the SSW Test. First, a brief overview of the test design and scoring procedure is provided for the reader who has not had the benefit of a workshop or practical experience. This overview also summarizes information for those who have practiced the SSW Test and have attended at least one SSW workshop. The following two sections deal with the development of the test and specific parameters which have been evaluated with respect to its administration. A section covering advanced use has been included to emphasize important aspects of the test which have appeared in various places. The last three sections provide literature dealing with specific types of patients—hearing loss and dialect, children, and adults.

Although this book is an attempt to compile information relating to the entire scope of the SSW Test, some significant contributions which have appeared as chapters in other books have not been included here. Only reference to these works is provided, since they tend to be easily available.

It is hoped that this collection of material stimulates thought and interest for it is the clinician who can make additional contributions to this intriguing area of audiology. As for the SSW Test, it is our hope that its adulthood is as exciting as its earlier years.

Dennis Arnst
Jack Katz

Acknowledgements

For permission to reprint the materials in this book the editors wish to thank each author and the following publishers and journal editors:

The Almqvist and Wiksell Periodical Company   For permission by the publisher and the authors to reproduce the following articles from *Scandinavian Audiology*: "Clinical validity of Central Auditory Tests" (1975) by J. Jerger and S. Jerger; Normal Adult performance on a Temporally Modified Staggered Spondaice Word Test" (1980) by M. L. Matthies and D. C. Garstecki.

Annals of Otology, Rhinology, and Laryngology   For permission granted by Ben H. Senturia, M.D., Editor and the authors to reproduce the following articles: "Staggered Spondaic Word Test: Support" (1971) by R. F. Balas; "A Staggered Spondaic Word Test for Detecting Central Auditory Lesions" (1963) by J. Katz, R. A. Basil, and J. M. Smith.

American Medical Association   For permission granted by the publisher and the authors to reproduce the following articles from *Archives of Otolaryngology*: "Reversible Neuro-audiologic Findings in a Case of Right Frontal Lobe Abscess with Recovery" (1980) by F. E. Musiek and E. Sachs; "Central Auditory Dysfunction Among Chronic Alcoholics" (1980) by J. B. Spitzer and I. M. Ventry.

American Speech-Language-Hearing Association   For permission granted by the publisher and authors to reproduce the following articles from the *Journal of Speech and Hearing Disorders*: "The SSW Test: An Interim Report" (1968) by J. Katz; "SSW and Dichotic Digit Results Pre- and Post-commissurotomy: A Case Report" (1979) by F. E. Musiek and D. H. Wilson; "Central Auditory Nervous System Dysfunction in Echolalic Autistic Children" (In Press) by A. Wetherby, R. Koegel, and M. Mendel. And the following articles from the *Journal of Speech and Hearing Research*: "Lead and Lag Effect Associated with the Staggered Spondaic Word Test" (1976) by B. Freeman and D. Beasley; "Central Auditory Function in Stutterers" (1978) by J. W. Hall and J. Jerger.

Cortex   For permission granted by E. Capitani, M.D., Managing Editor and the authors to reproduce the following article: "A Study of Three Tests of Central Function with Normal Hearing Subjects" (1968) by M. Brunt and C. P. Goetzinger.

Creative Age Publications   For permission granted by the publisher and the authors to reproduce the following articles from *Audiology and Hearing Education:* "The New SSW Test (List EE) and the CES Test" (1980) by D. W. Johnson and R. E. Sherman; "Diagnostic Significance of the Type A Pattern" (1980) by J. R. Lucker.

Journal of Auditory Research   For permission granted by J. D. Harris, Ph.D., Editor and the authors to reproduce the following articles: "The Articulation Function of a Staggered Spondaic Word List for a Normal Hearing Population" (1965) by R. F. Balas and G. R. Simon; "The Use of Staggered Spondaic Words for Assessing the Integrity of the Central Auditory Nervous System" (1962) by J. Katz; "The Hebrew Version of the Staggered Spondaic Word (SSW) Test" (1976) by B. Keydar and J. Katz; "Effects of Age and Sex on Dichotic Listening: The SSW Test" (1977) by C. McCoy, M. Butler, and J. Broekhoff; "The Effects of Practice on 8–10 Year Old Children Using the Staggered Spondaic Word Test" (1979) by S. B. Minetti and J. H. McCartney.

Journal of Otolaryngology   For permission granted by Peter Alberti, M.D., Editor and the authors to reproduce the following article: "Audiological Tests for Evaluation of Central Auditory Disorders" (1977) by R. G. Winkelaar and T. K. Lewis.

The Professional Press, Inc.   For permission granted by the publisher and the authors to reproduce the following article from the *Journal of Learning Disabilities:* "Central Auditory Dysfunction in Learning Disabled Children" (1975) by J. H. Stubblefield and C. E. Young.

The University of Nebraska Press   For permission granted by M. Sullivan, M.A., Editor and the authors to reproduce the following article from *Central Auditory Processing Disorders:* "New Developments in Differential Diagnosis Using the SSW Test" (1975) by J. Katz and G. Pack.

The Williams and Wilkins Company   For permission granted by the publisher and the authors to reproduce the following articles from *Ear and Hearing:* "The Staggered Spondaic Word Test: A Normative Investigation of Older Adults" (1980) by J. D. Amerman and

M. M. Parnell; "The Use of the Staggered Spondaic Word and Competing Environmental Sounds Tests in the Evaluation of Central Auditory Function of Learning Disabled Children" (1981) by D. W. Johnson, M. L. Enfield, and R. E. Sherman; "Errors on the Staggered Spondaic Word (SSW) Test in a Group of Adult Normal Listeners" (1981) by D. Arnst.

The Editors are also indebted to the support and encouragement of IRMA and CHARLENE.

Contributors

Dorothy (Haberkamp) Air, Ph.D.
University of Cincinnati
Division of Audiology and Speech
Pathology
Department of Otolaryngology and
Maxillofacial Surgery
Cincinnati, Ohio

James D. Amerman, Ph.D.
University of Missouri
Speech and Hearing Clinic
Columbia, Missouri

William B. Arndt, Ph.D.
University of Missouri
Department of Psychology
Kansas City, Missouri

Dennis J. Arnst, Ph.D.
Veterans Administration Medical
Center
San Francisco, California

Robert F. Balas, Ph.D.
University of Wisconsin, Stevens
Point
School of Communicative Disorders
Stevens Point, Wisconsin

Rocco A. Basil, M.A.
Private Practice
Wellsburg, West Virginia

Glen M. Baquet, M.S.
University of Alabama
Audiology Service
University, Alabama

Daniel S. Beasley, Ph.D.
Memphis State University
Speech and Hearing Center
Memphis, Tennessee

Jan Broekhoff, Ph.D.
University of Oregon
Speech Pathology and Audiology
College of Education
Eugene, Oregon

Michael A. Brunt, Ph.D.
Illinois State University
Department of Speech Pathology
and Audiology
Normal, Illinois

Stephanie Bryant (Minetti), M.A.
Private Practice
Professional Audiology
Sacramento, California

Myrtice Butler, Ph.D.
University of Oregon
Speech Pathology and Audiology
College of Education
Eugene, Oregon

Denise L. Cafarelli, M.S.
Cleveland Clinic Foundation
Department of Otolaryngology and
Communicative Disorders
Cleveland, Ohio

Mary Collard, M.A.
Cleveland Clinic Foundation
Department of Otolaryngology and
Communicative Disorders
Cleveland, Ohio

Janet L. Conant, M.A.
California State University,
Sacramento
Department of Speech Pathology and
Audiology
Sacramento, California

Philip C. Doyle,M.A.
University of California, Santa
Barbara
Speech and Hearing Center
Santa Barbara, California

Michael Dybka, Ph.D.
San Jose State University
Department of Special Education
Audiology and Speech Pathology
San Jose, California

Mary L. Enfield, Ph.D.
Bloomington Public Schools
Minneapolis, Minnesota

Ora Eschenheimer, M.S.
Mount Sinai Medical Center
New York, New York

Barry A. Freeman, Ph.D.
Private Practice
Memorial Hospital
Clarksville, Tennessee

Dean C. Garstecki, Ph.D.
Northwestern University
Department of Communicative
Disorders
Evanston, Illinois

Cornelius P. Goetzinger, Ph.D.
University of Kansas Medical Center
Audiology Clinic
Kansas City, Kansas

Sheila Goldman, M.S.
Casa Colina Hospital
Department of Speech Pathology
Pomona, California

James W. Hall, III, Ph.D.
University of Pennsylvania School of
Medicine
Department of Otorhinolaryngology
Human Communication
Philadelphia, Pennsylvania

Brenda K. Harder, M.A.
Arizona State University
Audiology Clinic
Tempe, Arizona

David Hicks, M.A.
Private Practice
East Bay Audiology and Speech
Pathology Services,Inc.
Berkeley, California

James Jerger, Ph.D.
Baylor College of Medicine and the
Methodist Hospital
Department of Otorhinolaryngology
and Communicative Sciences
Houston, Texas

Susan Jerger, M.S.
Baylor College of Medicine and the
Methodist Hospital
Department of Otorhinolaryngology
and Communicative Sciences
Houston, Texas

David W. Johnson, M.S., M.A.
University of Minnesota Medical
School
Minneapolis, Minnesota and
Department of Otolaryngology
Hennepin County Medical Center
Minneapolis, Minnesota

Jack Katz, Ph.D.
State University of New York
at Buffalo
Department of Communicative
Disorders and Sciences
Amherst, New York

Bilha Keydar, M.A.
ENT Department
Meir General Hospital
KFAR SAVA, Israel

Robert Koegel, Ph.D.
University of California, Santa
Barbara
Speech and Hearing Center
Santa Barbara, California

Deanie (Kushner) Vogel, Ph.D.
Audie Murphy Memorial Veterans
Hospital
San Antonio, Texas

Deborah A. Larkins, M.A.
Cleveland Clinic Foundation
Department of Otolaryngology and
Communicative Disorders
Cleveland, Ohio

Terry K. Lewis, M.A.
Saskatchewan Hearing Aid Plan
Saskatoon, Saskatchewan
Canada

Paul R. Lohnes, Ph.D.
State University of New York at
Buffalo
Department of Educational
Psychology
Amherst, New York

Julie Lukas, M.S.
Phoenix, Arizona

Jay R. Lucker, Ed.D.
Educational Audiologist
Greenburgh Central School
District #7
Hartsdale, New York

Melanie L. Matthies, M.A.
University of Illinois
Department of Speech and Hearing
Sciences
Champaign, Illinois

James H. McCartney, Ph.D.
California State University,
Sacramento
Department of Speech Pathology and
Audiology
Sacramento, California

Carolyn McCoy, Ph.D.
University of the Pacific
Department of Communicative
Disorders
Stockton, California

Maurice Mendel, Ph.D.
University of California, Santa
Barbara
Speech and Hearing Center
Santa Barbara, California

Frank Musiek, Ph.D.
Dartmouth Medical School
Section of Otorhinolaryngology and
Audiology
Dartmouth-Hitchcock Medical
Center
Hanover, New Hampshire

Dean Kent Myrick, M.S.
Speech and Language Pathology
Orleans Parish School District
New Orleans, Louisiana

Richard H. Nodar, Ph.D.
Cleveland Clinic Foundation
Department of Otolaryngology and
Communicative Disorders
Cleveland, Ohio

Gary Pack, M.D.
Menorah Medical Center
Department of Neurology
Kansas City, Missouri

Martha M. Parnell, Ph.D.
Speech and Hearing Services
Springfield Public Schools
Springfield, Missouri

Richard K. Peach, M.A.
Northwestern University
Department of Communicative
Disorders
Evanston, Illinois

Lynn (Price) McDonald, M.A.
Northern New Mexico Rehabilitation
Center
Department of Audiology
Las Vegas, New Mexico

Steven J. Rawiszer, M.A.
Hearing Conservation Specialist
State Department of Health Services
Maternal and Child Health Branch
Sacramento, California

Floyd Rudmin, M.S.
McGill University
Toronto, Canada

Ernest Sachs, Jr., M.D.
Dartmouth Medical School
Section of Neurosurgery
Dartmouth-Hitchcock Medical
Center
Hanover, New Hampshire

Frank E. Sansone, Ph.D.
Southern Connecticut State College
Audiology and Speech Pathology
New Haven, Connecticut

Robert E. Sherman, Ph.D.
Office of Planning and Development
Hennepin County Government
Center
Minneaplis, Minnesota

George R. Simon, Ph.D.
Veterans Administration Medical
Center
Denver, Colorado

Joen M. Smith, M.A.
Tulane University
New Orleans, Louisiana

Jaclyn B. Spitzer, Ph.D.
Veterans Administration Medical
Center
Cleveland, Ohio

James H. Stevens, Ph.D.
Bishop Clarkson Memorial Hospital
Otoneurologic Service
Omaha, Nebraska

James H. Stubblefield, Ph.D.
Northern Arizona University
Hearing Clinic
Flagstaff, Arizona

Martha Todebush, M.S.
Private Practice
Audiological Services of San
Francisco
San Francisco, California

Ira M. Ventry, Ph.D.
Teachers College
Columbia University
Department of Speech Pathology
and Audiology
New York, New York

Amy Wetherby, M.A.
University of California, San
Francisco
School of Medicine
Department of Otolaryngology
Speech Pathology and Audiology
San Francisco, California

Donald H. Wilson, M.D.
Dartmouth Medical School
Section of Neurosurgery
Dartmouth-Hitchcock Medical
Center
Hanover, New Hampshire

Richard G. Winkelaar, M.A.
Foothills Hospital
Audiology Department
Calgary, Alberta
Canada

C. Ellery Young, Ed.D.
Oregon College of Education
Speech Pathology and Audiology
Monmouth, Oregon

Introduction

To write this introduction I have reflected on the more than 20 years of the Staggered Spondaic Word (SSW) Test. The exercise has been both rewarding and interesting. I have tried to pick out important factors and events that have resulted in our present use and understanding of the procedure. When one considers our lack of knowledge at the time the SSW Test was conceived, it is surprising that the test contained the qualities to survive two decades of use. Its success can be traced to certain characteristics of the procedure as well as to some outside influences.

In the early 1960s, I (and most audiologists) understood little about brain and brainstem dysfunction, dichotic listening, and the broad implications of central auditory testing. We were intrigued that "temporal lobe tumors" produced an aberrant effect on certain speech tests and that it occurred in the ear opposite the lesion. It was also mystifying that the contralateral effect could be observed whether the lesion was on the left (language dominant) or right side. Despite our lack of sophistication, it is gratifying that subsequent research has not nullified most of our early concepts and observations. More recent findings tend to support, refine, clarify, and explain the original work. In part this is a tribute to the magnificent organization of the central nervous system (CNS).

Early research demonstrated the value of central auditory procedures, but the application of this information for clinical purposes was rather slow. So gradual has been the growth of interest that we still have not reached the pinnacle, some 25–30 years after the famous report by Bocca and his associates. Most of the hurdles that had discouraged audiologists from using central auditory nervous system (CANS) procedures have been eliminated or significantly reduced. Audiologists (a) were typically untrained in the anatomy and physiology of CANS; (b) had very little mention of these disorders in their class lectures and outside readings; (c) lacked practical clinical procedures with normative data; and (d) had no supervised testing experience.

To make the move toward central testing even less hospitable, there was little demand for audiologists to identify or to locate central auditory problems. In fact, quite to the contrary, many considered this change in orientation to be of questionable propriety. To alter the scope of audiology from the ear alone to an expansion encompassing the entire system was threatening to some. They felt that it might be outside of the legitimate province of the audiologist or that it would jeopardize our relationship with our otological colleagues. Many people wondered who would come to an audiologist for evaluation of CNS dysfunction when they could have an EEG, brain scan or arteriogram. Sometimes I hear the same concerns now with regard to Computerized Tomography (CT) and Positron Emission Tomography (PET) scans, but the referrals continue to increase as does our referral base.

We no longer hear concerns about propriety or hurting our relationship with other professionals. The American Speech, Language and Hearing (ASHA) and other groups have acknowledged our role in the evaluation of central auditory function. Over the years training institutions have done much to prepare their students for an expanded role in evaluating the auditory system. Graduate programs are placing increasing emphasis on the anatomy and physiology of CANS in their curricula. The evaluation of central function is often included when covering the audiological test battery. More and more institutions are offering courses dealing exclusively with central auditory disorders and tests. Currently, graduate programs are making an effort to provide central testing experiences for their students in audiology.

The work in acoustic reflex and Auditory Brainstem Response (ABR) testing has had a beneficial effect on the SSW and other behavioral procedures. The physiological methods have drawn the close attention of audiologists to the CNS. Thus, behavioral tests geared to the evaluation of the brainstem or even the brain have become more appropriate and necessary.

Audiologists have done much to "retool" themselves even though central disorders were not covered in their graduate training. They have many sources of information to prepare themselves in the evaluation of central auditory function. There has been a considerable growth in the number of articles, papers, and seminars devoted to CANS. We hope that this book will help both students and professionals already working in the field to gain a wealth of information about at least one test.

As audiologists have become more involved in central auditory evaluations, there has been reciprocal interest by other professions and the public at large. Most audiologists have a ready market for their services by the time they are ready to provide them. Others must call attention to the service and do some preliminary education. Otologists and neurologists have simply expanded the types of referrals that they had made in the past. Also, audiologists with a broader view of auditory disorders are now more likely to employ a central component in their test battery when they see patients for whom the peripheral evaluation has not sufficed. The responsiveness of the medical community has been fostered not only because we have demonstrated our capabilities in evaluating central disorders, but also because of the reports appearing in their own journals. Often it has been because of the encouragement of our professional colleagues that audiologists have sought further training.

Speech–language pathologists, school personnel, and others have been clamoring for help with the communicatively handicapped and with learning disabled children. Professionals who work with such children have long realized that a large percentage of them have significant auditory processing deficits. These children frequently do not hear their own speech errors, cannot differentiate similar sounds, have difficulty learning phonics, or cannot understand what is said when there is background noise present. When professionals referred these children to an audiologist or a physician for evaluation, they were told in many cases that hearing was essentially normal. Since the auditory problem could not be attributed to a peripheral hearing loss, it was logical that the professionals concluded the difficulty to be in auditory perception. The audiologist may be surprised to find that by the time he is ready to test, counsel, and provide other services to the communicatively and learning disabled that he has an eager and waiting population with which to work.

From a professional point of view the audiologist is now in a good position to assemble a battery of central auditory tests. Presently, there is an array of auditory procedures to evaluate: (a) brain disorders in adults, (b) brainstem dysfunction, and (c) central auditory functions in children with learning and communication problems. The SSW Test has made a significant contribution in each of these three areas.

It is safe to say that the SSW Test has influenced the development of central auditory evaluation and has been influenced by it in return. It was one of the earliest procedures used in the United States and continues to be an important instrument for measuring central dysfunction. Unlike most audiologic procedures, the SSW was slow to be widely accepted and understood but its use by audiologists and other professionals has grown steadily. The greatest burgeoning of interest has occurred over the past five years. The test seems to contain many of the important characteristics necessary in meeting our present diagnostic and remediation needs. As you learn more about it, you may find that it has many facets that are not widely used but have great implications for the future.

The SSW Test sprang up in a moment of inspiration one day in August 1960. Since then it has been studied by a large number of researchers and clinicians. The new information has led to a series of refinements and expansions which have added importantly to our original conceptions. Many articles and chapters have been written about the test, making it the most studied central auditory procedure. It has become the subject of many Master's theses and doctoral dissertations and the number of reports on it at conferences and symposia have increased dramatically in recent years. I have given 80 SSW workshops in the past 15 years and believe that these three-day intensive programs are the most effective way of mastering the test.

One of the strengths of the SSW Test is that it is a multidimensional procedure. It contains various component parts and can be viewed across selected parameters. In this sense the SSW is a battery of central subtests, some of which tap overlapping functions while others challenge unique processes. The various types of SSW scores and response biases will be covered in this book.

The SSW Test should not stand alone. Rather, it is to be given as part of a larger audiologic battery of standard and special tests. It is not possible to differentiate a central problem from a peripheral one if the raw SSW is viewed in isolation. Central problems may compound the dysfunction that is associated with peripheral loss and vice versa. Therefore, it is necessary to evaluate both systems in order to understand the auditory problem. There is far too much overlap and mutual interdependence between the peripheral and central auditory systems to completely ignore one of them.

Audiologists not only compare the SSW with peripheral tests but also to other central procedures. This gives the tester confidence when different tests support one another. Unique information from some of the special features of the methods can also be obtained. Recently, the SSW has been compared with another central test, the Competing Environmental Sound (CES) Test. CES was developed specifically as a companion procedure to the SSW. Like the SSW, it is a dichotic procedure, but the competing sound signals are, for example, music and the slamming of a door. Similarities and differences between the tests can provide localizing information that is not obtainable from either procedure alone. CES is still an experimental approach but it appears to contain useful information.

During the early phases of the SSW we had no conception of the test's potential, no idea what was important, nor to a great extent what it was we were testing. We understood that temporal lobe tumors could be located with the use of "sensitized" speech tests (e.g., filtered speech or binaural integration tasks), but had no assurance that a binaural separation test would be an appropriate challenge to higher cortical functions (especially if the disorder was not associated with a tumor). I was not aware of the dichotic work going on at the same time in Germany and Canada. After recording the original SSW tape, I was quite concerned that the test would not be an effective challenge to anyone because it was so easy. The "easiness" feature is one of the important attributes of the test. I associate the value and success of the SSW with several factors: (a) very good fortune; (b) ease and simplicity; (c) binaural competition and complexity; (d) counterbalancing; and (e) longevity.

The SSW Test has benefited abundantly from good luck. For example, it was fortuitous that the staggered spondaic words were roughly comparable in intelligibility to W-22 words for patients with peripheral losses. We did not foresee this, but were quick to take advantage of it. This fortunate coincidence permits us to utilize the SSW Test with patients who have hearing losses. The subsequent corrections of the SSW scores then led to other important contributions, such as distinguishing between inferior and superior brainstem disorders.

It was indeed good fortune to learn critical information at critical times. Dr. William Hardy, who was a site visitor on a research grant application, told me that I would not learn much about the SSW Test if I simply tested a large group of right and left hemisphere patients as I had planned. He suggested that I test a small group of patients who had small and well localized lesions to learn what the test was telling us. This advice was extremely important to the life and usefulness of the test. It is likely that I would have given up in hopeless confusion had I proceeded with the crude evaluation of large groups at the outset. I did not realize that SSW Test performance varies considerably from one region to the next in the same hemisphere. Therefore, there would have seen a lack of consistency within the hemisphere groups and considerable overlap in performance of right and left hemisphere cases. With patients having large lesions to the CNS, the specific clues that suggest certain loci of dysfunction would not have been uncovered.

I was very lucky that Dr. Arthur Epstein (Tulane School of Medicine) volunteered to be the neurological consultant for an early SSW study. His insights helped dispel the notion that the SSW is a *temporal lobe* test. He found the test was not specifically sensitive to disorders of the temporal lobe, but rather to the auditory reception region (Heschl's Gyrus). He pointed out that those cases showing the large peaks of errors in the ear contralateral to the brain lesion were the ones that had auditory reception involvement. Thus, from 1964 on we studied brain dysfunction as involving either auditory reception or nonauditory reception. While other CANS tests might indeed tap temporal lobe function as a whole, the SSW Test has different signs for the anterior and posterior regions.

The SSW is an easy test to take, especially if you have a normal CANS. Sometimes the listener is not aware that the competing words overlap in time. A number of factors contribute to the ease of the procedure. The test is made up of familiar spondaic words (the component monosyllables have a high frequency of usage in English). The words are spoken slowly, distinctly, and at a comfortable listening level (50 dB SL). Part of the simplicity lies in the fact that the listener need only remember two (albeit compound) words. The feature of brevity is also deserving of mention. The test tape runs 7½ minutes, but in routine cases the testing and scoring take 10–15 minutes. Because of the ease and simplicity, the SSW test can be used with many populations including children, mentally handicapped, and hard of hearing individuals.

While there is no major challenge from the acoustics of the SSW nor the type of speech material, the demands on the CNS come from the binaural competition and the complexities of the test. By demanding simultaneous information presented to the two ears, a considerable challenge is placed on CANS. In addition, there are noncompeting words that the listener must deal with in each ear. A pause between the two connected monosyllables creates somewhat of a memory factor for some pathological cases. It is perhaps because of the binaural presentation and the complexity of the task that we see peculiar types of responses on the SSW. No doubt the word reversals that we see in the test responses can be attributed to this challenge.

Counterbalancing is another intrinsic characteristic of the test. The counterbalancing of odd and even numbered items turned out to be quite valuable. Half of the items begin with the first monosysllable to the right ear (right-ear-first) and half start with the first word to the left ear (left-ear-first). When deciding to counterbalance the items, I had no reason to believe that some people would actually perform differently on those two halves of the test. But that's exactly what happened. This provides us with localizing information when seen in brain lesion cases. These response biases seem to provide processing pattern information in learning disabled children.

The counterbalancing also permits us to compare performance on the first spondees versus the second spondees without regard to the ear making the error. Thus, we can look at what might be considered a memory factor by seeing the number of errors on the first word (half of the first words were to the right and half to the left), the second word, and so on. A third type of response bias that can be obtained because of the counterbalancing is the Type A pattern. This will be discussed in some detail in this text. Response bias is one of the unique contributions of the SSW Test. It can tap functions that are far removed from what we consider the auditory cortex and even beyond the temporal lobe itself.

While longevity is not an internal characteristic of the SSW Test, it is, nevertheless, an important one. The longer the existence of a test, the more time one has to work out the bugs and to discover its strengths.

Fortunately, the growth of interest in the test was slow. This permitted early researchers and clinicians plenty of time to understand it and work out the corrections, rules, and localizing signs.

There is already a large compendium of information about the SSW Test, but there remains much to be worked out. The strong evidence of the test's effectiveness makes it even more valuable to refine, clarify or expand. Other important SSW findings need to be replicated. Audiologists have thus far put the test to excellent use. Speech–language pathologists and psychologists have also found important applications for it in their own work.

I am pleased how often the SSW Test seems to seek out important and sometimes elusive information. One cannot help but be impressed how it goes about unobtrusively gathering clues, up to the last item. When the test is scored, it is ready to turn over all of its valuable finds. Of course, like every test, this procedure has its shortcomings and problems. To learn what is presently known about the test one must invest time and thought. Just like the genie of old, the SSW Test will only serve fully those who have mastered it.

Jack Katz

Contents

3 Acoustic and Psychoacoustic Factors

6 Use of the Staggered Spondaic Word Test and Competing Environmental Sounds Test with Children

7 Use of the Staggered Spondaic Word Test with Adult Populations

Although the Staggered Spondaic Word (SSW) Test is relatively short (40 items administered in approximately 10 minutes), it contains much valuable information related to processing in the entire auditory system—the peripheral mechanism, the subcortical pathways, and the cortex. As a result, it can be used to understand many types of disorders in many types of populations. The SSW is part of a test battery and should not be used in isolation. Moreover, the complexity of the many interconnections within the central auditory nervous system should be kept in mind as results are being evaluated.

This Overview has been written for readers with varying amounts of background with the SSW Test. For those who have plunged in and weathered at least one SSW workshop and have several test administrations "under their belts," this chapter should be a summary. For those who are still testing the waters and have little or no experience with the SSW Test, this chapter should serve as an organizational framework for exploring the many dimensions involved in the test and the system it taps.

Test Paradigm

The SSW Test is a dichotic listening task involving two spondee words partially overlapped in time. It is often referred to as a "double simultaneous stimulation test"—both ears receive different words at approximately the same time. The

1

Overview of the Staggered Spondaic Word Test and the Competing Environmental Sounds Test

Dennis Arnst

FIGURE 1.

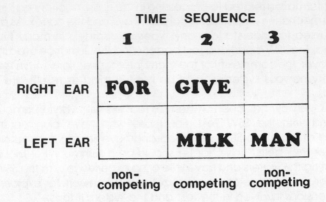

task of the patient is to repeat the entire set of words as it is presented. In order to offset the right ear advantage effect which is inherent in dichotic stimulation tasks, the spondee words on the SSW Test have been overlapped only partially. As can be seen in Figure 1, the first spondee is presented to one ear while the second spondee is presented to the other ear with a slight delay. Consequently, the first spondee leads the second. This arrangement of words introduces competing and noncompeting items for both the right and left ears.

During the test, word pairs are alternated between ears. First one ear receives the leading spondee, and on the next itme the other ear receives it. This alternating sequence provides counterbalancing for presentation of the test items as shown in Figure 2. When the word pair sequence is started in the right ear, it is referred to as the **right-ear-first** or **REF condition**. When started in the left ear, the sequence is referred to as the **left-ear-first** or **LEF** condition. Even-numbered items on the SSW Test are presented to one ear first (e.g., right ear) while the odd-numbered items are presented to the other ear first. Beginning the test in the right ear or the left ear has no effect on results; however, it is important to record this information to avoid reversing results and invalidating the interpretation.

Background Information

Test equipment and set-up

The equipment required to administer the SSW Test includes the following:

    a. Dual-channel audiometer
    b. Compatible, dual-channel tape recorder/player
    c. SSW/CES tapes
    d. Test forms

FIGURE 2.

SSW TEST: TIME SEQUENCE

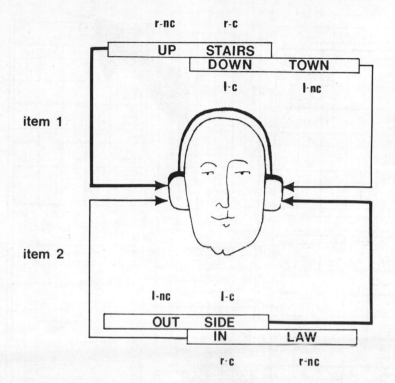

Before administering the SSW Test, five preliminary steps should be carried out:

1. Calibrate the tape with the VU meter.
2. Select REF or LEF conditions and indicate the choice on the score sheet (see Figure 3).
3. Listen to the tape under earphones to verify that the ear choice coincides with the output.
4. Complete the pure tone and speech audiometry summary section on the score sheet (see Figure 3).
5. Mark out inappropriate REF/LEF condition on page two and three of score sheet (see Figure 4).

These steps will help insure that the test is being presented in the prescribed manner.

FIGURE 3.

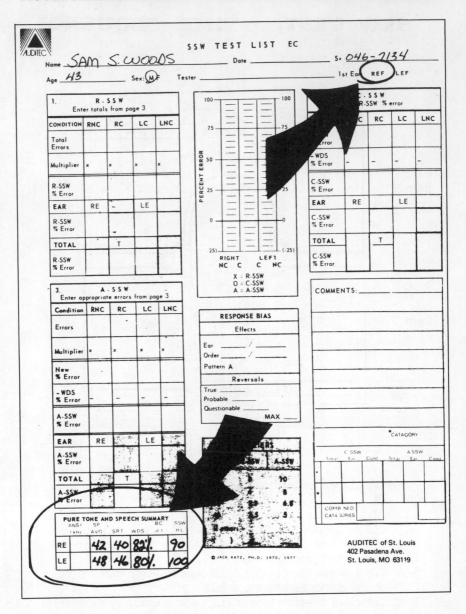

Overview of the SSW Test and CES Test

FIGURE 4.

Top of Page 2

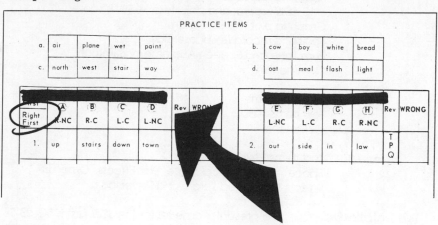

PRACTICE ITEMS

a.	air	plane	wet	paint

b.	cow	boy	white	bread

c.	north	west	stair	way

d.	oat	meal	flash	light

First Right First	(A) R-NC	(B) R-C	(C) L-C	(D) L-NC	Rev	WRONG
1.	up	stairs	down	town		

	(E) L-NC	(F) L-C	(G) R-C	(H) R-NC	Rev	WRONG
2.	out	side	in	law	T P Q	

Bottom of Page 3

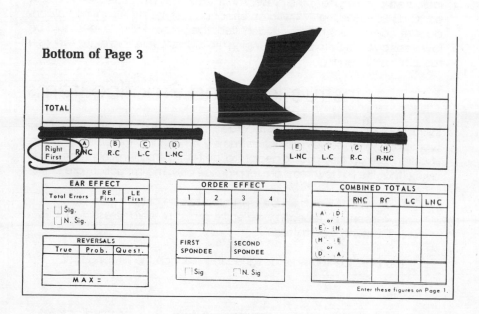

TOTAL									
Right First	(A) R-NC	(B) R-C	(C) L-C	(D) L-NC			(E) L-NC	(F) L-C	(G) R-C	(H) R-NC

EAR EFFECT			
Total Errors	RE First	LE First	
☐ Sig.			
☐ N. Sig.			

ORDER EFFECT			
1	2	3	4

FIRST SPONDEE		SECOND SPONDEE	
☐ Sig		☐ N. Sig	

COMBINED TOTALS			
	RNC	RC	LC	LNC
(A) (D) or (E) (H)			
(H) (E) or (D) (A)			

REVERSALS		
True	Prob.	Quest.

MAX =

Enter these figures on Page 1.

Dennis Arnst

5

The Response Form consists of the following:

Page 1   Patient identification
           Space to calculate raw (R-SSW) score, corrected
             (C-SSW) score, and adjusted (A-SSW) score
           Graph to plot the SSW-gram
           Space to record Response Bias
           Pure Tone and Speech Audiometry Summary
           Comments

Page 2   Practice items
           Test items 1–20
           Comments

Page 3   Test items 21–40
           Space to record/calculate Ear Effects, Order Ef-
             fects, Combined Totals, and Reversals

Presentation level.   The presentation level for the SSW Test is 50 dB-SL
re: the **three frequency pure tone average** (PTA). If tolerance problems are
indicated by the patient, the presentation level may be decreased to as low
as 30 dB-SL regarding PTA with no effect on test results. Also, when a conductive component has been identified, the presentation level should be
lowered to 30 dB-SL to avoid changing the dichotic task to a diotic task as a
result of cross-hearing.

Instructions and Practice Items

Instructions for the SSW Test are recorded on tape and are followed by four
word pairs, which serve as practice items. It is helpful to the patient if the instructions are outlined prior to beginning the test. The patient should be made
aware that the first few items are for practice only. The instructions are simple:

1. Groups of words will be presented to one or both ears.
2. Respond by repeating the entire group of words presented.
3. Guessing is permitted.

The practice items are designed to introduce the listening task.

Assuming a REF presentation, the practice items are presented as follows:

a) airplane   right ear
    wet paint   right ear

b) cowboy   left ear
    white bread   left ear

Overview of the SSW Test and CES Test

| c) northwest | right ear |
| stairway | left ear (not overlapped) |

| d) oatmeal | left ear |
| flash light | right ear (not overlapped) |

These practice items are designed to orient the patient to the fact that words will be presented to one or both ears. Test items 1 and 2 (upstairs–downtown; outside–inlaw, respectively) contain the easiest word pairs on the test.

Recording Patient Responses
Errors

The Response Form has all the word pairs arranged in sequence by monosyllable for each spondee word. A space to total the number of errors is provided to the right of each item (see Figure 5). Recording the responses of the patient is accomplished with a set of symbols which will permit a replication of the person's response to the stimulus. If all monosyllables are repeated accurately, nothing is marked on the test items, but a dot (•) is placed in the error column. If any of the monosyllables are repeated incorrectly, a horizontal line is drawn through the word(s) with the error. The type of error is also indicated above the incorrect response. The scoring symbols used to record the patient's incorrect responses are shown in Figure 6 and are summarized below:

Item	Error	Symbol
1	none	DOT in the error column
2	omission	line through the incorrect word; DASH above error
3	substitution	line through the incorrect word; substituted WORD above error
4	distortion	line through the incorrect word; error written in PHONETICS above error
5	"Don't Know"	line through the incorrect word; "DK" written above error

These symbols are used as the patient repeats each of the test items. As soon as the word pair has been scored, the total number of errors is indicated in the Error Column (see Figure 6). Omissions, substitutions, distortions, and "DKs" are the **only four errors** recorded on the SSW Test.

Response Form.   The form used to record the patient's responses has been prepared as follows (see Figure 5):

FIGURE 5.

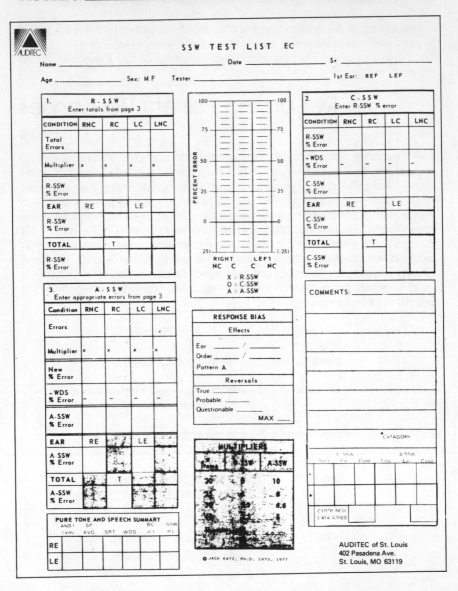

Overview of the SSW Test and CES Test

PRACTICE ITEMS

a.	air	plane	wet	paint
c.	north	west	stair	way

b.	cow	boy	white	bread
d.	oat	meal	flash	light

Left First / Right First	L-NC (A) / R-NC	L-C (B) / R-C	R-C C / L-C	R-NC D / L-NC	Rev	WRONG
1.	up	stairs	down	town	T P Q	
3.	day	light	lunch	time	T P Q	
5.	corn	bread	oat	meal	T P Q	
7.	flood	gate	flash	light	T P Q	
9.	meat	sauce	base	ball	T P Q	
11.	house	fly	wood	work	T P Q	
13.	sun	day	shoe	shine	T P Q	
15.	back	door	play	ground	T P Q	
17.	snow	white	foot	hall	T P Q	
19.	blue	jay	black	bird	T P Q	
SUM						

	R-NC E / L-NC	R-C F / L-C	L-C G / R-C	L-NC H / R-NC	Rev	WRONG
2.	out	side	in	law	T P Q	
4.	wash	tub	black	board	T P Q	
6.	bed	spread	mush	room	T P Q	
8.	sea	shore	out	side	T P Q	
10.	black	board	air	mail	T P Q	
12.	green	bean	home	land	T P Q	
14.	white	walls	dog	house	T P Q	
16.	school	boy	church	bell	T P Q	
18.	band	saw	first	aid	T P Q	
20.	ice	land	sweet	cream	T P Q	
SUM						

COMMENTS: _____

_____

_____

_____

_____

Dennis Arnst

PAGE 3

	A	B	C	D	Rev	WRONG		E	F	G	H	Rev	WRONG
21.	hair	net	tooth	brush	T P Q		22.	fruit	juice	cup	cake	T P Q	
23.	ash	tray	tin	can	T P Q		24.	nite	light	yard	stick	T P Q	
25.	key	chain	suit	case	T P Q		26.	pluy	ground	bat	boy	T P Q	
27.	corn	starch	soap	flakes	T P Q		28.	birth	day	first	place	T P Q	
29.	day	break	lamp	light	T P Q		30.	door	knob	cow	bell	T P Q	
31.	bird	cage	crow's	nest	T P Q		32.	week	end	work	day	T P Q	
33.	book	shelf	drug	store	T P Q		34.	wood	work	beach	craft	T P Q	
35.	hand	ball	milk	shake	T P Q		36.	fish	net	sky	line	T P Q	
37.	for	give	milk	man	T P Q		38.	sheep	skin	bull	dog	T P Q	
39.	race	horse	street	car	T P Q		40.	green	house	string	bean	T P Q	
SUM Page 3							SUM Page 3						
SUM Page 2							SUM Page 2						
TOTAL							TOTAL						

Left First	L-NC (A)	L-C B	R-C C	R-NC (D)				R-NC (E)	R-C (F)	L-C (G)	L-NC (H)		
Right First	R-NC	R-C	L-C	L-NC				L-NC	L-C	R-C	R-NC		

EAR EFFECT				ORDER EFFECT					COMBINED TOTALS				
Total Errors	RE First	LE First		1	2	3	4			RNC	RC	LC	LNC
☐ Sig. ☐ N. Sig.									A-(D or E-(H				
REVERSALS				FIRST SPONDEE		SECOND SPONDEE			H-E or (D-A				
True	Prob.	Quest.											
MAX =				☐ Sig ☐ N. Sig					Enter these figures on Page 1.				

Overview of the SSW Test and CES Test

FIGURE 6.

PRACTICE ITEMS

a.	air	plane	wet	paint
c.	north	west	stair	way

b.	cow	boy	white	bread
d.	oat	meal	flash	light

Left First	L-NC	L-C	R-C	R-NC		
Right First	Ⓐ R-NC	Ⓑ R-C	Ⓒ L-C	Ⓓ L-NC	Rev	WRONG
1.	up	stairs	down	town	T P Q	●
3.	day	light	day ~~lunch~~	time	T P Q	/
5.	corn	dK ~~bread~~	oat	meal	T P Q	/

	R-NC	R-C	L-C	L-NC		
	E L-NC	F L-C	G R-C	H R-NC	Rev	WRONG
2.	out	side	~~in~~ —	law	T P Q	/
4.	wash	t⌐ᴈ	black	board	T P Q	/
6.	bed	spread	mush	room	T P Q	●

Word Sequence Changes.

The sequence in which the word pair is repeated is also important. Although it is not counted as an error, the way in which the patient changed the sequence of the test item needs to be represented. The order in which each monosyllable is repeated is indicated by numbering 1–4. If the sequence is correct as presented, no numbering is required (see Figure 7).

FIGURE 7.

PRACTICE ITEMS

a.	air	plane	wet	paint
c.	north	west	stair	way

b.	cow	boy	white	bread
d.	oat	meal	flash	light

Left First	L-NC	L-C	R-C	R-NC		
Right First	Ⓐ R-NC	Ⓑ R-C	Ⓒ L-C	Ⓓ L-NC	Rev	WRONG
1.	up	~~stairs~~ —	down	town	T P Q	/
3.	day 3	time ~~light~~ 4	lunch 1	time 2	Ⓣ P Q	/

	R-NC	R-C	L-C	L-NC		
	E L-NC	F L-C	G R-C	H R-NC	Rev	WRONG
2.	out 1	side 4	in 3	law 2	Ⓣ P Q	●
4.	wash 2	cloth ~~tub~~ 3	black 1	~~board~~ — 4	T P Q	2

Item 1 shows an omission but no sequence change. Item 2 shows no errors were made on the monosyllables, but the sequence was changed. Item 3 shows a substitution error and a sequence change. Item 4 shows an omission, a substitution, and a sequence change. In all these examples, the order of repetition is indicated by numbers below the monosyllable.

Whenever the word sequence has been changed and no more than one error has been made, the rearrangement of the sequence is known as a **reversal.** Items 2 and 3 are reversals; because item 4 contains **two** errors, it is not. Reversals are indicated in the REV box at the left of the error column (see Figure 7).

Several other symbols have been developed to reflect the patient's response pattern during the test. These are summarized in Table 1 along with each of the other symbols discussed in this section. A complete review of the response symbols is also provided in the **SSW Workshop Manual.**

Scoring: Tallying Responses

SSW scores are based on the number of errors. A **quantitative** evaluation of the patient's performance is made by evaluating the errors in each of the the listening conditions–right noncompeting (RNC), right competing (RC), left competing (LC), and left noncompeting (LNC). Errors are totaled for each of the listening conditions for both REF and LEF presentations. The Response Form provides space to calculate the total errors (see Figure 5).

A **qualitative** evaluation of the patient's performance is also made, based on the total errors in the (a) REF versus LEF listening conditions, (b) the first spondee versus second spondee presentation, and (c) by changing the word sequence (reversals). Collectively, these three types of errors are known as **response bias.** Space for tallying these errors is also provided on the Response Form.

Eight Cardinal Numbers

The total numbers of errors made in each of the listening conditions REF and LEF are known as the **eight cardinal numbers**. These numbers can be found on page 3 of the Response Form (see Figure 8).

Columns A–D represent errors in the four listening conditions presented REF; columns E–H represent errors in the listening conditions presented LEF. All other scores on the SSW Test can be determined with these eight numbers. It is often helpful to preserve the eight cardinal numbers for future reference when reporting test results. Note that columns E–H represent the listening conditions in reverse order compared to A–D. The order change is due to the REF/LEF presentation randomization as shown in Figure 8.

Combined Totals

In order to obtain the total number of errors in each listening condition, the

TABLE 1.
SSW Scoring Symbols

	Response	Marking
1.	No error on any word	Dot (·) in error column
2.	All mistakes (except word order)	Draw a horizontal line *through* word
3.	Word omission	Dash *above* word omitted
4.	Substitution	Write in substitution *above* stimulus word
5.	Distortion	Write in distortion *above* stimulus word
6.	Patient indicates the presence of a word but cannot repeat the stimulus	Enter DK *above* stimulus word
7.	Addition or omission of a final *s*	No error; diagonal mark (/) through sound omitted or at place were sound added
8.	Different word order	No error; enter numbers (1–2–3–4) indicating order in which patient repeated stimuli *below* stimulus words
9.	Reversal	No error; abnormal word sequence and no more than one error in the stimulus sequence; indicate reversal in REV column on score sheet
10.	Intrusive word (patient adds extra word to stimulus sequence	No error; insert a caret where the word was added and write word *above* symbol (e.g., "cat")
11.	Need to replay stimulus item	No error; enter R in stimulus I.D. number box
12.	Fast start; quick response	No error; enter Q in stimulus I.D. number box
13.	Delay in response	No Error; insert X to indicate where delay occurred
	If item was scored incorrectly,	circle the word and indicate "OK."

FIGURE 8.

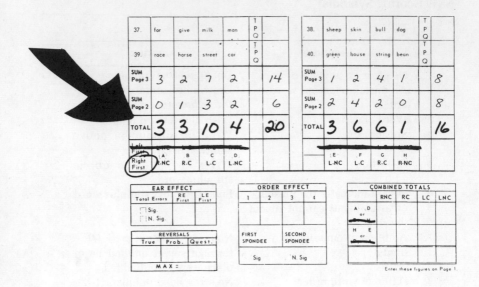

37.	for	give	milk	man	T P Q		38.	sheep	skin	bull	dog	T P Q
39.	race	horse	street	car	T P Q		40.	green	house	string	bean	T P Q
SUM Page 3	3	2	7	2	14		SUM Page 3	1	2	4	1	8
SUM Page 2	0	1	3	2	6		SUM Page 2	2	4	2	0	8
TOTAL	3	3	10	4	20		TOTAL	3	6	6	1	16

| Left First | A R-NC | B R-C | C L-C | D L-NC | | E L-NC | F L-C | G R-C | H R-NC |
| Right First | | | | | | | | | |

EAR EFFECT				ORDER EFFECT				COMBINED TOTALS				
Total Errors	RE First	LE First		1	2	3	4		RNC	RC	LC	LNC
☐ Sig. ☐ N. Sig.								A D or				
REVERSALS				FIRST SPONDEE		SECOND SPONDEE		H E or				
True	Prob.	Quest.										
MAX =				Sig		N. Sig		Enter these figures on Page 1.				

FIGURE 9.

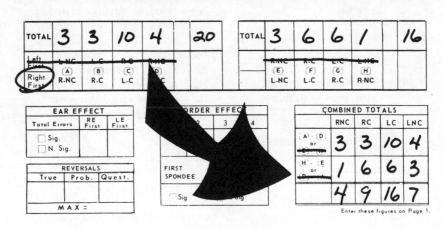

TOTAL	3	3	10	4	20		TOTAL	3	6	6	1	16
Left First	L-NC	L-C	R-C	R-NC			R-NC	R-C	L-C	L-NC	
Right First	A R-NC	B R-C	C L-C	D L-NC			E L-NC	F L-C	G R-C	H R-NC	

EAR EFFECT				ORDER EFFECT				COMBINED TOTALS				
Total Errors	RE First	LE First				3	4		RNC	RC	LC	LNC
☐ Sig. ☐ N. Sig.								A (D) or	3	3	10	4
REVERSALS				FIRST SPONDEE				H E or	1	6	6	3
True	Prob.	Quest.							4	9	16	7
MAX =				☐ Sig				Enter these figures on Page 1.				

eight cardinal numbers need to be arranged so all errors in the RNC, RC, LC, and LNC can be combined. Space is provided on page 3 of the Response Form for this purpose (see Figure 9).

Note that the first row contains the errors from columns A–D and the second row contains the errors from the columns H–E **in that order**. It is necessary to rearrange the last four cardinal numbers so each listening condition can be tallied. If this change were omitted, RNC errors from the REF half of the test

Overview of the SSW Test and CES Test

FIGURE 10.

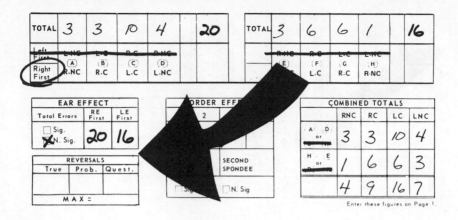

would be added with the LNC errors from the LEF half of the test. The net effect would be to miscalculate the errors and consequently, misinterpret the results.

Response Bias: Ear Effect

Response Bias is based on the **type** of errors made on the SSW Test. **Ear effects** reflect the errors made in the REF versus LEF conditions. The total errors in columns A–D are the REF errors; errors in columns E–H are the LEF errors. Significant ear effects are obtained when the difference between REF and LEF is greater than or equal to five (see Figure 10).

Reponse Bias: Order Effect

Order effects are based on the number of errors on the first spondee versus the second spondee. The total errors in columns A, B, E, and F are first spondee errors; errors in columns C, D, G, and H are second spondee errors. Significant order effects are obtained when the difference between first and second spondee errors is greater than or equal to five (see Figure 11).

Response Bias: Reversals

Reversals represent changes in the word pair sequence made by the patient. The total number of test items for which the sequence was changed is reported as reversals. Any item with two or more errors (i.e., omission, substitution, distortion, or **dk**) despite a sequence change, **cannot** be counted as a reversal. Although some early attempts were made to categorize the type of reversal (i.e., true, partial, questionable), current practice has found that ap-

FIGURE 11.

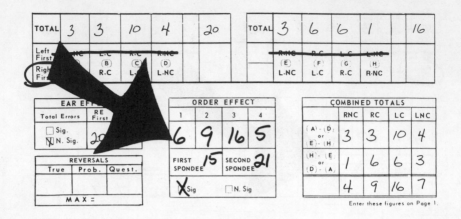

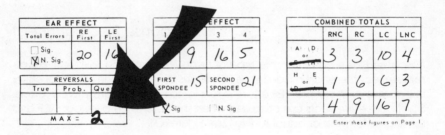

FIGURE 12.

proach unnecessary. Changes in word sequence are now identified solely as "reversals" (see Figure 12).

Scoring: Calculating SSW Scores

Raw (R-SSW) Scores

The **raw** SSW score, or R-SSW, represents the percent error for each of the listening conditions (RNC, RC, LC, LNC) based on the Combined Totals determined on page 3 of the Response Form (lower right-hand corner). Each of the values is transferred to the R-SSW Calculation Block on the front page of the Response Form (upper left-hand corner) in the appropriate space for each listening condition (see Figure 13).

FIGURE 13.

COMBINED TOTALS				
	RNC	RC	LC	LNC
(A) - (D) or (F) - (C)	3	3	10	4
(H) - (E) or (B) - (C)	1	6	6	3
		4	9	16	7

Enter these figures on Page 1.

1.	R - S S W Enter totals from page 3			
CONDITION	RNC	RC	LC	LNC
Total Errors	4	9	16	7
Multiplier	x	x	x	x
R-SSW % Error				
EAR	RE		LE	
R-SSW % Error				
TOTAL		T		
R-SSW % Error				

To determine the percent error score, each total score is multiplied by 2.5 (i.e., 40 items x 2.5 = 100%). (A convenient multiplication table is provided in the **SSW Workshop Manual.**) Rounding is permissible to the nearest even number to eliminate the decimal. Once the percentage scores have been calculated for each of the four listening conditions, the two right-ear conditions are averaged for the **right ear R-SSW score.** The same procedure is followed for the two left-ear conditions. Right and left EAR scores are then averaged for the **total R-SSW score** (see Figure 14).

FIGURE 14.

1.	R - S S W Enter totals from page 3			
CONDITION	RNC	RC	LC	LNC
Total Errors	4	9	16	7
Multiplier	x25	x25	x25	x25
R-SSW % Error	10	22	40	18
EAR	RE		LE	
R-SSW % Error	16		29	
TOTAL		T		
R-SSW % Error		22		

FIGURE 15.

1.	R - S S W Enter totals from page 3			
CONDITION	RNC	RC	LC	LNC
Total Errors	4	9	16	7
Multiplier	×.25	×.25	×.25	×.25
R-SSW % Error	10	22	40	18
EAR	RE		LE	
R-SSW % Error	16		29	
TOTAL		T		
R-SSW % Error		22		

2.	C - S S W Enter R-SSW % error			
CONDITION	RNC	RC	LC	LNC
R-SSW % Error	10	22	40	18
- WDS % Error	-	-	-	-
C-SSW % Error				
EAR	RE		LE	
C-SSW % Error				
TOTAL		T		
C-SSW % Error				

Corrected (C-SSW) Scores

The **corrected** SSW scores, or C-SSW, are calculated to account for peripheral distortion (i.e., cochlear hearing loss). To determine C-SSW scores, the R-SSW scores for each listening condition are transferred to the appropriate space on the C-SSW Calculation Block on the front page of the Response Form (upper right-hand corner; see Figure 15).

Next, the percent Error scores for the Word Discrimination Scores (WDS) are determined for each ear and subtracted from R-SSW (see Figure 16). In the

FIGURE 16.

2.	C - S S W Enter R-SSW % error			
CONDITION	RNC	RC	LC	LNC
R-SSW % Error	10	22	40	18
- WDS % Error	-8	-8	-20	-20
C-SSW % Error	2	14	20	-2
EAR	RE		LE	
C-SSW % Error				
TOTAL		T		
C-SSW % Error				

FIGURE 17. ═══════════════════

2.	C : S S W Enter R-SSW % error			
CONDITION	RNC	RC	LC	LNC
R-SSW % Error	10	22	40	18
- WDS % Error	-8	-8	20	-20
C-SSW % Error	2	14	20	-2
EAR	RE		LE	
C-SSW % Error	8		9	
TOTAL		T		
C-SSW % Error		8		

example, WDS –right ear = 92%; WDS –left ear = 80%. Therefore 8% was subtracted from the R-SSW scores for the right ear and 20% was subtracted from the R-SSW scores for the left ear. The difference is the C-SSW score. Once the C-SSW scores have been determined for each listening condition, right ear conditions can be averaged for the **right ear C-SSW score** and the left ear conditions can be averaged for the **left ear C-SSW score**. The EAR scores are then averaged for the **total C-SSW score** (see Figure 17).

Response Bias

Response bias is calculated from the eight cardinal numbers and reflects values combining the total number of errors, **not** percentage error scores. These values are determined from the information provided on page 3 of the Response Form.

Ear effects are calculated by adding the total number of errors in the REF versus LEF presentations. For REF errors, sum the errors in columns A–D; for LEF errors sum the errors in columns E–H. The results are entered in the Ear Effect box. Order effects are the total errors in columns A, B, E, and F compared with the errors in columns C, D, G, and H. These values are entered in the Order Effect box. Reversals are simply the number of times the patient changed the order of a word pair. The total number of reversals is entered in the Reversal box.

After the Response Bias has been calculated, each score is transferred to the front page of the Response Form to facilitate interpretation (see Figure 18).

Dennis Arnst

FIGURE 18. ════════════════════════════════════

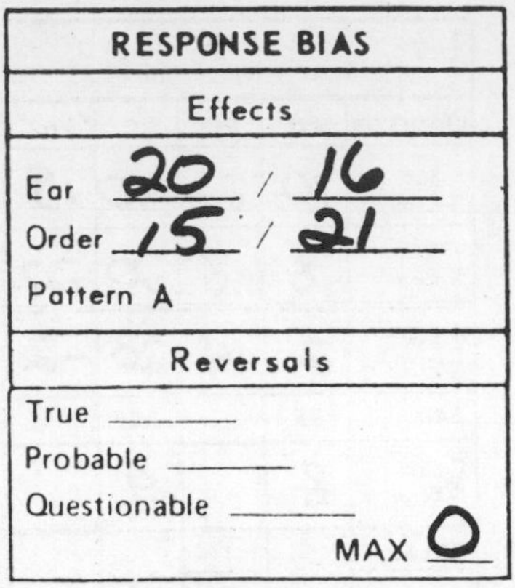

RESPONSE BIAS
Effects
Ear **20** / **16**   Order **15** / **21**
Pattern A
Reversals
True _____   Probable _____   Questionable _____   MAX **O**

Scoring: Analysis of SSW Scores

The SSW-Gram

After the R-SSW, C-SSW scores, and the Response Bias have been calculated, the **SSW-gram** is prepared. R-SSW results for each listening condition are plotted on the graph using an "X"; C-SSW results are plotted on the same graph using an "O" (see Figure 19). R-SSW scores are connected with solid lines; C-SSW scores are connected with broken lines. The resulting graph reflects condition scores and is useful in interpreting test results.

TEC Analysis

In order to classify performance, Total, Ear, and Condition scores are compared with the norms established for the SSW Test. This process is known as the **TEC analysis**. Representative scores are used to place the patient's performance on the continuum from normal to severe. The range of scores and the corresponding performance category are shown in Table 2.

To do the TEC analysis, the Total score and the Ear and Condition scores are selected and compared with performance categories. For both the Ear and Condition results, the score with greatest number of errors is selected and used for the TEC analysis. Also, whenever there are negative numbers, both the most positive and most negative number are included in the analysis. For example, if the C-SSW Ear scores were right = 22 and left = 12, the right ear score (i.e., 22) would be used in the TEC analysis. If the Condition scores for C-SSW were RNC = 8, RC = 26, LC =12, and LNC = 4, the RC score (i.e., 26) would be selected. On the other hand, if the Condition scores were RNC = –12, RC = – 2, LC = 6, and LNC = – 14, the LNC score (–14) and the LC score (6) would both be used in the TEC analysis. The representative scores are transferred to the TEC Analysis Block in the lower right-hand corner on the front page of the Response Form (see Figure 20).

FIGURE 19.

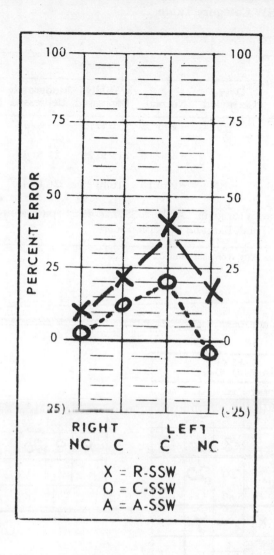

TABLE 2.
C-SSW/A-SSW Category Table

	Categories				
	Over-Corrected	Normal	Mildly Depressed	Moderately Depressed	Severely Depressed
Total	−5	−4 to 5	6 to15	16 to 35	36 to 100
Ear	−7	−6 to 10	11 to 20	21 to 40	41 to 100
Condition	−10	−9 to 15	16 to 25	26 to 45	46 to 100

Boundaries for given C-SSW/A-SSW scores. Separate information is provided for Total, Ear, and Condition scores.

* From: Jack Katz, *SSW Workshop Manual*, 1979

FIGURE 20.

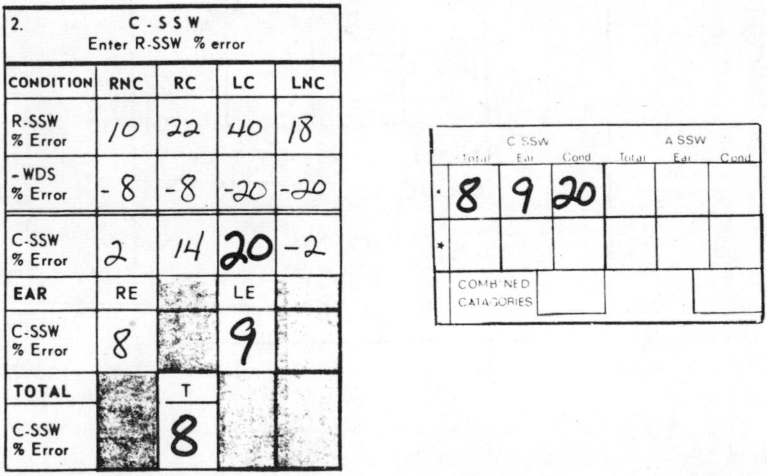

When the scores have been selected, each is compared with the performance ranges in the normative table (see Figure 22). An appropriate label for the corresponding category is entered. Finally, to determine the overall TEC category or the representative SSW category, the results are combined according to the following rules:

Overview of the SSW Test and CES Test

FIGURE 21.

	C SSW			A SSW	
Total	Ear	Cond	Total	Ear	Cond
8	9	20			
*Mi	N	Mi			
COMBINED CATAGORIES	Mi				

1. If all categories are the same, use the common category (e.g., Mi, Mi, Mi = Mi).

2. If different categories are represented, use
   a) the most common category (e.g., Mi, Mo, Mo = Mo)
   b) the median category (e.g., Mi, Mo, S = Mo)

3. If an overcorrected category is present, include it as part of the final SSW score (e.g., Mi, Mi, Mo–O = Mi–O).

4. Ignore normal (N) findings in combined categories (e.g., N–O = O; N–Mo = Mo).

The SSW category is representative of the quantitative aspects of the test.

Ear and Order Effects

Whenever the difference between the two scores of the Ear Effect and/or Order Effect is five or greater, a significant Response Bias effect has been identified. The standard convention for reporting these results is based on the number pairs and either "Low/High" or "High/Low." These terms reflect the score in the pair with the greatest errors (high) and the fewest errors (low). For example:

Ear 14/24 = Low/High (L/H)
Order 12/6 = High/Low (H/L)

It is important to remember that ear and order effects are based on total errors and do not represent percentage error scores.

Reversals have no special classification. Any change in sequence which qualifies as a reversal is simply totaled and reported and one number. Taken together, Response Bias is used in the qualitative analysis of the SSW Test.

Adjusted (A-SSW) Score

The **adjusted-SSW** score, or the A-SSW, is the last aspect of the test to be analyzed. It assesses performance related to Heschl's gyrus (the primary auditory reception area) and is based on the patient's best performance. The A-SSW score is calculated using the part of the test with the least number of errors. A survey of the Ear and Order Effects will locate the scores to be used.

The A-SSW serves as a conservative estimate of the the integrity of Heschl's gyrus. It attempts to eliminate confusing influences from other processing deficits. The A-SSW score is calculated **only** when the following conditions are met: (a) the C-SSW score (combined category) is **Moderate** or **Severe**; (b) a signficant Ear or Order Effect is present; and (c) a cortical dysfunction is suspected.

The basis for the A-SSW score is the Response Bias showing the least number of errors. Both Ear and Order Effects are considered. To select the proper Response Bias, the following rules are applied:

1. If Ear Effect is significant and Order Effect is not, adjust for Ear Effect.
2. If Order Effect is significant and Ear Effect is not, adjust for Order Effect.
3. If Ear and Order Effect are significant, adjust for the Response Bias with the least number of errors.

After the proper Response Bias has been identified, the appropriate values are chosen from the eight cardinal numbers. For example, if the eight cardinal numbers = 4–13–13–7 (REF) and 6–19–12–8 (LEF), Ear Effect = 37/45 and Order Effect = 42/40. Ear Effect is significant (L/H) and Order Effect is not significant. The least number of errors were made in the REF presentation (37) and the first four cardinal numbers (4–13–13–7) would be selected to calculate the A-SSW. Other examples for selecting the appropriate scores to determine A-SSW are shown below:

Eight Cardinal Numbers	Response Bias		Numbers to select* (RNC–RC–LC–LNC)
	Ear Effect	Order Effect	
5–7–15–6; 6–18–11–7	33/42 (L/H);	36/39 (ns)	5–7–15–6
16–20–8–7; 14–18–11–9	51/52 (ns);	68/35 (H/L)	9–11–8–7
4–4–9–4; 14–16–2–2	21/34 (L/H);	38/17 (H/L)	2–2–9–4

*Note: The order in which the errors are arranged must be RNC–RC–LC–LNC

After the appropriate numbers have been selected, they are entered under the correct listening conditions on the A-SSW Calculation Block (front page, lower left-hand corner of the Response Form). Because only half of the items are being considered in the A-SSW, the multiplication factor for the percent error is five. When the percent error score is obtained, the correction procedure is again applied by subtracting the percent error from the WDS. A-SSW Ear scores are determined by averaging the right and left listening conditions; the total A-SSW score is obtained by averaging the Ear Scores (see Figure 22). Finally, a TEC analysis for the A-SSW is done following the same rules as used with the C-SSW scores.

At this point the patient's responses have been recorded, tallied, and scored. The important components of the SSW Test have been analyzed and are ready for interpretation.

Interpretation

Interpretation of the SSW Test is not a simple task. It involves a systematic review of scores and careful integration of all available information. Some basic rules to be kept in mind before finalizing the results on the SSW Test include the following:

1. All aspects of the SSW Test must be evaluated together; R-SSW, C-SSW, Response Bias, and A-SSW (when appropriate) cannot be used in isolation. The strength of the test lies in the fact that the information provided by all aspects of the test tend to build.

2. SSW results must be interpreted in the context of the complete audiometric test battery, including the case history.

3. SSW Test results reflect an **area of dysfunction** rather than being lesion-specific. A given finding is not exclusively associated with a specific pathology.

These guidelines provide an important basis for evaluating test scores and should be carefully considered with each patient.

The SSW-Gram

In general, the SSW-gram is the first consideration of the test results since it provides a graphic overview of the patient's performance. The SSW-gram summarizes the patient's (a) performance across listening conditions; (b) compares scores in competing and noncompeting conditions; (c) compares ear scores; and, (d) compares results evaluating peripheral, central pathway, and cortical components.

Performance in the competing items will usually show the greatest number of errors since these test conditions stress the central auditory nervous system most. A **peak** in performance (error score) is usually found in either the right or left competing condition. However, it is possible to have a fairly equal number of errors scored in both RC and LC.

Dennis Arnst

FIGURE 22.

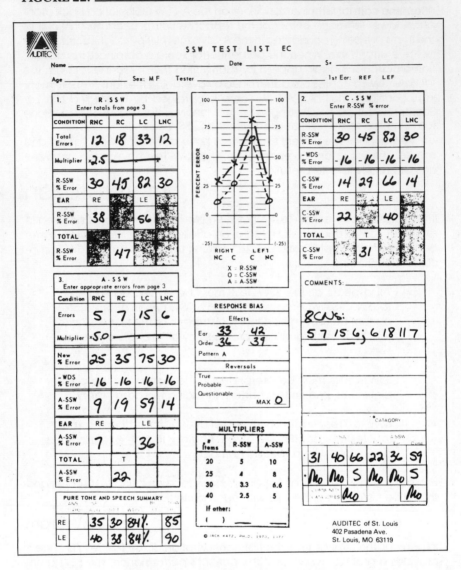

Whenever a **Moderate** or **Severe** category is obtained for one or both ears, the peak is associated with dysfunction in Heschl's gyrus, the upper brainstem area, or the corpus collosum/anterior commissure area. The side of the auditory nervous system involved is usually reflected in the contralateral ear scores in cortical problems and in the ipsilateral ear scores for areas at the brainstem and below. These results are shown in Table 3. Evaluation of peaks is accomplished by inspecting the SSW-gram and the C-SSW Ear scores.

TABLE 3. ━━━━━━━━━━━━━━━━━━━━━━━━━━━━━

Summary of data presented by Katz

Group	N	C-SSW (Ear Scores) ipsilateral	contralateral
Unilateral cochlears	22	0.3	1.3
VIIIth nerve	5	−28.0	−1.0
Low brainstem	3	−13.0	−1.0
High brainstem	4	53.0	4.0
Auditory reception (AR)	15	17.0	52.0
Nonauditory reception (NAR)	24	2.0	8.0

Note: AR = involvement of Heschl's gyrus
           NAR = cortical involvement, but not involving Heschl's gyrus

* Short Course—Localizing Auditory Disorders of the Brain and Brainstem ASHA Convention, Houston, Texas, November 1976

In comparing the R-SSW and the C-SSW results on the SSW-gram, peripheral involvement can be identified.

If R-SSW = C-SSW (Figure 3)	minimal peripheral factor involved, result usually associated with AR or NAR problems
If R-SSW is poorer than C-SSW (Figure 4)	a significant peripheral factor is present; may reflect cochlear, VIIIth nerve, or low brainstem dysfunction

(Note: AR problems involve Heschl's gyrus; NAR problems involve cortical areas outside the superior temporal lobe)

Comparison of the C-SSW and A-SSW results on the SSW-gram is also helpful in evaluating the status of Heschl's gyrus (AR).

FIGURE 23.

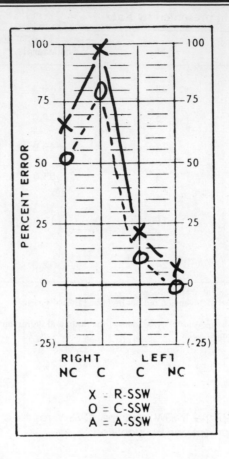

If C-SSW and A-SSW
= Mo or S   (Figure 25)

Heschl's gyrus is most
likely site (see use of CES
p. 34) for differentiation of
corpus collosum from AR)

If A-SSW = Mi
(Figure 26)

Heschl's gyrus not the
primary area of involve-
ment; problem may be
close but not directly in the
primary auditory cortex

If A-SSW = N

results usually associated
with NAR problems

FIGURE 24.

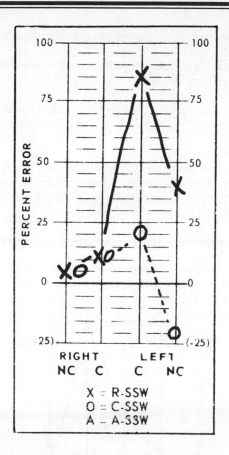

Since the A-SSW score is calculated when a **Moderate** or **Severe** score has been obtained, these results are typically suggestive of cortical problems. Careful consideration of Response Bias is especially necessary in NAR cases to assist in localizing the dysfunction. Furthermore, peak errors in AR cases are highly indicative of the hemisphere of involvement; NAR cases do not accurately predict which side of the cortex is injured. Cross-checking SSW results with scores on the Competing Environmental Sounds (CES) Test (see p. 34) will aid in identifying the hemisphere for NAR cases.

TEC Analysis

The TEC category (combined) is a guide to the severity of performance. Usually, the more severe the category, the more likely the possibility that the patient has a cortical dysfunction. Although age and increased amount of hearing loss are complicating factors, the SSW Category follows a systematic pattern. A summary of data reported by Katz is provided in Table 4.

Generally, the following observations can be made:

1. The probability of obtaining a **Moderate** or **Severe** SSW result in cases of cochlear hearing loss is very low.

2. The chance of obtaining an overcorrected score in cochlear hearing loss is fairly high and is more prevalent in unilateral cases.

3. The greater the overcorrected score, the greater the possibility of VIIIth nerve involvement. A small overcorrected score is more likely consistent with low brainstem or cochlear hearing loss cases.

FIGURE 25. ═══════════════════════════════

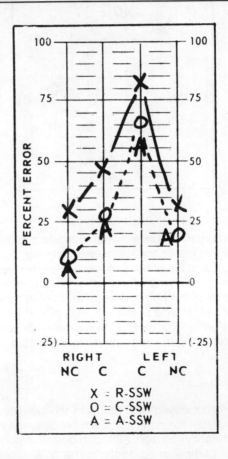

Overview of the SSW Test and CES Test

FIGURE 26.

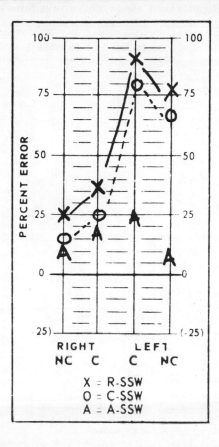

4. **Moderate** and **Severe** SSW scores in the presence of retrocochlear signs (often mild in nature) are consistent with high brainstem dysfunction.

5. NAR cases need careful evaluation, since Normal and Mild scores are common and may be disregarded or mislabeled as cochlear problems. CES results can aid in identifying the involved hemisphere.

6. AR cases clearly fall into the Moderate and Severe categories.

The most important fact to consider in light of these results is that the **SSW categories are not mutually exclusive with respect to dysfunction.** Overlap in terms of absolute value of a test score is possible. Consequently, a combination of factors needs to be considered when evaluating results. These influences include age, hearing loss, history, special audiometric tests,

TABLE 4.
Combined TEC Results for Cases with Various Sites of Lesion (in %)

Group	Over-corrected	Normal	Mild	Moderate Severe
Normal N = 25	–	100	–	–
Conductive N = 17	6[a]	82	12[b]	–
Cochlear Bilateral N = 42	38[c]	52	10	–
Unilateral N = 22	54[d]	14	27	4
Retrocochlear N = 14	64[e]	–	–	36[f]
Auditory Reception N = 12	–	–	8	92[g]
Nonauditory Reception N = 19	5[i]	47	42	5

The lesions did not always conform neatly to the assigned category.

[a] This S did have slightly elevated B/C scores.
[b] Possibly with a presentation level of 30 dB SL fewer conductive hearing loss cases would have scored mild TEC
[c] 2 S's were O-mi.
[d] 1 S was O-Mi.
[e] 1 S was O-Mi; 1 S was O-Mo.
[f] 1 S was O-Mo.
[g] 1 S had O-Mo with a bilateral S-N loss.
[h] NAR excludes corpus collosum & ant. comm. cases.
[i] This S had an S-N overlay.

*Data from Katz, SSW Workshop Manual, 1979.

and Response Bias. Moreover, it is important to remember that a **normal** SSW category does not imply lack of dysfunction. A normal result can be found in cases with cochlear hearing loss, NAR dysfunction, as well as perfectly unaffected auditory processing.

Response Bias

The patient with purely peripheral or purely central problems can demonstrate response bias. In addition, the locus of cortical problems is often reflected in the Response Bias result. Ear and order effects can be used to differentiate anterior from posterior dysfunction. Reversals aid in identifying problems in an area along the central fissure and the anterior temporal lobe (the Reversal Strip). In general, significant Reponse Bias can be interpreted as follows:

Anterior Bias   Ear L/H
                             Order H/L
                             Reversals

Posterior Bias   Ear H/L
                             Order L/H

Anterior bias is related to problems centered in the frontal or anterior temporal lobe; posterior bias relates to problems centered around Heschl's gyrus (the primary AR areas) and the temporo-parietal areas.

Reversals are related to disorders involving the pre motor and pre-and post-central gyri areas and the anterior temporal lobe immediately below. This section of the cortex has been identified by other researchers (Luria 1970 and Effron 1963) in cases with auditory sequencing problems, and for purposes of the SSW Test has been labeled the **Reversal Strip.** The greater number of reversals is associated with dysfunction above the Sylvian fissure and the smaller number below (in the temporal lobe). Six reversals is con-

TABLE 5. ▬▬▬▬▬▬▬▬▬▬▬▬▬▬▬▬▬▬▬▬▬▬▬▬▬▬▬

Response Bias on the SSW Test in Various Pathological Groups

Group	N	% with Rev	M for S's with Rev's	% with EAR	% with ORDER
Conductives	15	40	8	20	7
Cochlear	63	21	2	16	28
Unilateral	22	36	3	14	27
Bilateral	41	12	1	17	29
Retrocochlear	14	7	1	15	29
AR	12	33	5	50	43
NAR	18	44	12	17	28

*From: Katz, SSW Workshop Manual, 1979.

sidered the demarkation point. Because of the location of the Reversal Strip, reversals tend to be considered a mid-cerebral or anterior sign and frequently are associated with Ear L/H and Order H/L types of Response Bias.

Typically, significant ear and/or order effects are associated with cortical processing problems. However, care must be taken when evaluating Response Bias, since peripheral and brainstem disorders may interject bias in the results. Consequently, significant ear and/or order effects which occur in the absence of **Moderate** or **Severe** C-SSW **and** A-SSW results (combined category) cannot be attributed to AR dysfunction. Furthermore, if significant ear and/or order effects occur with **Normal** or **Mild** C-SSW (combined category) results, involvement of NAR aspects of the cortex can only be implicated if there is no hearing loss in the speech frequencies. However, it would be inappropriate to dismiss significant Response Bias with a **Mild** C-SSW and hearing loss. In such cases, review of the case history, extended interview of the patient, and other test results should be consulted before ruling out the possibility of a NAR problem.

A summary of Response Bias on the SSW Test in various pathological groups is provided in Table 5.

Type A / Type B Patterns

A peculiar response pattern has been identified and found to occur in individuals with sound symbol association problems. The **Type A pattern** refers to the arrangement of errors reflected in the eight cardinal numbers. One of the error columns appears inordinately large. To be classified as a Type A pattern, one of the cardinal numbers must be, (a) twice as large as each of the others, (b) at least three points greater, and must (c) occur in column B or F. The **Type B pattern** is similar. The eight cardinal numbers meet the same criteria, except the results occur in column C or G.

Both special patterns are thought to occur as a result of delays in processing time, which precipitates the build up of errors in one of the competing listening conditions. Each of these patterns has been found in children and adults with frontal and/or temporo-parietal dysfunction. Significant Response Bias typically occurs with a Type A or B pattern. It may be due to the unusual distribution of errors and not the usual processing difficulties. When there is a significant Type A or B pattern, ear and order effects are meaningless in locating the site of dysfunction.

The Competing Environmental Sounds (CES) Test

The **Competing Environmental Sounds (CES) Test** is a companion evaluation procedure to be used with the SSW Test. It was designed to assess auditory processing problems associated with the right hemisphere, since disorders involving the right Heschl's Gyrus and some corpus collosum or anterior commissure areas produce similar results. Auditory information

FIGURE 27.

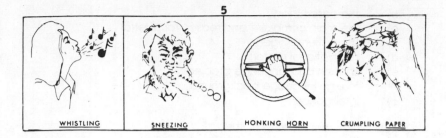

received by the right hemisphere (non-language specific) cannot be forwarded for processing in the left hemisphere (language specific) when the corpus collosum and/or anterior commissure is involved. Consequently, peak errors occur for both types of problems in the left ear.

The CES contains a series of environmental sounds (e.g., door slamming, water running, children playing, dog barking) presented dichotically. Patients are asked to select the two sounds perceived from a series of four pictures (see Figure 27). Comparison of errors on the CES is made with the R-SSW for the right and left ears. Eight SSW/CES comparisons are made, four of which suggest right hemisphere dysfunction and four of which suggest left hemisphere dysfunction. These comparisons are shown in Table 6.

SSW/CES comparisons 1–8 are the mathematical computations required to evaluate the two sets of results. The scores needed include the following:

A	=	RSSW right ear
B	=	RSSW left ear
C	=	CES errors right ear
D	=	CES errors left ear
ΔR	=	A–C (Right RSSW–Right CES)
ΔL	=	B–D (Left RSSW–Left CES)

Comparisons O and 9–14 are the theoretical constructs differentiating the various types of problems the procedure attempts to define.

The exact impact of the CES Test is being evaluated currently and at this point in time needs to be defined more clearly.

Suggested Order of Interpretation

To avoid missing important information or drawing inappropriate conclusions regarding significant results, the following procedure for evaluating SSW results is recommended:

Step 1–Consider all of the following information:

a)   the case history
b)   the main complaint and reason for referral
c)   the patient's age
d)   motivational factors
e)   speech and language problems
f)   foreign language background
g)   intelligence

Step 2–Consider hearing status:
      Normal
      Conductive
      Sensory-neural
Step 3–Consider SSW Test results:
      Eight cardinal numbers
      SSWgram
      R-SSW vs. C-SSW
      C-SSW vs. A-SSW (when appropriate)
      TEC category

TABLE 6.
SSW/CES Comparisons for Right-handed (presumably left hemisphere-dominant) Patients

Number	Locus	Comparison
0	C	SSW ↓ LE & CES ↓ RE
1	R	$(B + C) \geqslant (A + D) + 10$
2	L	$(A + D) \geqslant (B + C) + 10$
3	R	$\Delta_R - \Delta_L \leqslant -10$
4	L	$\Delta_R - \Delta_L \geqslant 0$
5	R	$(A + B) - (C + D) \leqslant -10$
6	L	$(A + B) - (C + D) \geqslant 25$
7	R	$(A + B) - (C + D) \leqslant -25$
8	L	$(A + B) - (C + D) \geqslant 40$
9	R-AR	SSW & CES ↓ LE
10	L-AR	SSW & CES ↓ RE
11	R-AR + C	SSW ↓ LE & CES ↓ Bilaterally
12	L-AR + C	SSW ↓ Bilaterally & CES ↓ RE
13	R-NAR	SSW okay & CES ↓ Bilaterally
14	L-NAR	SSW ↓ Bilaterally & CES okay

C ≐ auditory commissural fibers (corpus collosum or anterior commissure

↓ ≈ 20% or more errors

okay ≈ normal (mild?)

Note: These comparisons are based on theoretical considerations (comparisons 0, 9–14; Katz, 1974) and observations (comparisons 1–8; Katz, Kushner, and Pack, 1975). Validation and cross-validation are still required, respectively.

TABLE 7. ▬▬▬▬▬▬▬▬▬▬▬▬▬▬▬▬▬▬▬▬▬▬▬▬▬▬▬▬▬

Most Common SSW Results in Various Groups

Group	TEC Categories	Response Bias	Audiometric Results
Normal	N	none	normal
Conductive	N, (Mi)	reversals (Ear Effect)	air-bone gap, etc.
Cochlear bilateral	N, O, (Mi)	Order Effect (Ear Effect, reversal[s])	cochlear signs
Cochlear unilateral	O, Mi, (N)	reversals, Order Effect	cochlear signs
VIIIth nerve & low brainstem	O ipsilaterally	Order Effect (Ear Effect), usually an absence of reversals	retrocochlear signs with depressed WDS
High brainstem	S, Mo ipsilaterally	(Same as above)	mild retrocochlear signs
Cerebellum	perhaps any category, depending on site	perhaps any bias including reversals	often retrocochlear
Auditory reception	S, Mo contralaterally	Ear Effect or Order Effect, reversals	often high frequency loss, somewhat depressed WDS in contralateral or both ears
Nonauditory reception (excluding J below)	N, Mi a peak of errors cannot be relied on to locate site of dysfunction	reversals, Order Effect, (Ear Effect)	normal
Corpus collosum/ anterior commissure	(Presume) Mo, S R-handers peak LE on SSW & RE on CES	will depend on which other centers are involved. More likely posterior signs with CC and anterior signs with AC	normal

This table shows the typical performance for patients with relatively "pure" problems. In various areas of the central system (e.g., corpus collosum) lesions to various locations may have no auditory effects at all. For both TEC categories and response bias, underlining indicates greater than 50% of the cases; parentheses indicates 10–25%; the rest are in between 25–50%.

(From: Katz, SSW Workshop Manual, 1979.)

Step 4–Consider
      Response Bias
      Ear Effects
      Order Effects
      Reversals

The information provided by each one of these steps is usually additive; however, due to the internal dynamics of the SSW Test, some signs can offset each other. It is imperative that all the results be carefully evaluated before a diagnostic conclusion is drawn. A summary of the most common SSW results in various types of problems is presented in Table 7.

A Final Thought About the SSW Test

Information on the SSW Test is becoming more readily available. Research studies, workshops, conferences, lectures, and clinical discussion can provide assistance for anyone who is interested. Ease and confidence with the SSW Test comes with practice and experience. But, before attempting to put the test into clinical use, it is strongly recommended that a group of normal-hearing individuals and a group of patients with sensory-neural hearing loss be evaluated. This practice will permit understanding of test administration, scoring, and some of the underlying principles. Next, to "fine tune" the interpretation process, patients with known and well localized lesions should be tested. These trial cases will ease the transition into the clinic.

Finally, the Staggered Spondaic Word Test is sensitive to dysfunction throughout the auditory system. Its internal dynamics and structure make it impossible for interpretation to be simplified to a single table of results for easy reference. Performance categories cannot be defined, so they are lesion specific and used without consideration of a wide range of information. Because the auditory system does not function simplistically, it is unrealistic to assume that any assessment tool designed to evaluate it can.

Enjoy the challenge both can provide!

The idea of the Staggered Spondaic Word (SSW) Test was conceived in 1960. At that time, audiologists were primarily concerned with otosclerosis, as well as noise-induced hearing loss. The area of differential diagnosis of VIIIth nerve versus cochlear problems was just beginning to heat up. To put the study of central auditory disorders in perspective, the Short Increment Sensitivity Index SISI Test of cochlear function had just recently been reported in the journals by Jerger, Harford, and Shedd. That test was not yet in general use because most clinics did not have equipment to provide the SISI signal. On the other hand, Békésy audiometers were available in many universities and some clinics but it was only in 1960 that Jerger proposed his classification system for the Békesy audiogram.

It was in this milieu that the SSW Test sprung up; however most audiologists did not take notice of central testing at the time. Even if they did, they were unable to utilize techniques that appeared in the literature due to a lack of proper equipment. Most audiologists had one-channel audiometers (not adequate for binaural fusion or dichotic tests), which were connected to phonographs (and not tape players). If a tape player was available, it was invariably a single-channel instrument.

The first article on the SSW Test appeared in the **Journal of Auditory Research** in 1962 and it is also the first article in this chapter (with updated information). The article was written to simply introduce the test. Because of our rather limited knowledge at that time, only concepts were given, without detailed accounts of expected results and diagnostic applications. J. Donald Harris, the editor of that journal, requested illustrative cases to show how the test could be used and these were appended at the end of the article.

In 1963 the second SSW article was published (Katz, Basil, and Smith), based in part on two Masters' theses. The research was carried out at Northern Illinois University. Although it was evident from the literature that tem-

2

Development
of the Staggered
Spondaic Word Test

poral lobe tumor cases showed adverse effects in the ear contralateral to the lesion, it was a shock to discover the same type of results with skull trauma cases. The fact that trauma would produce an effect similar to a brain tumor was only one aspect. The greater element of disbelief came from seeing the scar in the temporal lobe region and finding the ear near the scar to be quite normal. The influence was on the **opposite** ear. Also the high correlation and close similarity between the raw SSW score and the word discrimination score (WDS), led the way to the correction factor that was used in subsequent research and in clinics around the country.

By the time the third article appeared in 1968, the SSW Test had been in use for seven years in both laboratories and clinics. The test was found over and over again to be useful in differentiating disorders of the auditory reception (AR) centers from nonauditory reception (NAR) center involvements of the brain. This was a new concept in audiology literature and for this reason, perhaps, was not immediately grasped. This third article underscored the importance of the Corrected SSW (C-SSW) score, mentioned peculiarities in conductive and Meniere's cases on the test, and provided tentative norms on which to judge AR and NAR-type performance.

The next paper in this chapter is by Brunt and Goetzinger. It was the first to compare the SSW with other central tests. It was carried out on normal listeners. At that time, the Rush Hughes Test was probably the most used central auditory procedure. Among other things it benefited by being commercially available on a phonograph disc and required only a single-channel presentation. The third test, Kimura's competing digits, was being used by a number of researchers but enjoyed very little clinical use in this country.

Brunt and Goetzinger found the SSW Test to be less challenging to normals than the other two tests. Herein lies one of the important features of the SSW—it tends not to be challenging to normals, but is "set" at a level of difficulty that will be demanding of those who have CANS problems. Among normal control subjects, we consistently find few errors and a small range of variation. This is true not only for the "supra normal" subjects (e.g., young college students) but also for a cross section of the community including older individuals, those with somewhat lower intelligence, and those with variations in hearing. Because of this feature we would be less concerned about contamination from extraneous factors when testing a typical population than we would with procedures that are more demanding.

Support for the SSW Test as a procedure that differentiates AR from NAR disorders is reported in the next article. Balas used his own version of the SSW for his study. It is perhaps because of differences in the speaker, the recording technique, or the overlap that the results are in the same direction but less depressed than other tests by Katz or Jerger and Jerger (1975).

Additional support for the SSW Test as a measure of CANS problems comes from the work of Jerger and Jerger. These authors used several pathological populations and central tests to study the validity of CANS procedures and found the SSW Test to be particularly helpful in identifying brain disorders; however they noted that it was less sensitive in the determination of brainstem involvement than synthetic sentence identification (SSI) when there was ipsilateral competition finding considerable scatter in the SSW performance in these cases. We think that the wide scatter noted in this study may be a further strength of the SSW Test. In 1970, Katz reported that patients with upper brainstem lesions had highly positive C-SSW scores and those with lower auditory brainstem involvement had over-corrected scores. This can serve to differentiate upper and lower brainstem disorders. It is quite possible that the wide variations noted by Jerger is an indication of the various loci of dysfunction in their brainstem group.

The final article in this section is a recent one published by Arnst. It evaluates previous data obtained with normal listeners and the types of errors made by this group.

The Use of Staggered Spondaic Words for Assessing the Integrity of the Central Auditory Nervous System

Jack Katz, Ph.D.

Introduction

Audiological measures for localizing lesions in the peripheral hearing mechanism are presently more precise and reliable than those which have been designed to assess impairments in the central auditory pathways. Bocca, Calearo and Cassinari (1954) presented a preliminary report on a method of identifying temporal lobe tumors. Since that time there has been considerable interest in the higher auditory functions from both theoretical and diagnostic points of view. The attention focused on this complex area of the central nervous system has led to several new theoretical concepts and clinical methodologies which offer potential value (see Refs. 1, 3, 7, 10, 11, 13, 16, 17). Further contributions of audiology to the localization of central nervous system pathology will probably result from the addition and refinements of test procedures which reliably indicate the site of lesion.

The literature consistently reveals that conventional pure-tone and speech audiometry do not identify "cortical hearing" impairments. Audiologically, hearing disorders of this type may be uncovered by demanding the evaluation of unusually difficult material by the patient. In so doing, a heavier burden is placed upon the higher auditory mechanism. Weakness in integrative behavior is manifested in the in-

J. Auditory Res., 2, 1962, 327-337

ability to utilize the stimuli appropriately. Bocca and his associates have presented logical arguments for employing disorted speech stimuli in an effort to compel the use of integrative or synthetic processes of the central auditory system. These investigators employed several techniques for distorting speech material. They have utilized methods of (a) low frequency spectrum attenuation, (b) speech acceleration, and (c) speech switched periodically from ear to ear at a rapid rate.

Matzker (1959, 1960) employed two speech procedures: a rapid switching technique, and a frequency filtering method; he also investigated a pure-tone localization test. His results support the conclusions of Bocca. Matzker indicates that audiological procedures may be of considerable importance in diagnosing and locating disorders of the central nervous system. Walsh and Goodman (1955) and Miller (1960) studied the PB word lists and found that under certain conditions cortical damage could be inferred. Jerger (1960), and Jerger, et al (1961) utilized versions of several of the test procedures of Bocca, Matzker, and Walsh and Goodman. The resultant assessment battery included difficult speech measures and two types of sound localization methods.

Analysis of the literature suggests that there are three or four general approaches to identifying central auditory lesions with speech stimuli. (a) One method is to challenge the higher pathways of hearing by presenting less than a complete message to a subject and thus require the use of synthetic processes. This category includes methods which delete segments of a verbal message or limit its frequency spectrum. (b) Another means of affecting a breakdown of a "hidden" hearing disorder is to administer more than the required amount of information. In this case it is necessary for the subject to separate and integrate the stimuli into meaningful and non-meaningful portions. This may be illustrated by competing message techniques, in which irrelevant information is presented to the contralateral ear, or by the use of a background noise. (c) A third general technique of assessing central functioning is a complex presentation of speech. This method provides all of the information which is necessary and sufficient to supply the correct answer; however it is transmitted in a complicated manner. Tests which rely upon rapid ear-to-ear switching, and accelerated or decelerated spech are illustrative of the complex presentation method. (d) A fourth approach combines two or more individual procedures in order to obtain a more demanding test.

Limitations of Current Difficult Speech Techniques

Several promising audiological procedures and variations have been proposed for signifying lesions of the central nervous system. However, most often it is not clear from these measures at what level in the pathways the breakdown occurs. In addition, etiological groups are not necessarily consistent in their test behavior. Thus, improved specificity and reliability are of major importance to present-day investigators.

It is logical to assume that speech material which is ambiguous or has few distinguishable elements will suffer considerable loss of intelligibility when "sensitized" by any of the current difficult-speech methods. These subtle stimuli which are then further processed by any of the current techniques become particularly incomprehensible to individuals lacking central integrity. This inability is primarily demonstrable in the ear contralateral to the affected hemisphere. But even though at first glance such an approach seems ideal, nevertheless, methods which employ ambiguous speech stimuli incorporate an element of undesirability. The more precarious or unstable the speech material, from the standpoint of intelligibility, the greater the probability of artifacts due to individual differences which may be totally unrelated to central disturbance.

Since most of the techniques investigated to date have employed relatively unstable speech stimuli, namely, English monosyllabic words or their equivalents, it is not surprising that consistent normative data are lacking. As a result of the heterogeneity of the test items, and of the great amount of variability among individual listeners, little emphasis in difficult-speech tests has been placed on the absolute test score. Rather, in cases of suspected unilateral central pathology the performances for the two ears are compared wherever the test's structure permits. In some cases the analysis of some assessment procedures is necessarily based on a comparison of separate unilateral test conditions with a binaural condition.

Because of the expenditure of testing time necessary to cope with factors of unreliability, investigators have been unable to shorten their diagnostic measures. Several researchers have utilized rather extensive test batteries to provide the added reliability and accuracy in diagnosis. Since all of these approaches tend to be time-consuming, they may increase the possibility of psychological and physiological fatigue in the patient.

In addition to variables inherent in particular subjects such as age, intelligence, attention span, etc., most of the current methods are difficult to interpret in the presence of peripheral aural pathology. Since peripheral hearing loss has an unpredictable influence upon the test procedures, the possibility of confounding important information concerning the status of "cortical hearing" is enhanced. Particular uncertainty and equivocal findings would arise when distortions, such as reduced word discrimination ability, could be demonstrated by conventional techniques.

One would hesitate on the basis of current techniques to make a diagnosis with individuals exhibiting less than normal hearing for the frequencies within the speech range and also very good word discrimination ability. With few exceptions the distorted-speech techniques employ ambiguous, unstable speech stimuli. It can be seen that without material which is impervious to individual differences and unscathed by peripheral auditory distortions, serious limitations are placed on the procedure. Stable speech stimuli might provide greater certainty in diagnosis because of the likelihood of clearcut normative data and relative resistance to associated or coincidental auditory deviations of a peripheral nature.

Recent work by Calearo and Lazzaroni (1957) and by Bocca (1961) tends to show that improved test reliability occurs with more stable speech material. A group of normally-hearing individuals with considerable scatter on tests of intelligence, vocabulary, and memory were administered a switched-speech test using Italian trisyllabic words and short sentences. The findings of this investigation revealed that the three variables studied did not affect test results. There was evidence of excellent integrative ability for each of the three subgroups in the study. Any switching rate from one ear to the other was found to be acceptable. Bocca suggests that Calearo's test for the detection of malingering, which utilizes short sentence material, is an excellent tool for identifying higher auditory lesions. The switched-speech test may also provide greater specificity in diagnosis.

Stability of Speech Materials

The difficulty in identifying a word is related to considerations of familiarity, phonetic structure, length, stress, part of speech, etc. (see Giolas (1960) and Owens (1961) for discussion). If the word has rare usage, ordinary sound elements, and a common pattern it will be more difficult to identify. Thus a commonly used word with unique structure and stress will be intelligible at a weaker level than an unfamiliar word with less specific features. For these reasons English monosyllabic words require greater sound intensity for reception than short sentences or spondaic words. For the purpose of this study, spondaic words are those composed of two monosyllabic words with equal stress on each. Spondaic words and sentences contain greater redundancy and therefore much information can be omitted without noticeable reduction in intelligibility.

The stability of spondaic words is revealed by the fact that there is a reliable relationship between their reception thresholds and puretone thresholds in the speech frequencies. Even at intensity levels only slightly above the average threshold for the speech frequencies, nearly perfect intelligibility of spondaic words may be expected. This relationship is essentially unaltered when auditory sensitivity is reduced. This estimate is also appropriate even in cases in which moderate difficulty in discriminating monosyllabic words is present. This stability, common to spondaic words, provides a high degree of test-retest reliability (see Ref. 5). Differences as small as four or five db in spondaic word reception thresholds may be considered significant. It appears likely that the advantages in Calearo's switched-speech test are due to the use of more stable speech stimuli.

The Staggered Spondaic Word (SSW) Test

General Description

A staggered spondaic word (SSW) test has been devised which approaches the problem of assessment of the central pathways in a manner similar to that of Calearo and Bocca. Some new features are present in the SSW test which accentuate its potential value. The SSW test incorporates the stability of English spondaic words and the demanding features of a competing message technique in order to study insufficiency of the higher auditory nervous system. In addition, further "sensitization" is obtained by the introduction of two complex presentation methods. The proposed test requires that the patient attend first to one side, then to both sides *simultaneously* and then only to the second side, with different information presented concurrently to each ear. The procedure requires no more than 20 minutes and offers both quantitative and possibly important qualitative information.

Test Pattern

Specifically, the author proposes partial overlapping of words presented separately to each ear. That is, two spondaic words such as *upstairs* and *downtown* are combined to form one item. *Upstairs* is transmitted to the right ear and *downtown* to the left. The test provides competition, or concurrent stimuli in the two ears, for the monosyllabic words trials *stairs* and *down*, while trials *up* and *town* are presented normally, in a non-competing fashion. The program of transmission of the item may be clarified by the following diagram:

Ear	Time		
	1	2	3
Right	up –	stairs	
Left		down –	town

The two spondaic words which comprise each item in the SSW test were chosen on the basis of the following criteria:

1. Fairly familiar words.
2. Competing trials of approximately equal duration.
3. Noncompeting trials form a third spondaic word.

Two practice items precede the actual test items. The practice items are similar to the test items except that they do not overlap in time. The carrier phrase "Are you ready" introduces each item and is presented to the ear which will receive the initial word. The ear receiving the first word is alternated.

Administering the Test

The test material is delivered separately to each ear by use of the two channels of a stereophonic tape recorder which are led independently to a pair of earphones. The tape recorder also provides independent volume control for each ear and permits the precise time relationship between the words to be preserved. Each ear is stimulated at a constant level above its individual threshold. It is not yet clear which particular threshold is most appropriate. It may be that the average threshold for pure tones in the speech range (500, 1000 and 2000 cps) or perhaps just the threshold for 1000 cps may be preferred to the speech reception threshold for spondaic words (see Jerger (1960) Ref. 8 and Miller (1960) for discussion). However, in order to avoid possible inaccuracies it might be safest to employ the speech reception threshold.

The subject might be instructed:

> You will hear a series of words. Listen carefully and repeat **all** of the words that you hear. You will have plenty of time to respond, so just say the words as accurately and as clearly as possible. Do not respond until all of the words are presented. If you are not quite sure of a word, take a guess. Now tell me what you are going to do.

Analyzing Test Data

The structure and composition of the SSW test is such that it can provide various quantitative and qualitative bases for analyses. The 40 items, which represent 160 monosyllabic words or 160 bits of information, may be scored and scrutinized in several different ways. Diversified data concerning a symptom would thus be provided by the complex response pattern. For example, by tabulating the percentage of correct responses for the right ear with and without competition, and the left ear in noncompeting and competing conditions, nine meaningful percentages may be obtained. The total percentage correct indicates an individual's overall success on the test. A comparison between the 80 words presented to the right ear and the 80 presented to the left ear is most revealing with cases having unilateral lesions. Differences between competing and noncompeting trials may be considered separately for each ear, or together in cases of bilateral disorders. Analyses of these scores may indicate error patterns on the SSW test which may be due to peripheral distortions and those to central disturbance. The analysis of error pattern on the four possible monosyllabic responses to each item, regardless of the ear affected, could be expected to offer further versatility and diagnostic power to the SSW test.

There are 16 ways in which a patient can respond to each test item, ranging from all four monosyllabic words correct, to all incorrect. At the present time one might with due caution suggest that the individual who consistently responds incorrectly to, for example, the third monosyllabic word is functioning differently from one who consistently fails both the second and third words, or indeed from a patient who demonstrates no consistent error response. Further reliability might result from a pattern analysis based on operationally related response categories. Thus, by combining similar error patterns the score obtained would be based on a sample size from two to seven times the original number for any one error-type.

From the foregoing it may be inferred that the test procedures which supply only one or at the most a few sensitive scores representing an individual's entire response to difficult speech material may ignore important variations among etiological groups. On the one hand, test procedures which supply several scores can offer a wealth of opportunities for exploration by the diagnostician. We can but assume that lesions at various points in the higher auditory pathways will produce different effects on auditory perception, even if they are only subtle changes. One is encouraged in this assumption by the specificity of audiological procedures for the analysis of peripheral disorders. On the basis of such previous experience it would be logical to assume that variations in central functioning will manifest themselves, just as have peripheral lesions, with the advent of more sophisticated diagnostic techniques.

Case Studies

Six case studies are presented here to indicate the performance trends of normal subjects and of selected central- and peripheral-disturbance groups. These individuals are thought to be rather representative of their subgroups. Information concerning the speech average for pure tones, speech reception threshold, discrimination score and Staggered Spondaic Word Test results are shown in Table 1.

Discussion

The case studies presented provide some insight into the sensitivity and versatility of the SSW test. The patients who represent groups of central lesions demonstrate considerable difficulty on the test. It is indeed remarkable that these individuals who behave so normally on conventional audiometric measures should show such marked deviations from normal subjects on the SSW test. Case 2, of unilateral central trauma, demonstrates the vivid effect upon the contralateral ear, while the homolateral ear yields almost normal data. This contralateral affectation is consistently revealed in tests of higher auditory behavior.

It is of interest to note that the competing condition tended to be more difficult for all subjects. Nevertheless, the contrast between the competing and noncompeting conditions were most striking with central dysfunction. Although, Case 5, with peripheral damage, had a poor SSW score for the right ear, he differed from the other subjects by exhibiting a discrimination loss for conventional words and difficulty on the non-competing trials as well. We might infer that moderate discrimination losses will reflect themselves on both competing and non-competing words on the SSW test. The incorrect responses of patients with central dysfunction on the proposed test might be expected to be far out of proportion to the discrimination loss particularly for the non-competing trials.

Information concerning the reliability, the effects of age, and the effects of intelligence on the SSW test is not available at the present time. However, there is reason to be optimistic concerning these factors. Children as young as eight years of age have been administered the test and have shown normal adult responsiveness. This technique has not been given to children younger than eight years of age.

It is of value to describe the ease with which normal subjects perform on the SSW test. Individuals without significant neurological or otological histories make very few mistakes. In fact, sophisticated listeners often challenge the statement that the two competing trials completely overlap one another; but the timing accuracy of the tape recording is easily verified. The reason for this auditory illusion remains unexplained; it is perhaps related to the facility with which the intact brain is in fact able to handle competing or even conflicting information presented simultaneously at the two ears.

TABLE 1.
Case Studies of Six Patients Given the Staggered Spondaic Word Test

					SSW Test		% Correct
	Ear	PT AVE	SRT	DS	Non-Com.	Com.	Total

	Ear	PT AVE	SRT	DS	Non-Com.	Com.	Total
Case 1. Normal (control) male, 12 yrs. No significant medical history	R	-10		100	100	98	99
	L	-10		100	100	98	99
	Mn	-10		100	100	98	99
Case 2. Trauma (central) male, 24 yrs. Fell from a fast moving vehicle on right side of head at age 5. Unconscious 8 days. Residual scars on right side of head only (temporal, parietal and occipital regions).	R	-10	-4	100	98	92	95
	L	-10	-6	100	90	62	76
	Mn	-10	-5	100	94	77	86
Case 3. Cerebral Palsy (central) female, 11 yrs. Predominantly, right spastic involvement	R	0	6	100	98	30	54
	L	-3	4	100	100	70	85
	Mn	-2	5	100	99	50	74
Case 4. Older Age (central) male, 60 yrs. No significant medical history.	R	-5	0	100	98	52	75
	L	-3	0	100	100	70	85
	Mn	-4	0	100	99	61	80
Case 5. Sensory-Neural Hearing Loss (Peripheral) male, 39 yrs. Noise exposure in service in WW II.	R	13*	10	72	72	58	65
	L	10*	8	84	100	92	96
	Mn	12	9	78	86	75	80
Case 6. Conductive Hearing Loss (Peripheral) male, 42 yrs. Progressive hearing loss found to be otosclerosis.	R	26**	28	100	100	100	100
	L	40**	36	100	100	98	99
	Mn	33	32	100	100	99	100

*   For 2 best frequencies
** Approximately 30 db air-bone gap
PT AVE : Mean Threshold at 500, 1000, and 200 cps
SRT   : Speech Reception Threshold for spondees
DS   : Discrimination Score for live voice PB W22 lists at 40 db above SRT
Staggered Spondee Word Test Results at a Level 30 db above SRT
   Noncompeting condition : Monosyllables (Times 1 and 3)
    Competing condition : Monosyllables (Time 2)
        Total   : Percentage correct of all monosyllables

Summary

An audiological technique termed the Staggered Spondaic Word (SSW) Test is proposed for the assessment of lesions in the higher auditory pathways. This "competing-message" technique employs bilateral, partially overlapped spondaic words.

Spondaic words are employed in order to utilize their ability to pass through the peripheral auditory mechanism comparatively unscathed by concomitant or coincidental hearing loss and/or distortion. The stable speech material should also provide greater intra- and inter-subject consistency within various auditory disorder groups.

The SSW test offers the diagnostician many sources of information concerning the individual's ability to cope with a speech stimulus presented in a complex manner. The brevity of the complete SSW test (20 min.) renders it feasible as a potential clinical tool. On the basis of the analysis of early test results with various populations, no serious alterations in the theory underlying the proposed test have been necessary.

References

1. Bocca, E. Factors influencing binaural integration of periodically switched messages. *Acta Oto-laryngol.*, 1961, 53, 142–144.

2. Bocca, E., Calearo, C. and Cassinari, V. A new method for testing hearing in temporal lobe tumours; preliminary report. *Acta Oto-laryngol.*, 1954, 44, 219–221.

3. Bocca, E., Calearo, C., Cassinari, V. and Migliavacca, F. Testing "cortical" hearing in temporal lobe tumours. *Acta Oto-laryngol.*, 1955, 45, 289–304.

4. Calearo, C. and Lazzaroni, A. Speech intelligibility in relation to the speed of the message. *Laryngoscope*, 1957, 67, 410–419.

5. Epstein, A. and Hopkinson, N. T. Personal communication.

6. Giolas, T. "An Investigation of the Effects of Frequency Distortion upon the Intelligibility of Monosyllabic Word Lists and a Sample of Continuous Discourse." Ph.D. Dissertation, University of Pittsburgh, 1960.

7. Jerger, J. Audiological manifestations of lesions in the auditory nervous system. *Laryngoscope*, 1960, 70, 417–425.

8. Jerger, J. Observations on auditory behavior in lesions of the central auditory pathways. *Arch. Oto-laryngol.*, 1960, 71, 797–806.

9. Jerger, J., Mier, M., Boshes, B. and Canter, G. Auditory behavior in parkinsonism. *Acta Oto-laryngol.*, 1960, 52, 541–550.

10. Lucas, A. Transitory phenomena in audiometric diagnosis. *Ann. Otol., Rhinol., Laryngol.*, 1961, 70, 669–676.

11. Matzker, J. Two new methods for the assessment of central auditory functions in cases of brain disease. *Ann. Otol., Rhinol., Laryngol.*, 1959, 68, 1185–1197.

12. Matzker, J. Der heutige Stand der Diagnostik cerebraler Hörstörungen. *H.N.O.*, Berlin, 1960, 8, 97–109.

13. Matzker, J. and Welker, H. Die Prufung des Richtungshörens zum Nachweis und zu topischen Diagnostik von Hirnerkrankungen. *Z. Laryngol. Rhinol.*, 1959, 38, 277–294.

14. Miller, M. H. Audiologic evaluation of aphasic patients. *J. speech hearing Dis.*, 1960, 25, 333–339.

15. Owens, E. Intelligibility of words varying in familiarity. *J. speech hearing Res.*, 1961, 4, 113–129.

16. Sanchez-Longo, L. P., Forester, F. M. and Auth, T. L. A clinical test for sound localization and its applications. *Neurology,* 1957, 7, 655–661.

17. Walsh, T. and Goodman, A. Speech discrimination in central auditory lesions. *Laryngoscope,* 1955, 65, 1–8.

A Staggered Spondaic Word Test for Detecting Central Auditory Lesions

Jack Katz, Ph.D.   Rocco A. Basil, M.A.   Joen M. Smith, M.A.

The staggered spondaic word (SSW) test has been recently proposed as a measure of central integrity. The present report concerns a pilot investigation of this procedure with patients having various types of auditory disturbances and with normal subjects.

In 1954, Bocca, Calcaro and Cassinari[2] published their initial findings of an audiological method for establishing the presence of temporal lobe tumors. Since conventional audiometric techniques are not sensitive to 'cortical' hearing disorders, they sought to challenge the functional integrity of higher auditory centers through the use of distorted speech stimuli. They state:

> "Following a logical line of thought, we decided to sensibilize the vocal audiometric tests by making words less

Ann. Otol. Rhinol. & Laryngol., 72, 908–917, 1963.

easily recognizable, in order that their correct perception should involve psychic integration to a higher extent. If the assumption that the psychic function of hearing being localized in or near the cortex is correct, then the test devised by us should give the opportunity of exploring the cortical auditory areas, and as a consequence, be the most adequate means of testing hearing in the cases where only the higher stations of the auditory pathway are functionally impaired." (p. 220)

The work of Bocca and his associates provided the ground work for a number of studies employing distorted or difficult speech.[1 5 7 8 9] The various methods which were utilized demonstrated that speech tests were sensitive indicators of the presence of lesions in the higher auditory mechanism when portions of the message were deleted, when superfluous information was introduced, when the stimulus material was presented in a complex manner or, no doubt, when combinations of these methods may have been used. Since each of the above criteria may be met by any number of individual procedures or ramifications, an infinite variety of potential measures of central auditory integrity are available.

It is of considerable value, for purposes of localizing unilateral cortical hearing impairments, that the inability to cope with difficult test material resides primarily in the ear contralateral to the affected hemisphere. Investigators have consistently found this contralateral affectation in using diagnostic measures of central lesions in spite of normal or nearly normal bilateral responses on conventional audiological tests.

Because monosyllabic words are easily rendered unintelligible in the presence of disorders affecting the sensorineural transmission of auditory stimuli, they tend to increase the probability of indicating any type of disorder. Thus, test results might well reflect differences in peripheral hearing or even vocabulary. Recently, there has been a tendency to place a heavier emphasis upon reliability and stability in the construction of cortical hearing tests.[1 3 6]

In order to insure greater reliability in central auditory assessment one might employ selected polysyllabic words or short sentence material. These stimuli are more unmistakable than monosyllabic words and, therefore, tend to yield fainter reception thresholds along with greater consistency. Calearo has employed short sentences in his test of higher auditory function. This stable-stimulus approach has proved itself to be quite resistant to individual differences.[1] Another approach may be that of using spondaic words since it has been shown that they offer high test-retest reliability.[4]

The Staggered Spondaic Word (SSW) Test

Katz[6] has recently proposed the use of the SSW test as a measure of central integrity. The stimulus material and the structural makeup of this procedure might well provided a reliable and versatile means of investigating higher auditory behavior. Methods for assessing cortical hearing which are oblivious to peripheral hearing loss or to other unrelated individual differences have important attributes for clinical diagnosis. Procedures with high reliability are of considerable value for both clinical and research purposes. In addition, techniques which provide a number of independent scores are potentially capable of offering finer distinctions among various sites of lesions. For the above reasons the SSW test may furnish some desirable features to the test procedures presently available.

One might suspect high test-retest and odd-even reliability and the capacity to withstand peripheral distortions when spondaic words are used (for the purposes of this investigation spondaic words are those composed of two monosyllabic words which are spoken with equal stress). The organization of the proposed test permits comparisons of several auditory operations. Most importantly, each ear may be analyzed separately in both normal and difficult speech conditions within each test item. Nevertheless, the SSW test takes no more than 20 minutes and appears to maintain the interest of the subjects.

Specifically, the SSW test is composed of 40 items. Each item is made up of two spondaic words such as *upstairs* and *downtown*. One spondee is presented to each ear in a partially overlapping fashion. That is, the second monosyllable of the initial spondaic word and the first monosyllable of the second spondaic word are transmitted simultaneously to the opposite ears. The ear receiving the initial word is alternated. The presentation of an item may be diagrammed as follows:

	Time Sequence		
	1	2	3
Right ear	up	– stairs	
Left ear		down	– town

Experimental Design

Equipment

A Korting model MT-158 stereophonic tape recorder was employed for the recording and playback of the SSW test. The output was fed through a pair of matched TDH-39 earphones. Each channel of the tape recorder was calibrated separately from 40 to 90 db SPL at 1000 cps in 5 db steps. Calibrated, commercially available instruments were used for the standard hearing tests.

Audiological Procedures

Normal subjects were screened at 10 db between 250 and 8000 cps at octave intervals. For these individuals speech reception thresholds were assumed to be 0 db SL and word discrimination for W-22 words to be about 100 per cent. All experimental group subjects in this investigation were administered threshold tests for air and bone conducted pure tones and live voice speech reception thresholds and W-22 word discrimination lists.

Prior to the evaluation of test subjects it was necessary to establish the appropriate level at which the SSW test should be presented. The 50 db dial reading was chosen because at this volume young normal individuals had essentially no difficulty with the test material. Both experimental and control subjects were administered the test at the dial reading 50 db above their 1000 cps threshold in the particular ear.

Phase I. A group of twenty university and high school students, having a mean age of 20, with normal hearing and reporting no significant otological or neurological history were utilized as the control population. They were instructed to repeat *all* of the words that they heard. Each of the 160 monosyllabic word trials was scored independently as being correct or incorrect regardless of the order in which it was repeated. The results were divided into four categories:

TABLE 1. ━━━━━━━━━━━━

Mean Number of Errors for the Control (Normal), Trauma (Central), Conductive (Peripheral), and Sensory-Neural (Peripheral) Groups on the SSW Test

Group	N	Right NC	Right C	Left C	Left NC	Sum Right	Sum Left	Total
Normal	20	.6	.8	1.1	.0	1.4	1.1	2.6
Trauma	6	3.3	7.3	8.0	2.7	10.7	10.7	21.3
Conductive	5	.2	2.2	2.0	.0	2.4	2.0	4.4
Sensory-Neural	10	9.4	13.5	12.1	5.6	22.9	17.7	40.6

Development of the Staggered Spondaic Word Test

1. The words presented to the right ear without a competing message in the contralateral ear (RNC).
2. The words presented to the right ear with simultaneous competition in the contralateral ear (RC).
3. The words presented to the left ear with simultaneous competition in the contralateral ear (LC).
4. The words presented to the left ear without a competing message in the contralateral ear (LNC).

The control group repeated 3,149 monosyllables correctly and 51 incorrectly. Thus, better than 98 percent of the responses on the SSW test were correct. The 20 normal individuals ranged from zero to nine errors. Five subjects had no errors and only two had more than five errors. It was noted that a few of the normals had difficulty at first so two practice items were inserted at the beginning of the test. About half of the control group and all of the subjects in the other gorups received the practice items. It is apparent from Table 1 that no particular ear or condition suffered especially on the SSW test although the left non-competing condition (LNC) received no errors.

It was of interest to note the facility with which the control group was able to respond to the test material. Some subjects were convinced that the competing words were not completely overlapped. Nevertheless, it was a simple matter to demonstrate that the words were indeed simultaneous. There appeared to be no difference in the performance of the high school and university students.

In addition, a number of children eight years old and above were assessed with the same procedure. They responded in essentially the same manner as the control group. From this observation it appears that age, as young as eight years, is not a significant factor.

Phase II.   This portion of the investigation was concerned with subjects suffering from probable unilateral brain damage due to head injury. Six subjects met the criteria of a history of unilateral physical trauma to the head, scars on that side of the head and paralysis contralateral to the affected hemisphere or both. The group had a mean age of 21.5 years. The subjects had normal pure-tone thresholds between 250 and 8000 cps and normal results on the conventional speech tests of hearing. SRT's of 2 and 1.7 db were obtained for the contralateral and homolateral ears, respectively. Word discrimination was 99.7% in each ear (Table 2).

The unilateral trauma group had a mean error of 21.3 on the SSW test. Table 1 indicates the mean number of incorrect responses presented for the right and left ear without consideration of the affected hemisphere. The left side was traumatized in four of the six cases. These

TABLE 2.

Mean Pure-Tone Averages for the Speech Frequencies (500, 1000 and 2000 CPS), Speech Reception Thresholds, and Word Discrimination Scores for the Right and Left Ears

SPEECH AVERAGE Group	RE	SRT LE	RE	LE	DISCRIMINATION RE	LE
Normal	0 *	0	0 *	0	100%	100%
Trauma	−6.3	−3.5	3.7	0	99.7%	99.7%
Conductive	30	33	33.6	34.8	95.2%	96.8%
Sensory-Neural	20.7	23.9	21.2	23.5	80.4%	78.8%

*Speech averages, SRT's and word discrimination scores for the Normal group were assumed.

are plotted by the percentage of incorrect responses in Figure 1. More significant information is obtained when the data are re-organized into contralateral and homolateral ears. This is shown in Table 3 and presented graphically in Figure 2. It can be seen that of the more than 21 average errors only 5.8 were in the homolateral ear. Five of the six subjects obtained total scores of 17 or more. The total number of incorrect responses for the unilateral trauma group ranged from 5 to 36. It is of interest to note that the errors in the contralateral ear ranged from 5 to 25. In each case contralateral ear was obviously poorer and for that ear the competing trials suffered to a greater extent than did the noncompeting trials. This tendency supports the earlier literature since the contralateral ear appears most severely affected in cases of central disturbance.

Phase III. The conductive hearing loss group which was composed of five subjects had a mean age of 24 years. The average speech reception threshold for the group was about 34 db with 95 and 97 per cent discrimination in the right and left ears, respectively. Since the subjects performed in such a normal fashion on the SSW test, additional data were not collected on conductive ears (Tables 1 and 2). This finding serves to support the hypothesis that the SSW test is not affected by reduced sensitivity per se.

Phase IV. The effect of depressed word discrimination ability was assessed by employing a group of 10 subjects with sensory-neural losses. The mean age of this group was 30 years. Speech reception thresholds ranged from 2 to 52 db with means of 21 and 24 db for the

FIGURE 1. ━━━

The percentage of errors for the normal (control), unilateral head trauma (central), sensory-neural (peripheral), and conductive (peripheral) groups on the competing and noncompeting items for the right and left ears on the SSW test.

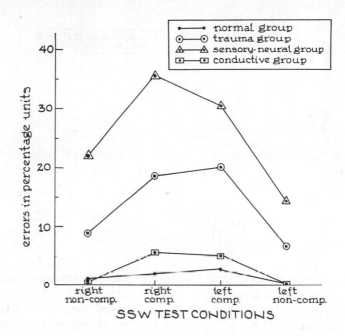

━━━ normal group
⊙━━⊙ trauma group
△━━△ sensory-neural group
▣━━▣ conductive group

errors in percentage units

SSW TEST CONDITIONS

right non-comp. · right comp. · left comp. · left non-comp.

TABLE 3. ━━━

Means for the Unilateral Trauma (Central) Group for the Standard Audiometric Tests and the SSW Test for Contralateral and Homolateral Ears

		Contra-lateral	Homo-lateral	Total
Standard Test	Speech Average	−4.7 db	−5.2 db	
	SRT	2 db	1.7 db	
	Discrimination	99.7%	99.7%	
SSW Test	Noncompeting	4.5	1.5	6.0
	Competing	11.0	4.3	15.3
	Sum	15.5	5.8	21.3

FIGURE 2.

The percentage of error for unilateral head trauma (central) group for the ear contralateral and homolateral to the damaged side for both competing and non-competing message conditions.

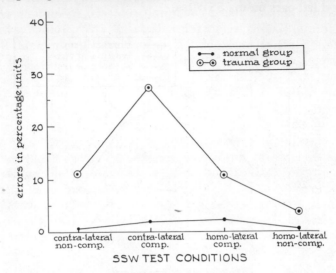

right and left ears respectively. Discrimination scores ranged from 56 to 100 per cent in the right ear with a mean of 80 per cent and ranged from 28 to 100 per cent in the left ear with a mean of 79 per cent (Table 2).

This sensorineural group was assumed to represent peripheral lesions. The group was made up of individuals with losses due to acoustic trauma, ototoxicity and familial factors. This group had a mean of 40.6 errors on the SSW test ranging from 6 to 112 incorrect responses. A strong positive correlation was suspected between the word discrimination score on the W-22 lists and the SSW score. Statistical evaluation bore out this finding. A Pearson r of .93 was obtained. This suggests that a large portion of the variance observed on the SSW test is attributable to differences in intelligibility. Although this finding is somewhat disappointing in light of our desire to have a test which is free from peripheral distortion, the high correlation between the two measures permits an estimate of the amount of error attributable to peripheral lesions.

Another means of distinguishing between difficulty due to peripheral and central lesions might be the ratio of noncompeting and competing conditions in the affected ears. The tendency for individuals with central lesions (head trauma) to adequately handle noncompeting signals in the contralateral ear is obvious (Figure 2). This is not the case with peripheral distortion as shown in Figure 1. The sensory-neural group exhibited difficulty in both conditions.

Development of the Staggered Spondaic Word Test

Summary

The purpose of this pilot study was to investigate the value of the staggered spondaic word (SSW) test as a measure of central dysfunction. Twenty normal hearing (control) subjects, six unilateral head trauma (central) subjects with normal hearing, five conductive (peripheral) hearing loss subjects and ten sensory-neural (peripheral) hearing loss subjects were given standard audiological tests as well as the SSW test.

The individuals with unilateral head trauma exhibited considerable difficulty on the SSW test especially in the ear contralateral to the injury. These findings agree with the results found by other investigators using different tests of higher auditory function and thus tends to support the theoretical considerations upon which the present test is based. Control subjects had essentially no difficulty on the proposed test. Children as young as eight years of age responded without apparent difficulty. Patients with conductive hearing losses behaved as did the normals on the SSW test. This suggests that hearing loss per se is not sufficient to interfere with the analysis of CNS function. Individuals with sensorineural hearing losses along with word discrimination losses of a moderate to severe degree demonstrated reduced ability on the SSW tests. Thus, it appears that the SSW test, in its present form, is resistant only to mild or perhaps moderate peripheral distortions. Two methods are suggested to distinguish the peripheral SSW errors from those of a central origin.

It is concluded on the basis of the present investigation that the SSW test appears to offer a number of important features which may be of both clinical and experimental value.

References

1. Bocca, E.: Factors Influencing Binaural Integration of Periodically Switched Messages. Acta Oto-laryngol. 53:142, 1961.

2. Bocca, E., Calearo, C., and Cassinari, V.: A New Method for Testing Hearing in Temporal Lobe Tumours; Preliminary Report. Acta Oto-laryngol. 44:219, 1954.

3. Calearo, C., and Lazzaroni, A.: Speech Intelligibility in Relation to Speed of the Message. Laryngoscope 67:410, 1957.

4. Epstein, A., and Hopkinson, N.T.: Personal communication.

5. Jerger, J.: Observations on Auditory Behavior in Lesions of the Central and Auditory Pathways. A. M. A. Arch. Otolaryngol. 71:797, 1960.

6. Katz, J.: The Use of Spondaic Staggered Words for Assessing the Integrity of the Central Auditory Nervous System. J. Auditory Res. 2:327, 1962.

7. Matzker, J.: Two New Methods for the Assessment of Central Auditory Functions in Cases of Brain Disease. Annals of Otology, Rhinology and Laryngology 68:1185, 1959.

8. Miller, M. H.: Audiologic Evaluation of Aphasic Patients. J. Speech Hearing Dis. 25:333, 1960.

9. Walsh, T., and Goodman, A.: Speech Discrimination in Central Auditory Lesions. Laryngoscope 65:1, 1955.

Author's Note:

This was the first article to present group data on the SSW Test as well as some early observations. The data and most of the observations have stood up over time. It should be pointed out that all of the SSW data are raw SSW results. The findings in this study led to the corrected SSW scores. Another change that we have made since this article is that Right NC and Right C are averaged and not totaled to get the Right Ear score. The Right and Left Ear scores are averaged to get the Total score.

There were no established normative data for adults and, therefore, any comparisons with normal adult performance must be considered of a general nature. Since that time we have established norms for adults and have a better idea about the performance of children. In the article we noted that children as young as eight years of age performed much like adults. This is quite true, but we cannot expect all normal eight year olds to do so.

The SSW Test: An Interim Report

Jack Katz

Over the past 20 years there has been a gradual refinement in the audiologic diagnosis. Prior to World War II hearing loss was dichotomized
into either conductive or nonconductive categories. New techniques
now permit a finer and more reliable assessment of the auditory system
from the outer ear to the cortex of the brain. Some procedures have
provided diagnostic information for as much as two decades while
others have quickly fallen into disuse. The purpose of this paper is to
report on the present status of the Staggered Spondaic Word (SSW) Test
as a measure of central auditory dysfunction (Katz, 1962). The "central
auditory" area is the primary auditory reception center of the cerebral
cortex, which encompasses the superior temporal gyrus, bilaterally,
particularly the middle and posterior portions.

The Study of Auditory Problems

Since 1954 there has been considerable interest in locating auditory
disorders at the cortical level. Two general methods have been used.
First, Bocca, Calearo, and Cassinari (1954) drew attention to the value
of specialized speech tests in identifying "hidden" hearing loss. Later,
Sanchez-Longo, Forester, and Auth (1957) demonstrated that tests of
sound localization could also indicate a central auditory lesion. The

Journal of Speech and Hearing Disorders May 1968, Vol. 33, No. 2

present review deals with speech techniques used to designate central auditory dysfunction.

"Cortical" hearing tests show the defect in the ear contralateral to the affected hemisphere. This contralateral phenomenon has been demonstrated in all clinical studies whether or not the hemisphere dominant for language was impaired. This is probably because the majority of the fibers arising from one cochlea course to the opposite temporal cortex (Rosenzweig, 1951).

The successful use of central auditory tests in Europe (Bocca, Calearo, Cassinari, and Migliavacca, 1955; Matzker and Welker, 1959) and the United States (Walsh and Goodman, 1955; Goldstein, Goodman, and King, 1956) led to a proliferation of techniques (Calearo and Lazzaroni, 1957; Matzker, 1959; Feldmann, 1960; Jerger, 1960; de Quiros, 1961; Kimura, 1961; Katz, 1962; Berlin, Chase, Dill, and Hagepanos, 1965). Audiologists have gradually incorporated one or more of these tests into their clinical battery. Berlin et al. (1965) have shown fairly good agreement among various central auditory tests. This is substantiated by the experience of many clinicians; however, the correlation among these measures is far from perfect. It would appear unrealistic and perhaps undesirable to have complete agreement for the multitude of central tests. It is unlikely that the unilateral filtered speech tests patterned after the technique of Bocca et al. (1954) require the integrity of the same centers as tests based on separation of binaurally competing messages (Feldmann, 1960; Katz, 1962). Thus, a battery of central tests might sample the integrity of different auditory areas and thereby provide more specific localization of the brain dysfunction.

Four varieties of central speech tests are now in use. Distorted speech materials delivered in a monaural mode were the first central speech tests to be employed. The distortion may be accomplished by acoustic filtering, low fidelity, and other means. A second technique is time distortion. Speech which is speeded up or slowed down falls into this category. The third major category is that of supplementary messages, or integration. These methods usually require the listener to combine binaural sources of information in order to obtain an accurate response. A fourth approach to uncovering central auditory disorders is the competing message technique or separation. These methods are usually binaural. Independent signals are presented in an overlapped fashion. One or both of the messages may be required of the listener. These four groups of tests may have many modifications and combinations thus offering an infinite variety of techniques. Presumably, many cortical and subcortical centers might be identified by an appropriate assortment of auditory tests.

Since the earliest work with central auditory speech tests, there has been a gradual trend to include stable materials (Calearo and Lazzaroni, 1957; Feldmann, 1960; Kimura, 1961; Katz, 1962). By "stable materials" we mean clear, familiar speech containing considerable redundancy. These materials are less likely to be affected by peripheral hearing loss than are distorted monosyllables. In order to challenge the nervous system, complex presentations of material have come into use and therefore increase our ability to investigate the primary auditory system and, perhaps, areas of secondary function. Conceivably these procedures assess more abstract function than some of the earlier tests. In their chapter in *Modern Developments in Audiology* (1963), Bocca and Calearo provide an excellent and comprehensive review of the literature on central auditory processes.

The Staggered Spondaic Word Test

The SSW test was designed to evaluate central auditory impairment. The rationale for the technique appears elsewhere (Katz, 1962). The initial attempts to determine its value have been described by Katz, Basil, and Smith (1963), who found that the test differentiated normal listeners from those with histories of skull trauma. The ear contralateral to the damaged side gave the poorest results. This could not be accounted for on the basis of word discrimination score (WDS) or lack of hearing sensitivity. A group of patients with peripheral hearing loss and no known neurologic involvement were also tested. Their proficiency on the SSW test depended entirely on their word discrimination ability. The deviation from normal performance was eliminated by correcting the SSW score for the WDS. The W-22 WDS was simply subtracted from the SSW score in the same ear. This pilot investigation demonstrated the potential value of the SSW test in sorting central nervous system problems from those of peripheral hearing loss and from normals.

In 1965 Balas and Simon reported on the intelligibility of SSW items as a function of the level of presentation. Berlin et al. (1965) studied various central auditory procedures with a group of patients following temporal lobectomy. They found the SSW test to have considerable accuracy in indentifying the damaged hemisphere. Brunt (1965) used the SSW test with children having functional articulation disorders. Springer (1966) studied the value of this test with stutterers. In our own laboratories over 600 subjects—including normals and those with wide varieties of problems—have been evaluated. These subjects ranged in age from 5 to 80 years.

Test Description

In the SSW test, clear, relatively familiar spondaic words[1] are presented to each ear in a partially overlapped manner. A momentary pause separates the two individual monosyllables of each of the two spondees in a test item. An example of a test item is diagramed below:

	Time Sequence		
	1	2	3
Right ear	up	stairs	
Left ear		down	town

The listener is expected to repeat both spondees. The order in which he responds is noted but not considered in the scoring. Errors on the test constitute omissions, substitutions, or distortions of any monosyllable. A few very minor deviations are not penalized such as "white wall" instead of "white walls." Errors are marked on a score sheet and later analyzed.

Initially, the subject is given the following instructions:

You are going to hear some words which will be presented to one or both of your ears. The words will be presented in small groups. Just as soon as the group of words is completed, I would like you to repeat them all back to me. Take a guess if you are not quite sure of a word. Before each item you will hear the phrase, "Are you ready?" Please don't repeat this phrase, just the group of words that follow it.

Construction of Lists and Test Tapes

Familiar spondaic words were paired so that the first monosyllable (time sequence #1) and the last monosyllable (time sequence #3) formed a third spondaic word. This was done to increase the likelihood of the subject's missing one or both competing words. No attempt was made to match the length or phonetic content of the competing words in the item. The 40 items of the test were alternated so that the initial monosyllable was in the right ear for all odd items or vice versa.

The most successful method of producing an SSW tape was to use two monophonic tape recorders. Their outputs were led to a dual channel tape recorder through a Grason-Stadler Model 162 speech audiometer.

---

[1] "Spondaic word" in this case is used to refer to a combination of two monosyllabic words which are given equal stress. These words form a familiar combination such as *green bean*, *Sunday*, *baseball*, and *al(l)right*.

Development of the Staggered Spondaic Word Test

A dual channel storage oscilloscope was used to estimate the amount of overlap. However, the trained ear is usually able to judge the appropriate overlap without benefit of the oscilloscope.

Equipment and Procedures

The listener is seated in a quiet room or audiometric chamber. Earphones mounted in standard cushions or in circumaural muffs are placed on him. The rest of the audiometric equipment may be housed in an adjoining control room provided that the patient's face is visible and that clear monitoring of the responses is possible. Several suitable seating arrangements may be used in a one-room setup. The two-channel SSW tape is played on a compatible tape recorder. Each channel of the tape recorder is routed to a separate channel of a speech audiometer. The intensity is set to 50 dB HL (re: 22 dB SPL) when SRT is 0 dB HL or better. When one or both SRT's are poorer than zero the SSW test is presented at 50 dB SL in that ear. This level is expected to provide a maximum score (Balas and Simon, 1965; Katz and Olroyd[2]) and, therefore, deviations from normal performance cannot be attributed to lack of sensitivity. In some cases where there is a sharp drop in hearing within the speech frequencies (500, 1000, and 2000 Hz) the intensity of the signal may be increased to insure that the listener is not penalized for his peripheral hearing status. Rather large errors in intensity may be made without significantly affecting the test results. Of all the groups tested, the patients with conductive hearing loss appear to require the most care in setting the appropriate levels.

When health and comfort permitted, we administered pure tone threshold, SRT, and WDS tests, either recorded or live voice. In addition, patients with hearing loss were given ABLB, SISI, tone decay, median plane localization, Bekesy audiometry, and/or other tests as indicated. Presently, the SSW test is given in an IAC Model 1600 suite using an Ampex Model 602-2 tape recorder and a Grason-Stadler Model 162 speech audiometer, or a Viking 87 tape recorder associated with an Allison Model 22 audiometer.

Following the instructions, the patient is given a number of practice items to insure that he is capable of repeating the two-spondee answer. If he has difficulty with these easy items he has a second chance to listen and respond. If he repeats the carrier phrase or does not follow instructions he maybe reinstructed. Sometimes it is necessary to train the listener to wait for all of the words before responding. When a speech problem interferes with accurate assessment the patient may write his responses. The listener is given a liberal amount of time to respond, but is encouraged to answer promptly.

---

[2]Katz, J., and Olroyd, Marie, unpublished study, 1965.

SSW Lists

A number of SSW tapes have been produced in our laboratories. Despite the many differences in equipment, techniques, and speakers used, there is considerable similarity among the various recordings. The phonetic structure and degree of overlap of the competing monosyllables are probably of importance to the overall level of difficulty. Of course, familiarity and probability of occurrence of the word combinations also affect the listener's score.

We have used lists ranging from 20 items (List C-EC) to 80 items (List ED-2). Thus far, our 40-item (List EC) and 52-item (List 1 B) recordings have been most successful. These lists are long enough to give reliable information but short enough to avoid extreme fatigue and boredom. The first 80-item test (List ED-1) was too difficult for our normal subjects. This was probably due to the vocabulary level of some items and the extreme care which we took in overlapping the words. List ED-2 was not as difficult despite the use of these same word combinations. In this recording, less stringent overlap was demanded. When this test was used with groups of children, one or two items (e.g., *although-eyes right*) accounted for most of the errors. This was no doubt due to the improbable nature of the words for this population. The ED-2 list might have particular value as a research tool because it has been divided into two equated lists, with two scramblings of each (Turner, 1966).

List EC is our most useful clinical tape to date. Results on this list agree quite well with the other versions of the test. The speech is clear and contains a good signal-to-noise ratio. The C-EC list is made up of the 20 items of the 40-item EC list which have the simplest vocabulary. Therefore, this list might provide a better measure with young children than the other lists. Unfortunately, each error on a monosyllable has a 5% effect on the score. Thus, the variability among normal subjects may be rather wide. This EC and C-EC lists contain four practice items.

Scoring

Figure 1 shows the final page of an SSW scoring form. Note that columns A and H both represent right noncompeting (RNC) conditions, except that the errors tabulated in A were for items in which the right ear was first. Column H is for left-ear-first items. Columns B and G are right competing (RC) conditions, C and F left competing (LC), while D and E represent left noncompeting (LNC) conditions.

To facilitate scoring and terminology "SSW Score" will refer to the percentage of error, whether for a specific condition, ear, or for the total test. "Corrected SSW Score" (C-SSW Score) is designated as the percentage of error (SSW Score) minus the percentage of error on the

FIGURE 1.
The last page of an SSW record form.

	L-NC ~~ ~~ (A) R-NC	L-C (B) R-C	R-C (C) L-C	R-NC (D) L-NC		R-NC (E) L-NC	R-C (F) L-C	L-C (G) R-C	L-NC (H) R-NC
31.	bird	~~cage~~ *range*	crow's	nest					
32.						week 3	end 4	work 1	day 2
33.	book	shelf	drug	store·					
34.						wood	work	~~beach~~ —	craft
35.	~~head~~ *can*	~~bull~~ —	milk	shake					
36.						fish	net	sky	line
37.	for 3	~~give~~ *wish* 4	milk 1	man 2					
38.						sheep	skin	~~bull~~ *hot*	dog
39.	race	~~horse~~ [√ʒ]	street	car					
40.						green	house	~~string~~ *green*	bean
TOTAL (p.4)	1	4	0	0		0	0	3	0
p.3	1	4	1	0		1	0	4	0
p.2	0	3	0	0		0	1	5	1
p.1	1	3	0	0		0	0	3	·1
GRAND TOTAL	3	14	1	0		1	1	15	2
	R-NC ~~L-NC~~	R-C ~~L-C~~	L-C ~~R-C~~	L-NC ~~R-NC~~		L-NC ~~R-NC~~	L-C ~~R-C~~	R-C ~~L-C~~	R-NC ~~L-NC~~

W-22 word discrimination test. Thus, the listener is not penalized for auditory distortion which is primarily attributable to lesions below the level of the brain. With a W-22 score of 88%, 12% would be subtracted from the competing and noncompeting Raw SSW Scores for the particular ear of the listener. To obtain the Raw SSW Score for any one condition, we multiply the number of errors by 2.5, for a 40-item test. To calculate the SSW Score for one ear we multiply the number of errors in both conditions by 1.25 and for the entire test by 0.625 or simply 0.62.

SSW Norms

Table 1 shows the total C-SSW performance for various samples of normal subjects. Results for the ED-2 list were not included because the test appears too difficult for clinical purposes. From Table 1 we find the point which is two standard deviations above the various means ranges from 2.0 to 4.6. None of the 99 subjects exceeded to a total corrected SSW Score of 5. The same approach was employed to determine the upper limit of normal for either ear or for any one condition. A listener whose score exceeds these limits has not performed normally.

In defining normality we have attempted to establish a boundary which is based on both statistical as well as individual data. Because of the sparse population of patients with central auditory dysfunction the landmarks are based on individual performance alone. Figure 2 shows the C-SSW Scores for samples of subjects with well localized lesions in the central nervous system, subjects with lesions in the peripheral auditory system, and normals. The 10 normals were randomly drawn from the 99 control subjects described in Table 1. The central group was divided into patients with lesions in the auditory cortex ($N = 7$) and those whose cortical lesions spared the middle and posterior superior temporal gyrus ($N = 10$). These individuals had unilateral tumors or vascular lesions. The patients with hearing loss were divided into sensory-neurals ($N = 14$) and conductives ($N = 9$). They were diagnosed as having peripheral hearing loss and normal central nervous systems.

Our preliminary criteria for designating a patient with central auditory dysfunction is 15 for the total corrected score, 20 for either ear, and 25 for any condition. Between the upper limit of normal and the lower limit of central auditory dysfunction is the mild error range which includes 30% of the remaining pathological subjects. Mild C-SSW Scores have been noted in the central nonauditory group, which is free from hearing loss, and the two peripheral hearing loss groups. Table 2 summarizes the C-SSW Score criteria presently used in evaluating adult performance on the SWW test.

TABLE 1. ▬▬▬▬▬▬▬▬▬
Mean Corrected SSW Scores and Standard Deviations for Various Age Groups and Lists

Study	N	List	Age	Age Range	Corrected SSW Score	S.D.
Katz, Basil, and Smith (1963)	20	1A	20	14–28	− .4	1.5
Katz and Fishman (1964)	10	1B	22	20–24	.8	1.9
Goldman and Katz (1965)	24	1B	24	18–39	− .3	2.2
Katz and Fishman (1964)	20	1B	39	30–49	1.3	1.9
Katz and Myrick (1965)	10	C-EC	23	19–29	−1.3	2.2
Brunt and Katz (1967)	15	EC	38	16–55	−3.2*	2.6

* This lower mean is attributable to poorer WDS than the older groups.

TABLE 2. ▬▬▬▬▬▬▬▬▬
Upper Limits for Corrected SSW Scores

C-SSW	Normal	Mildly Abnormal	Moderately Abnormal	Severely Abnormal
Total Score	5	15	35	100
Ear Score	10	20	40	100
Condition Score	15	25	45	100

Analysis of the SSW Test

Performance of patients between 12 and 60 years of age having reasonably normal intelligence may be compared with the SSW limits noted above. Figure 2 shows that the scores might be profitably divided into four groups: moderate-severe, mild, normal, and possibly supranormal. The present discussion will involve only the first three categories.

Central Disorders

Definition   "Central disorders" refers to impairment of the cerebral cortex and subcortical areas, probably down to the level of the midbrain.

SSW Conditions.   The first analysis of the SSW test involves the performance on the four conditions (RNC, et al.). When the poorest C-SSW Score on any one condition does not exceed 15 this performance cannot be differentiated from normal. Thus we have strong assurance that there is no central auditory involvement, provided the ear and

FIGURE 2.
Total corrected SSW Scores for subjects with central nervous system disorders, hearing loss, and normal controls.

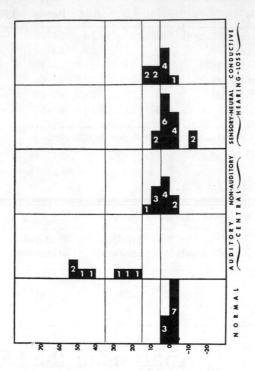

total scores are also within normal limits. Nevertheless, a patient with such a score might have a central nonauditory disorder. That is, he might have a cortical lesion outside the primary auditory centers of the brain.

A patient whose test results show a corrected SSW condition in excess of 25 very likely has central auditory dysfunction if lack of motivation and cooperation can be ruled out as major factors. When one side is affected to this extent the cerebral hemisphere contralateral to it should be suspected. A patient whose score falls between 16 and 25 on an SSW condition is not a normal listener; however, the score is not sufficiently severe to indicate central auditory impairment. Such an individual falls into the central nonauditory category provided that his hearing for speech is normal. At present we do not know what SSW results are obtained when the patient has a central nonauditory lesion as well as a hearing loss in the speech range.

SSW Ear Performance.   We can now analyze the SSW results for each ear in a manner similar to that used to study the various conditions. A C-SSW Score of 10 serves as the upper limit of normal. It has been our experience that ear performance is generally a more accurate indicator of central auditory function than either the SSW conditions or total score. Typically a patient who fails the ear analysis also fails the other two analyses. As in the case of a moderate or severe deviation in one of the SSW conditions, defective performance in one ear suggests that the dysfunction is in the contralateral hemisphere.

Total SSW Score.   Table 2 shows the limit of normal for total C-SSW to be 5. Since we have worked almost exclusively with unilateral central problems we do not know if some patients with bilateral nonauditory lesions are likely to exceed the central auditory limit of 15. For example, at present we have no way of knowing whether a patient with bilateral lesions in the frontal or occipital lobes would reveal scores suggestive of primary auditory disorder (16 or greater) or central nonauditory (15 or less). On the basis of the total C-SSW Score alone the specific hemisphere cannot be identified.

Response Bias.   Response bias refers to any one of a number of unlikely responses that persist in the patient's test performance. The first step is to look at the symmetry of columns A through H. It is presumed that a normal cooperative subject will make random errors when the items are right-ear-first as well as left-ear-first. We would become intrigued if the subject made seven errors but each of them occurred when the left ear was leading (e.g., A = 0, B = 0, C = 0, D = 0; E = 1, F = 3, G = 2, H = 1). The likelihood of this happening by chance alone is less than 1 in 100. This type of response bias is called an "ear effect." Ear effects and other response biases seem to have diagnostic significance whether or not the C-SSW Score exceeds the normal limits.

Another important response bias is the "order effect." This is seen when the patient makes more errors on the first spondee than on the second spondee or vice versa. For example, A = 3, B = 14, C = 2, D = 0; E = 4, F = 15, G = 4, H = 1; or 36 errors on the first spondee and 7 on the second. We can assume that such a distribution did not arise by chance. A third bias which is similar to the ear and order effects is the "pattern effect." This refers to two different configurations of errors for the right-ear-first items as opposed to the left-ear-first items.

The other major response bias noted to date is the "reversal." A reversal is any response by the patient in which all monosyllables are given correctly but in an order that differs from the one presented on the test tape. Instead of "up-stairs–down-town," for example, the patient responds "down-town–up-stairs" (3, 4, 1, 2).

A "partial reversal" is a response in which an item is repeated out of order but one of the monosyllables is also incorrect (e.g., "down-town–up-first").

Significance of Response Bias.　When response bias was originally observed it was thought to represent a confounding influence on the SSW test. It seemed to us that some type of nonauditory error was projected into the test. Recently, we realized that this error could be used as a qualitative method to analyze the patient's disorder. In addition, it is possible to "adjust" the SSW score for order or ear effect by eliminating the most deviant portion. The auditory response is considered the portion with the least error because we assume that the pure auditory lesion will lead to difficulty in the contralateral ear regardless of whether it is the first spondee, second spondee, right-ear-first, or left-ear-first. Thus, the most likely nonbiased sample of auditory performance is the best portion of the patient's responses. When there are 36 errors on the first spondee and only seven on the second, the patient is obviously capable of missing only seven monosyllables if the material is presented in a certain way. Therefore, we eliminate equally from the right and left ear conditions by using only the second spondee for purposes of calculation. The remaining errors are multiplied by 5 instead of 2.5 and corrected for WDS. We are finding that the specific order effect, ear effect, and reversal combinations seem to provide information regarding the site of lesion of some auditory and nonauditory involvements.

Peripheral Auditory Disorders

Definition.　The term "peripheral" for our purposes denotes the auditory system from the outer ear to the VIIIth cranial nerve, terminating at the cochlear nuclei. Since we consider "central" to involve only the brain, the brainstem is left as a transition area from the peripheral to central systems. Thus far, we have seen characteristics of both peripheral and central disorders on the SSW test in the patients with brainstem lesions. Due to the small sample of brain stem subjects in our population this area will not be covered in detail. Similarly, specific discussion of VIIIth nerve and cerebellar conditions will await further research.

SSW Correction.　Katz, Basil, and Smith (1963) reported that WDS correlates extremely well with the SSW results. They found $r = 0.93$ for a group of 15 subjects with either conductive or sensory-neural hearing losses. In our laboratory we compared SSW results and WDS for 15 patients with sensory-neural hearing loss in one or both ears. The Pearson product-moment correlation coefficient was 0.92. The mean WDS was 79% and the raw SSW result was 81% correct. It appears that the use of the correction for word discrimination loss is justified. When both central auditory and peripheral hearing loss are present, we assume that the WDS will account for the peripheral distortion, leaving the central portion for analysis.

Some patients with conductive losses and some diagnosed as having Meniere's disease perform more poorly on the SSW test than do others with peripheral hearing losses. Presumably, in the case of conductives, high presentation levels might stimulate the cochleas by bone conduction causing a diotic effect. Diotic presentation is more difficult than the typical dichotic mode (Goldman and Katz, 1966). Some type of "central masking," not unlike that described by Martin, Bailey, and Pappas (1965), might also be involved.

SSW deviations in some Meniere's patients suggests that there may be a greater central component in this disorder than is traditionally acknowledged. In support of such an explanation is the recent work by Barac, Hagbarth, and Stahl (1966), who demonstrated abnormal EEG's in Meniere's cases.

Pseudohypacusis. All tests which require the cooperation of the patient may be jeopardized to a greater or lesser extent by the individual with a nonorganic problem. Five patients suspected of having unilateral pseudohypacusis were administered the SSW test. After further testing four of the five revealed thresholds 50–100 dB more sensitive than their initial test performance. No effort was made to exact the "true" SSW responses. Rather the patients were left to respond as they wished. In some cases the presentation levels were below the admitted thresholds. Also, the possibility of true central auditory lesions was never ruled out in any of these cases.

The total C-SSW Scores were 3, 4, 19, 34, and 36. All but one of these patients showed bilaterally symmetrical results despite the claim of a unilateral hearing loss.

Validation of the SSW Test

In order to obtain information which would help to validate the SSW test we established blinded conditions for the neurologist, otologist, and audiologist. The neurologist was responsible for assessing the integrity of the central nervous system and the otologist for assessing the peripheral auditory system.

The neurologist indicated whether the primary auditory centers were affected. This was rated on a six-point scale from "definitely auditory" to "definitely nonauditory." The neurologist was guided in his diagnosis primarily by surgical or autopsy information, when available. In addition, radiologial studies were of particular significance in cases with vascular disorders.

From Figure 2 it is clear that the SSW test is capable of differentiating normal subjects from patients with central auditory disorders. The latter group appears also to be differentiated from the central nonauditory patients. This provides strong evidence that the SSW test is indeed assessing central auditory dysfunction. Figure 3 shows the raw, corrected, and adjusted SSW Scores for the 17 patients with cortical lesions, as a function of the neurologic diagnosis. An impressive relationship exists between the SSW and neurologic evaluations. Of the three methods employed the C-SSW Score seems to be the most useful, particularly if there is some degree of hearing loss present.

Misleading Findings

In six cases originally considered to have central damage in a known location the SSW findings did not agree with the neurological

FIGURE 3.
Total SSW Scores versus neurologic categorization of cortical lesions.

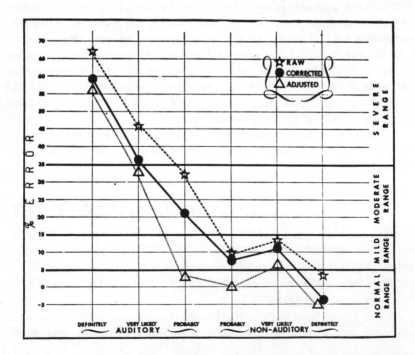

Development of the Staggered Spondaic Word Test

diagnosis. In two of these cases the retest demonstrated that the earphones had been reversed. In two other cases it was learned that there were other neurological impairments or a history of severe skull trauma. These previous insults accounted for the SSW findings. In the last two cases SSW results did not agree with the neurological diagnosis; however, the reasons for these discrepancies are not yet clear. In one case a patient with a left fronto-temporal isthmus mass exhibited normal SSW results. It was observed that this patient had ear and order effects. The total C-SSW Score was 4% and suggested that there was no central auditory dysfunction. The neurological diagnosis indicated that auditory centers were "probably" affected. This patient behaves more like those with central nonauditory problems on the SSW test. It is well to point out that this particular diagnosis was based on the pneumoencephalogram, carotid angiogram, EEG, and neurological evaluation and not surgical or autopsy findings. The individual will be followed to determine whether the neurological diagnosis or the SSW information provided the more accurate picture.[3]

In another patient more perplexing results were obtained. This 58 year old male was diagnosed as having a left fronto-parietal metastatic carcinoma. The diagnosis was based on a carotid angiogram, EEG, and neurological examination. A brain scan and sonogram were both negative. No surgical or autopsy confirmation have been obtained to date. The neurologist categorized the lesion as being nonauditory in nature. Both the initial SSW test and retest revealed a grossly abnormal pattern for the left ear with excellent test-retest reliability. The performance in the right ear was essentially negative. In this case two bizarre findings were observed. First, the patient showed signs of dramatic auditory dysfunction on the SSW test and, second, the dysfunction was in the homolateral ear. We would expect if the lesion actually involved auditory centers the breakdown would occur in the contralateral ear. On the other hand if the lesion was nonauditory we would expect very few errors on the SSW test. Because the results for this patient are so different from the others with central impairment it is our feeling that (1) other lesions or pressure might exist due to the carcinoma or, (2) the results might reflect some previous injury. Another factor might possibly have influenced the SSW findings in this case. While the patient had relatively normal hearing for speech he did exhibit an extensive sensory-neural loss primarily in the left ear beyond 1000 Hz. Other patients with both central auditory and peripheral hearing loss problems have shown both aspects in their SSW results. When word discrimination was accounted for the evidence of the central problems remained. Unfortunately, such was not the case with this patient. We

---

[3] A second staffing by another neurological consultant indicated the lesion to fall short of the auditory area. This agrees with the SSW finding.

will continue to follow him in order to determine whether the SSW test was indeed an inaccurate indicator of the patient's central auditory function.

Summary

The SSW test has been studied as a method for evaluating central auditory dysfunction in cases with cortical disorders, peripheral hearing loss, and normal subjects. A total Corrected SSW (C-SSW) Score of 5 represents the upper limit of normal performance while a score of 16 denotes the lower limit of central auditory dysfunction. The test might also provide qualitative information about the presence of central nonauditory dysfunction. On the basis of our experience with this test it appears to be both a practical and valid measure of central auditory dysfunction.

Acknowledgements

The author would like to thank the many people who have contributed to the development of the SSW test, and would like particularly to acknowledge Arthur W. Epstein, Consulting Neurologist, for his valuable suggestions and criteria used in these studies, and Marie Olroyd for testing, retesting, and following up numerous patients reported here. In addition, data included in this report represent the work of Howard Eldot, Lois Turner, Michael Brunt, and Carla Burgess. The author wishes to thank Wallace Rubin and Oscar Pinsker for otological evaluations and Wayne Hill, Eugene Baska, Arnold Schoolman, and Dewey Zeigler for neurological and neurosurgical evaluations and consultation.

This research was supported in part by Public Health Service Research Grant No. NB06518 from the National Institute of Neurological Disease and Blindness, and the United Cerebral Palsy Educational and Research Foundation Grant, T-146-64.

References

Balas, R. F., and Simon, G., The articulation function of a staggered spondaic word list for a normal hearing population. *J. aud. Res.*, 4, 285–289 (1965).

Barac, B., Hagbarth, K. E., and Stahl, J., EEG in Meniere's disease. *Acta Otolaryng.*, 62, 333–340 (1966).

Berlin, C. I., Chase, R. A., Dill, Anne, and Hagepanos, T., Auditory findings in patients with temporal lobectomies. *Asha*, 7, 386 (1965).

Bocca, E., Calearo, C., and Cassinari, V., A new method for testing hearing in temporal lobe tumours; preliminary report. *Acta Otolaryng.*, 44, 219–221 (1954).

Bocca, E., and Calearo, C., Central hearing processes. In J. Jerger (Ed.), *Modern Developments in Audiology*. New York: Academic Press (1963).

Calearo, C., and Lazzaroni, A., Speech intelligibilty in relation to the speed of the message. *Laryngoscope*, 67, 410–419 (1957).

De Quiros, J. B., Accelerated speech audiometry, an examination of test results. In *Translation of the Beltone Institute for Hearing Research*, No. 17 (1964). Based on Interpretacion de los resultados obtenidos conlogoandio-metria accelerada. *Revista Fono-audiologica,* 7, 128–164 (1961).

Feldmann, H., Untersuchungen zur Diskrimination differenter Schall-bilder bei simultaner, monauraler und binauraler Darbietung. *Arch Ohr. usw. Heilk. u. Z. Hals- usw. Heilk,* 176, 600–605 (1960).

Goldman, Sheila, and Katz, J., The SSW test: dichotic, diotic and monaural. Paper presented ASHA Convention, Washington, D.C., 1966.

Goldstein, R., Goodman, A., and King, R., Hearing and speech in in-fantile hemiplegia before and after left hemispherectomy. *Neurology,* 6, 869–875 (1956).

Jerger, J., Observations on auditory behavior in lesions of the central auditory pathways. *Arch. Otolaryng.,* 71, 797–806 (1960).

Katz, J., The use of staggered spondaic words for assessing the integrity of the central auditory nervous system. *J. aud. Res.,* 2, 327–337 (1962).

Katz, J., Basil, R. A., and Smith, J. M., A staggered spondaic word test for detecting central auditory lesions. *Ann Otol. Rhinol. Laryng.,* 72, 908–918 (1963).

Kimura, Doreen, Some effects of temporal lobe damage on auditory perception. *Canad. J. Psychol.,* 15, 156–165 (1961).

Martin, F. N., Bailey, H. A. T., and Pappas, J. J., The effect of central masking on threshold for speech. *J. aud. Res.,* 5, 293–296 (1965).

Matzker, J., Two new methods for the assessment of central auditory functions in cases of brain disease. *Ann. Otol. Rhinol. Laryng.,* 68, 1185–1197 (1959).

Matzker, J., and Welker, H., Die Prufung des Richtungshorens zum Nachweis und zur topischen Dia-gnostik von Hirnerkrankungen. *Z. Laryng. Rhinol. Otol.,* 28, 277–294 (1959).

Rosenzweig, M. R., Representation of the two ears at the auditory cortex. *Amer. J. Physiol.,* 167, 147–158 (1951).

Sanchez-Longo, L.P., Forester, F. M., and Auth, T. L., A clinical test for sound localization and its applications. *Neurology,* 7, 655–661 (1957).

Springer, Betty A., A comparison of the central auditory integrity of stutterers and nonstutterers on the staggered spondaic word test. Master's thesis, Vanderbilt Univ. (1966).

Turner, Lois K., A normative study on the SSW test for various age groups. Master's thesis, Univ. of Kansas (1966).

Walsh, T., and Goodman, A., Speech discrimination in central auditory lesions. *Laryngoscope,* 65, 1–8 (1955).

Author's Note:

Remarkably little has changed in the basic understanding and procedures that are used with the SSW Test since this article appeared in 1968. While there have been considerable refinements and extensions there, only a few updates are necessary.

Although it is not wrong to use the speech reception threshold as the basis for the 50 dB presentation level, it is more practial to employ the 3-frequency speech average. Fewer adjustments are needed for setting the levels when a person has a drop in hearing at 2000 and 4000 Hz.

It was not clear in the 1960s and early '70s how to deal with reversals. We were not sure if the varying sequencing problems that we noted were equivalent or indeed proper to score. In 1968 we were concerned with *true* and *partial* reversals. Later we looked at another variation, *questionable* reversals. After studying the problem for more than 10 years, I decided that the various types of reversals are essentially interchangeable. Thus, if a person reorders the sequence of the item in his response and gets all of the words correct, or if he makes one mistake and upsets the sequence these are equivalent reversals (although in the latter case he also shows an error). A reversal is also counted when a person alters the order of three words and omits a fourth (e.g., "stairs, town, up" for "upstairs, downtown").

I believe that brain and brainstem problems can be differentiated, but my terminology might be confusing. The central nervous system includes both the brain and the brainstem so at the present time when referring to the CNS, we do not exclude either of them. The brainstem continues to act like a transistion region between the peripheral auditory mechanism and the *brain*. What I referred to back in the 60s as *central auditory* can be more properly designated as *auditory reception*, and *nonauditory* is now *nonauditory reception*.

A Study of Three Tests of Central Function With Normal Hearing Subjects

Michael Brunt and Cornelius P. Goetzinger

Introduction

For many years investigators have attempted to develop methods to assess the integrity of the auditory pathways beyond the cochlear. Much interest has centered on establishing tests of the cerebral auditory areas, as routine pure tone and speech tests were found inadequate for this purpose. Bocca, Calearo and Cassinari (1954) reported on the use of filtered words to reveal temporal lobe tumours in patients who evidenced normal hearing on conventional tests. Since then, Bocca, Calearo, Cassinari and Migliavacca (1955), Calearo (1957), Calearo and Antonelli (1963) and Calearo and Lazzaroni (1957) have utilized a variety of "sensitized" speech tests to detect central auditory problems.

During the past decade several other investigators as Goetzinger and Angeil (1965), Jerger (1964), Katz (1962) have developed analogous tests. Generally, their results were similar to those of the Bocca-Calearo group. The methods which indicated cortical problems revealed reduced performance for the ear opposite the lesion. Such findings are thought to arise because the peripheral auditory mechanism is represented maximally in the contralateral temporal lobe (Rosenzweig, 1951).

Cortex 4, 288–297, 1968

As noted above some tests have presented a speech signal of reduced redundancy, as for example the filtered speech of Bocca, Calearo and Cassinari (1954), the accelerated speech of Calearo and Lazzaroni (1957), the interrupted speech of Bocca (1961), or the distorted speech of Goetzinger and Angeil (1965). In general, the specialized tests may be divided into three categories based on method of presentation. They are: 1) monaural, 2) binaural and 3) dichotic (competing message) tests.

Monaural Tests

In this type of test difficult speech material is presented monaurally. Results are similar for each ear in the case of normal subjects. However, an individual with cerebral auditory damage will perform significantly poorer in the ear opposite the lesion. Bocca, Calearo and Cassinari (1954) used syllabic phonetically balanced (PB) words routed through a 500 Hz low-pass filter. Patients with temporal lobe tumors showed reduced performance for the ear contralateral to the tumor. Calearo and Antonelli (1963), Linden (1964) and Jerger (1964) employed filtered speech procedures with similar results.

Goldstein, Goodman and King (1956) administered the Rush Hughes (RH) recordings of the Harvard PB words to four hemiplegics both before and after hemispherectomy. They noted that the subjects' errors were greater for the ear contralateral as compared to the ipsilateral to the lesion. Goetziner and Angell (1965) reported the use of a difference score between an easy and a difficult discrimination test (the CID W-22's and RH PB-50's, respectively) as an indication of cortical damage. A difference score of 30% or more was considered significant and was reflected in the ear opposite the lesion.

Binaural Tests

Generally these tests utilize speech stimuli of reduced redundancy. For example, in one of Matzker's (1959) tests a different frequency portion of each test word simultaneously reached the two ears. In one condition a low frequency portion of each test word was sent to one ear simultaneously with a high frequency portion of the same test word routed to the other. To be more explicit, the word to one ear was filtered through an 1815-2500 Hz band-pass while the second ear received the identical word via a 500-800 Hz band-pass. Either condition heard monaurally was poorly understood. However, when the pass-band were presented simultaneously to the two ears there was a significant increase in intelligibility for normal individuals but not for patients with central auditory problems.

Another variation of the binaural method is Jerger's (1964) SWAMI (speech with alternating masking index) test. In this procedure PB-50's were presented binaurally while white noise 20 dB above the subject's speech frequency average was alternated between ears. Only limited success was achieved with this method.

Dichotic (Competing Message) Tests

These tests have the common attribute that each ear receives a different message—a dichotic stimulus presentation. Furthermore, the stimuli are time sequenced so the stimulus items reach both ears simultaneously. Kimura (1961a, 1961b) employed a competing message test (a paired digit test originally designed by Broadbent (1956) to investigate the performance of normals and subjects with cerebral pathology at various levels. She found that individuals with brain injury did significantly poorer than normals. However, both for normals and for patients a laterality effect was observed. In general, each group performed better in the right ear.

Dirks (1964) investigated the performance of 24 normal hearing young adults on a competing word test. The stimuli consisted of 1000 Hz low-pass filtered PB-50 words with a rejection rate of 18 dB per octave. Each item consisted of a pair of words time sequenced so that they arrived at the ears simultaneously. In addition to this presentation, Dirks gave the lists monaurally. He also administered Kimura's competing digits. The competing PB-word condition as well as the competing digits of Kimura both revealed a laterality effect not observed in the monaural condition. The results for the dichotic tests with reference to ear dominance agreed with those of Kimura.

Katz (1962) designed the Staggered Spondaic Word Test (SSW) to detect central auditory lesions. The item presentation is similar to that of Dirks and of Kimura except that spondees are used as stimuli. Each test item consists of non-competing as well as competing conditions. Normal subjects have shown very few errors on the test (Katz, 1962, 1968a). In contrast, patients with confirmed cerebral auditory pathology, as temporal lobe damage, have exhibited reduced performance as compared to normals. Generally, performance was poorer for the ear opposite the lesion and most reduced for the competing condition.

Laterality Effect and Dichotic Auditory Tests

Kimura (1961a, 1961b) noted that on the competing digit test both normals and individuals with cerebral pathology showed a laterality effect, performance for the right ear being better than for the left. Furthermore, cerebral dominance for speech was determined in one group of 120 subjects by the Wada-Rasmussen (1960) sodium amytal test. The latter correlated highly with the competing message test. Thus, Kimura's technique seemed to reveal cerebral dominance for speech.

In contrast, Calearo and Antonelli (1963) pointed out that no laterality effect was evident in their study utilizing monaural sensitized speech tests. In reply, Kimura (1963a) stated that the laterality effect may only be revealed through a binaural competing message task.

As previously mentioned, Kimura's findings were substantiated by Dirks (1964) using the Kimura test and his own dichotically-presented filtered PB words. Again, a significant difference occurred favoring the right ear.

Unpublished studies by Brunt (1962) and Myrick (1965) on Katz's SSW test suggested that a laterality effect will be evidenced by children six to ten years of age. However, this effect gradually decreased with age. Katz remarked (1968a) that at age 12 years and older only a very minimal laterality effect is seen. It is also interesting to note that Kimura (1963b) found a laterality effect in children with her competing digit task.

Materials and Methods

Purpose of the Study

The primary purpose of this study was to investigate the laterality or dominance effect, particularly with reference to left cerebral dominance. As pointed out above there is still conflicting evidence as to the occurrence of this phenomenon.

Subjects, Equipment, and Methods

Sixteen individuals between the age of 16 and 37 years served as subjects. There were six males and ten females. The average age of the group was 27 years with a standard deviation of 4.8 years. Threshold measures were taken on each subject to assure normal hearing bilaterally. Normal hearing was defined as ISO air conduction thresholds no greater than 25, 20, 20, and 25 dB respectively, at frequencies of 500, 1000, 2000 and 4000 Hz.

Equipment

Pure-tone thresholds were measured on a Beltone 15C pure tone audiometer equipped with TDH-39 earphones mounted in MX-41/AR cushions. The speech tests were presented with an Ampex 401 stereo tape recorder routed through a Grason-Stadler speech audiometer (Model 162) equipped with earphones as above. Presentation levels for each year were independently controlled through the Grason-Stadler audiometer.

The Kimura and Dirks tests were dubbed from a tape which had been sent to the Kansas University Audiology Clinic by Dirks. The SSW test was a tape recording prepared by Katz.

Tests: Description and Administration

The Kimura test used in this study consists of pairs of digits presented simultaneously to the two ears. Each pair of digits is two different numbers and each test item comprises three digit pairs. For example, a subject might hear 1-5-7 in the right ear and 2-4-10 in the left ear. The digits one to ten are used as stimuli.

The test stimuli comprised the 18 items of the Kimura test which were found by Dirks (1964) to most clearly demonstrate the laterality effect. These items may also be divided into three subtests or sets of six items each on the basis of presentation method. Set I consists of presenting three digits to the right ear and three different digits to the left ear simultaneously in one second. Set II is the same with the exception that three seconds are taken to present each test item. In Set III each item is again administered in one second with the exception that one digit is repeated. For example, if 3-6-2 were heard in the right ear, 6-4-9 might be heard in the left.

The Kimura test was administered at 40 dB above the speech frequency average per ear in contrast to Dirks' (1964) level of 20 dB relative to the speech reception threshold.

This procedure was followed in an attempt to circumvent the laterality effect as noted by Dirks on the Kimura at levels 20 dB above the speech reception threshold. The subject was instructed to repeat all the numbers he heard. An error was counted for every number not repeated correctly.

Essentially the Dirks test consists of two filtered lists of PB words presented under dichotic conditions. There are 50 words per list. As in Dirks' (1964) study the lists were also given monaurally. For both conditions the test lists were administered 40 dB above the speech frequency average in contrast to Dirks' presentation at 20 dB relative to the speech reception threshold. The subject was instructed to repeat all the words he heard. Also, in contrast to Dirks' (1964) publication the tape as prepared by him for us utilized a 500 Hz low-pass filter rather than the 1000 Hz low-pass filter.

The Katz test consists of 40 test items, each of which incorporates two spondees. They are arranged so each ear is exposed to both noncompeting and competing conditions. For example, the right ear might receive the word "upstairs" and the left, the word "downtown." However, "up" would arrive alone at the right ear (Right Non-competing condition) with "stairs" and "down" simultaneously and respectively presented to the right (Right-Competing) and left (Left-Competing) ears. "Town" would then be heard alone in the left ear (Left Non-Competing condition). To avoid ear order effects the lead ear is alternately the right or left.

The results may be viewed as a total score on the 40 items. In addition, the competing versus non-competing items may be examined as well as performance for the right and left ears.

The test list used in this investigation was list EC, the current revision (1968). However, Katz notes that this and earlier versions have shown very similar results. The test was administered 50 dB above the speech frequency average per ear as suggested by Katz (1962). The subject was instructed to repeat all the words that he heard. An error was counted for each half-respondee not repeated.

For the three dichotic tests, stimulus lists were alternately presented to the right and left ears to minimize interlist variability. For the monaural Dirks presentation, the ear tested first was alternated between half of the subjects to reduce ear order effects. Each subject was tested individually in an IAC acoustic room, Model 403A. The experimenter and equipment, except for earphones, were located in a similar control room. The order of test presentation was as follows: 1) pure-tone test, 2) Kimura Competing Digit Test, 3) the Dirk's Filtered Words Test, and 4) the Katz Staggered Spondaic Word Test.

Results

Table 1 presents a summary of results on the Kimura test for two methods of scoring; namely, the total tests score and set results for combined ears.

A Friedman two-way analysis of variance (Siegel, 1956) revealed a significant difference for the means of the three sets. Examination of Table 1 indicates that the subjects performed poorest on the set III items (5.2). Next, the data for the total score were analyzed relative to specific ears. The mean number of errors for the right ear was 2.0 (SD of 3.1) as compared to a mean of 7.1 (SD of 6.0) for the left ear. The difference between ears of 4.1 is significant at the .01 level using the Wilcoxon matched-pairs signed Ranks Test (Siegel, (1956). This finding indicates that the subjects' performance was superior for the right as compared to the left ears on the Kimura test for the total test score.

It will be recalled that Dirks (1964), likewise, administered the Kimura test to a group of normal-hearing subjects. Suffice to say that our results with the Kimura Test, for total test scores, showing superior-

TABLE 1. ▬▬▬▬

Means and Standard Deviations of Errors on the Kimura Test for Total Scores and Set Scores

Type of scores	Errors	
	Mean	S.D.
Total	10.1	8.6
Set I	2.5	2.6
Set II	2.4	3.1
Set III	5.2	4.0

ity of the right over the left ears, confirmed the findings of Dirks. Furthermore, the percentages of correct responses in each ear for each study were similar. (Means Dirks, RE = 92.6, LE 86.4; means this study RE = 94.4, LE = 86.9). Thus, there appears to be a dominance effect on this test relative to total test scores.

As a next step in the analysis of the data, the Dirks Filtered Word Test was examined. In the monaurally presented condition the mean number of errors for the right ear was 33.2 (SD = 4.3) and for the left ear 34.8 (SD = 4.9). The difference of 1.6 was not statistically significant. Thus, no dominance effect occurred. In the dichotic condition of the same test the mean number of errors for the right ear was 42.8 (SD = 3.8) and for the left ear 42.8 (SD = 3.2), hence, identical. However, when the differences between the mean number of errors for the right and left ears were tested across conditions (RE for dichotic versus RE for monaural, and LE for dichotic vs LE for monaural) the mean differences between conditions were highly significant (RE, $t = 6.17$; LE, $t = 7.38$) for both ears. These results indicate that dichotically presented filtered speech is more difficult to discriminate than the same material monaurally presented.

Finally, the scores on the SSW test were analyzed. For the total SSW test score the mean percent correct was 96.9. Stated differently, the mean number of errors was 1.25 with a standard deviation of 1.2. The mean number of errors for the right ear was 0.3 (SD = 0.5) and for the left 1.0 (SD = 1.6). The small difference between ears of 0.7 was found to be significant at the .02 level using the Wilcoxon Matched-Pairs Sign-Ranks Test. Although this difference is minute, nevertheless there is right ear dominance. This finding is in the direction of Katz's observation that the laterality effect in individuals 12 years of age and older is small.

Results were also examined with reference to the competing and non-competing mono-syllable conditions of the Katz test. For the right ear no errors were found in the non-competing condition. A mean error of only 0.7% obtained in the competing condition. The left ear exhibited a mean of 0.3% error in the non-competing condition and a mean error of 2.7% in the competing condition. The differences between competing and non-competing conditions were significant for each ear using the Sign Test (right ear, $p = .031$; left ear, $p = .002$). Thus, the competing condition was more difficult for each ear. These findings are, therefore, consonant with our results for the Dirks test. In short, both tests demonstrated that the subjects found the competing condition more difficult than monaural listening.

Discussion

To summarize our results, a right ear dominance effect was demonstrated both for the Kimura and Katz tests. To be sure, in the latter instance the effect was not large. However, it reached statistical significance. With reference to the Dirks test there was no difference between the ears for the dichotic condition. The findings could suggest that demonstration of ear dominance is test dependent. Unquestionably, much more research is required in order to delimit the parameters which contribute to an understanding of cerebral function in this respect.

Summary

The purpose of the study was to investigate the cerebral dominance effect as reported by several investigators. A group of subjects with normal hearing were administered three tests purported to give some evidence of higher level auditory function. The tests were the Kimura digits, the Katz SSW and the Dirks filtered PB's tests. The results indicated a significant right ear dominance effect for the Kimura and Katz tests. No difference between ears was found for the Dirks test. The findings could suggest that demonstration of ear dominance is test dependent. However, additional research is needed to resolve the issue.

References

Bocca, E. (1961) *Factors influencing binaural integration of periodically switched messages*, "Acta Otolaryngol.," 53, 142–144.

—, Calearo, C., and Cassinari, V. (1954) *A new method for testing hearing in temporal lobe tumours, preliminary report*, "Acta Otolaryngol.," 44, 219–221.

—, —, — and Migliavacca, F. (1955) *Testing cortical hearing in temporal lobe tumours*, "Acta Otolaryngol.," 45, 289–304.

Broadbent, D. (1956) *Successive responses to simultaneous stimuli*, "Quart. Jour. of Exp. Psychol.," 8, 145–162.

Brunt, M. (1962) *Performance on three auditory tests by children with functional articulation disorders*, Unpublished Master's Thesis, University of Pittsburgh, Pittsburgh, Pennsylvania.

Calearo, C. (1957) *Binaural summation in lesions of the temporal lobe*, "Acta Otolaryngol.," 47, 392–395.

— and Antonelli, A. (1963) *Cortical hearing tests and cerebral dominance*, "Acta Otolaryngol.," 56, 17–26.

— and Lazzaroni, A. (1957) *Speech intelligibility in relation to the speed of the message*, "Laryngoscope," 67, 410–419.

Dirks, D. (1964) *Perception of dichotic and monaural verbal material and cerebral dominance for speech*, "Acta Otolaryngol.," 58, 73–80.

— (1967) Personal communication.

Ferguson, G. A. (1959) *Statistical Analysis in Psychology and Education*, McGraw-Hill Book Company, New York.

Goetzinger, C. P., and Angell., S. N. (1965) *Audiological assessment in acoustic tumors and cortical lesions*, "EENT Monthly," 44, 39–49.

Goldstein, R., Goodman, A. and King, R. (1956) *Hearing and speech in infantile hemiplegia before and after left hemispherectomy*, "Neurology," 6, 869–875.

Jerger, J. (1964) *Auditory tests for the central auditory mechanism*, in Neurological Aspects of Auditory and Vestibular Disorders, ed. by Fields and Alford, Charles C. Thomas Company, Springfield.

Katz, J. (1962) *The use of staggered spondaic words for assessing the integrity of the central auditory system*, "Jour. of Aud. Res.," 2, 327–337.

— (1968a) Personal communication.

— (1968b) *The SSW test: An interim report*, "Jour. of Speech and Hear. Dis.," 33, 132–146.

Kimura, D. (1961a) *Some effects of temporal-lobe damage on auditory perception*, "Can. Jour. of Psychol.," 15, 156–165.

— (1961b) *Cerebral dominance and the perception of verbal stimuli*, "Can. Jour. of Psychol.," 15, 166–171.

— (1963a) *A note on cerebral dominance in hearing*, "Acta Otolaryngol.," 56, 617–618.

— (1963b) *Speech lateralization in young children as determined by an auditory test*, "Jour. of Compar. Physiol. and Psychol.," 56, 899–902.

Linden, A., (1964) *Distorted speech and binaural speech resynthesis tests*, "Acta Otolaryngol.," 58, 32–48.

Matzker, J. (1959) *Two new methods for the assessment of central auditory functions in cases of brain damage*, "Annals of Otol., Rhinol. and Laryngol.," 68, 1185–1197.

Myrick, D. K. (1965) *Performance of normal children on a central auditory test*, Unpublished Master's thesis, Tulane University.

Rosenzweig, M. R. (1951) *Representation of the two ears at the auditory cortex*, "Amer. Jour. of Physiol.," 167, 147–158.

Siegel, S. (1956) *Nonparametric Statistics for the Behavioral Sciences*, McGraw-Hill Book Company, New York.

Wada, J., and Rasmussen, T. (1960) *Intracarotid injection of sodium amytal for the lateralization of cerebral speech dominance: Experimental and Clinical Observations*, "Jour. of Neurosurg.," 17, 266–282.

Staggered Spondaic Word Test: Support

Robert F. Balas, Ph.D.

While the informed student of audiology accepts the primitiveness of his diagnostic art, he is aware that the clinical potential of many "experimental" techniques has not been realized.[5] One area of interest, particularly since the work of Bocca's group[4] in Europe and a report by Goldstein et al.[6] in the United States, is the use of distorted speech tests designed to identify and provide information on the sites of lesions within the central auditory system. Comprehensive discussions of central auditory processes, tests, and test material have been furnished elsewhere.[2,3] Generally, however, pure tone and speech audiometry as they are commonly administered do not reveal a hearing deficit, yet the so-called central auditory tests consistently demonstrate reduced speech discrimination scores in the ear contralateral to the affected hemisphere. The purpose of this report is to present clinical results which tend to support the use of the Staggered Spondaic Word (SSW) Test as a measure of central auditory dysfunction.[8-10]

Katz[9] has provided an excellent review and description of the SSW test along with suggested methods of scoring and analyzing test results. *Briefly*, however, the SSW test is made up of relatively familiar, spondaic words which are presented partially overlapped in time to each ear. To clarify, the following is an example of a test item:

Annals of Otology, Rhinology and Laryngology, February, 1971 Vol. 80, No. 1, Page 32

| | Time Sequence | | |
	1	2	3
Right ear	up	stairs	
Left ear		down	town

Each monosyllable represents a condition. "Up" is in the right (ear) noncompeting condition (RNC), and "town" the left noncompeting condition (LNC). The noncompeting monosyllables (time sequence #1 and #3) form another spondaic word, in this example, "uptown." "Stairs" and "down" are in the competing conditions (RC and LC). The latter are presented to each ear simultaneously (time sequence #2). Forty items are employed. The patient is required to repeat or write both spondees or the four monosyllables in any order. The test is presented at 50 dB SL (re: average pure tone threshold, 500-2000 Hz) for each ear.[1]

SSW Score refers to the percentage of error, whether for a condition (RNC et al.) ear, or the total test. Omissions, substitutions or distortions of any mono-syllable constitute an error. Katz's[9] "Corrected SSW Score" (C-SSW Score) was used in this study. Table 1 shows Katz's preliminary criteria for evaluating adult performance on the SSW test.[9]

Figure 1 shows the total C-SSW Scores for a sample of patients with CNS disturbances and from normal subjects. The control group (C) consisted of 30 normals with an age range from 7 to 70 years and a mean of 34 years. The CNS groups consisted of: 1) patients with temporal lobe lesions (TLL) affecting the superior temporal gyrus, the primary auditory reception area ($N = 10$); 2) patients with cortical lesions (CL) not involving the superior temporal gyrus ($N = 15$); and 3) patients suffering from temporal lobe seizures (TLS, $N = 10$). The latter group was included since Jerger[7] reported reduced discrimination on a filtered speech test by an individual with temporal lobe epilepsy. Patients in the TLL group were selected on the basis of clinical (30%) or operative (70%) evidence demonstrating a *temporal lobe lesion* involving the primary auditory cortex. In four cases direct involvement, particularly of the middle and posterior portion, of the superior temporal

TABLE 1. ▬▬▬▬▬▬▬▬▬▬▬▬▬▬▬▬▬▬▬▬▬▬▬▬▬▬▬▬▬▬

Upper Limits for Corrected SSW Scores

C-SSW	Normal	Mildly Abnormal	Moderately Abnormal	Severely Abnormal
Total Score	5	15	35	100
Ear Score	10	20	40	100
Condition Score	15	25	45	100

FIGURE 1.

Total corrected SSW scores for patients with CNS disturbances and normal controls.

TABLE I

UPPER LIMITS FOR CORRECTED SSW SCORES

C-SSW	Normal	Mildly Abnormal	Moderately Abnormal	Severely Abnormal
Total Score •	5	15	35	100
Ear Score	10	20	40	100
Condition Score	15	25	45	100

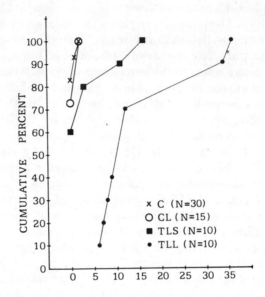

gyrus was questionable. According to the neurosurgeon, however, secondary damage as a result of surgical procedure was probable. Patients in the CL group had lesions primarily involving the *frontal*, *parietal*, or *occipital* lobes. In no case was there evidence of the lesion affecting the superior temporal gyrus. Most patients were virtually free of peripheral hearing impairment.

The total C-SSW Score for each patient in relationship to the upper limits of Katz's preliminary criteria shows that the normal controls (C), the central nonauditory patients (CL), and 80% of the patients with temporal lobe seizures (TLS) did not obtain a score exceeding 3. One patient in the latter group scored within the mild error range (6–15) and one in the "moderately abnormal" range (16–34). And only three central auditory patients (TLL) had scores suggesting involvement of the primary auditory cortex. The remaining seven patients performed

Development of the Staggered Spondaic Word Test

within the "mildly abnormal" range. The central nonauditory patients did as well as the normal controls. Forty percent of Katz's central nonauditory patients ($N = 10$) scored within the mild error range.[9] Our patients experienced less difficulty than those reported by Katz. Variables as type, site, size of lesion, resulting pressure, etc., or possible quality differences of the SSW tape, phonetic structure and timing of the overlapping monosyllables, and familiarity of the word combinations preclude definitive comparisons.

On the basis of total C-SSW Score, of course, the disturbed hemisphere cannot be identified. The four conditions (RNC et al.), particularly the competing conditions, as well as SSW ear performance should be analyzed. A patient who has a corrected SSW condition score exceeding 25, Katz suggests very likely has central auditory involvement. Sixty percent of TLL patients had scores greater than 25 in the competing condition in the ear contralateral to the affected hemisphere. Three patients scored in the severe range and three in the moderate range.

Summary

A Staggered Spondaic Word (SSW) tape was administered to patients with cortical disturbances and to normal subjects. The normal controls and patients with lesions primarily involving the frontal, parietal or occipital lobes and 80% of the patients with temporal lobe seizures scored within the "normal" range. Patients with temporal lobe lesions had greater difficulty, and the results tend to demonstrate the sensitivity of the SSW test in detecting central auditory dysfunction.

References

1. Balas RF, Simon GR: The articulation function of a staggered spondaic word list for a normal hearing population. J Auditory res 4:285–289, 1964

2. Bocca E: Distorted Speech Tests. In: Sensorineural Hearing Processes and Disorders. Graham AB (Ed), Boston, Little, Brown and Co., 1967, pp 359–370

3. Bocca E, Calearo C: Central Hearing Processes. In: Modern Developments in Audiology. Jerger J. (Ed), New York Academic Press, 1963, pp 337–370

4. Bocca E, Calearo C, Cassinari V: A new method for testing hearing in temporal lobe tumours. Acta Otolaryng 44: 219–221, 1954

5. Carhart R: Future horizons in audiologic diagnosis. Ann Otol 77: 706–716, 1968

6. Goldstein R, Goodman A, King R: Hearing and speech in infantile hemiplegia before and after left hemispherectomy. Neurology 6: 869–875, 1956

7. Jerger J: Audiological manifestations of lesions in the auditory nervous system. Laryngoscope 70: 417–425, 1960

8. Katz J: The use of staggered spondaic words for assessing the integrity of the central auditory nervous system. J Auditory Res 2: 327–337, 1962

9. Katz J: The SSW test: An interim report. J Speech Hear Dis 33: 132–146, 1968

10. Katz J, Basil R, Smith J: A staggered spondaic word test for detecting central auditory lesions. Ann Otol 72: 908–918, 1963

Clinical Validity of Central Auditory Tests

J. Jerger and S. Jerger

Six audiometric procedures were administered to seventy patients divided into seven groups: normal, eighth nerve, brain stem, temporal lobe, non-auditory CNS, aphasic, and amyotrophic lateral sclerosis (ALS). Pure-tone sensitivity was equated among groups. For the eighth nerve group, performance was consistently poor for all measures. For the brain stem group, performance was consistently depressed for difficult monotic speech tasks. For the temporal lobe group, performance was most severely affected for difficult dichotic speech messages. For the aphasic group, performance was generally poor for both monotic and dichotic speech procedures. For the non-auditory CNS and ALS groups, results were normal. Inter- and intra-group variability were substantial.

Introduction

In order to establish the validity of any proposed test procedure for the evaluation of auditory disorders, it is necessary to demonstrate (1) that the test yields the expected result in patients with auditory disorders and (2) that false-positive results usually do not appear in patients without auditory disorders.

In the case of central auditory disorder, we can identify at least four potential sources of error. First is the possibility that ill patients may perform poorly on difficult auditory tests due entirely to physical malaise rather than a central auditory problem. Second is the possibility that patients with *any* disorder of the central nervous system (CNS)

Scand Audiol 4: 147–163, 1975

may perform poorly on central auditory tests even though there is no direct involvement of the central auditory pathways per se. Third is the possibility that the presence of a language disorder in some patients with temporal lobe site may compromise the diagnostic value of degraded speech audiometry. Fourth, and finally, is the possibility that auditory test results may not be "site-specific" in some patients with either eighth nerve or brain stem auditory disorder because of secondary symptoms that masquerade as independent lesions. For example, is it possible for a patient with a brain stem disorder to show the same configuration of results as a patient with an eighth nerve site?

The present paper attempts to evaluate these potential sources of error by comparing the performance of groups of patients with central auditory disorders to the performance of patients in various control groups.

Method

Subjects

Seventy patients, tested by the Audiology Service, The Methodist Hospital, between 1968 and 1973, were divided into seven groups of ten patients each on the basis of the final medical diagnosis. Two were experimental groups composed of patients with either brain stem or temporal lobe disorders. Five were control groups divided into one normal group, one eighth nerve group, and three CNS groups.

Experimental groups

Brain stem   Site of lesion was confirmed surgically and/or radiographically in all 10 intra-axial brain stem patients. Final diagnosis from histopathologic report or pneumoencephalographic report was pontine glioma in 9 patients and arteriovenous malformation in 1 patient. Subjects were 2 females and 8 males. The average age was 26.0 years and ranged from 8 to 48 years. The brain stem lesion was primarily on the right side in 6 patients, primarily on the left side in 3 patients, and bilaterally symmetrical in 1 patient.

Temporal lobe.   Site of lesion was confirmed surgically and/or radiographically in 6 patients. Final diagnosis in these patients was astrocytoma in 2 patients, and either ependymoma, glioblastoma multiforme, glioma, or ischemia in the other four patients. The final medical diagnosis in the remaining patients was temporal lobe encephalopathy in 2 patients, temporal lobe embolyst in 1 patient, and skull trauma in 1

Development of the Staggered Spondaic Word Test

patient. Diagnosis was based on neurological findings, electrograms, clinical course, and history of onset. Subjects were 7 males and 3 females. The average age was 47.8 years and ranged from 24 to 63 years. The temporal lobe lesion was on the right side in 7 patients and on the left side in 3 patients. Patients in this group did not show any obvious language dysfunction accompanying the temporal lobe disorder.

Control groups

Normal.   Subjects were classified as normal on the basis of (1) hearing threshold levels less than or equal to 25 dB (ISO-64) between 250 and 4000 Hz, (2) normal findings on impedance audiometry, and (3) no evidence of intracranial disorder. Medical examination usually revealed a clinical history of dizziness and no other significant findings. Patients in this group did not have specific hearing complaints. Subjects were 6 females and 4 males. The average age was 41.1 years and ranged from 29 to 63 years. The purpose of the normal control group was to provide "baseline" information against which to compare the performance of the other control groups and the experimental groups. We referred all other test results to the data obtained in this normal group.

Eighth nerve.   Site of lesion was confirmed surgically in all patients. Final diagnosis from histopathologic report was acoustic neuroma in 5 patients, glomus jugularae tumor in 1 patient, cerebellopontine angle meningioma in 1 patient, cerebellopontine angle glioblastoma in 1 patient, jugular foramen neurofibroma in 1 patient, and clivus meningioma in 1 patient. Seven subjects were female and 3 were male. The average age was 40.7 years and ranged from 10 to 64 years. The lesion was on the right side in 5 patients and on the left side in 5 patients. The purpose of the eighth nerve control group was to determine whether eighth nerve auditory symptomatology may be confused with brain stem auditory symptomatology due to possible overriding secondary symptoms produced by either primary mass.

Aphasic.   All patients had a final medical diagnosis of aphasia. Histories revealed either a cerebrovascular accident or skull trauma. Eight patients were concurrently receiving aphasia therapy by the Speech Pathology Service of The Methodist Hospital. All of the 10 patients in this group could understand the verbal instructions for the audiometric tests. However, five patients were expressively impaired to the extent that speech tests involving oral repetition could not be carried out. The remaining five patients performed all speech tasks easily.

The length of time between the onset of the aphasia and the audiologic evaluation varied from 1 month to 28 years. Three patients were 1 to 3 months post-insult, three were 4 to 5 months post-insult, three were 10 to 12 months, and one was 28 years. Subjects were 5 females and 5 males. The average age was 46.5 years and ranged from 12 to 72 years. The purpose of the aphasic control group was to evaluate performance on speech intelligibility tests in patients with a language disorder in addition to possible temporal lobe disorder. We sought to determine whether auditory test results based on the perception of speech materials might be uniquely compromised by the presence of aphasia.

Non-auditory CNS.   Patients in this group had intracranial lesions that did not affect the central auditory pathways. Site of lesion was confirmed surgically and/or radiographically in all patients. Final diagnosis from histopathology, pneumoencephalography, or angiography was parietal glioblastoma in 1 patient, Arnold-Chiari malformation in 1 patient, pituitary tumor in 2 patients, midbrain glioma in 2 patients, vertebral artery aneurysm in 2 patients, parietal astrocytoma in 1 patient, and frontal falx meningioma in 1 patient. Subjects were 5 females and 5 males. The average age was 39.3 years and ranged from 22 to 53 years. The lesion was on the right side of the brain in 3 patients and on the left side in 3 patients. The remaining 4 patients had midline brain lesions. The purpose of the non-auditory CNS control group was to insure that abnormal test results were specific only to patients with direct involvement of the central auditory pathways.

ALS.   Patients in this group had amyotrophic lateral sclerosis (ALS), a degenerative motor neuron disease. Degeneration generally involves the Betz cells of the motor cortex, the motor nuclei of the brain stem, or the anterior horn cells of the spinal cord (Wolfgram & Myers, 1973). Subjects were 6 females and 4 males. The average age was 52.4 years and ranged from 31 to 66 years. The purpose of the ALS control group was to evaluate the effects on performance due to extreme physical malaise, (a characteristic of patients in this group), and to insure that "false-positive" results did not occur in patients with non-auditory brain stem disorders.

Test battery

Six audiometric test procedures were attempted on all patients. These procedures have been described in detail previously (Jerger & Jerger, 1974a) and are briefly summarized below.

Pure-tone sensitivity.   Threshold hearing levels (ISO-64) at octave frequencies between 250 and 4000 Hz were obtained by either conventional manual or Békésy techniques.

Békésy audiometry.   Sweep frequency tracings for interrupted and continuous signals were obtained over the frequency range from 200 to 8000 Hz. Frequency changed at a rate of one octave per minute. Intensity changed at a rate of 2.5 dB per second.

Acoustic reflex.   Acoustic reflex thresholds were measured at octave frequencies between 500 and 4000 Hz. Threshold levels were defined as the lowest hearing level (HL) in dB that produced reliable deflections of the balance meter when sound was presented to the ear opposite the ear containing the impedance bridge probe. The maximum intensity used to elicit reflex contractions was 110 dB HL.

PI-PB functions.   Performance-intensity functions for monosyllabic (PB) word lists (PI-PB) were constructed by presenting blocks of 25 words at each of several suprathreshold levels. Generally, performance was defined from that intensity level yielding 0 to 20% correct up to a maximum speech intensity of 110 dB sound pressure level (SPL). The patient repeated each word to a tester who scored it as correct or incorrect. White noise masking was presented to the nontest ear whenever the speech level was sufficiently intense to cross over and be heard in the nontest ear.

Synthetic sentence identification (SSI).   SSI materials (Jerger et al., 1968) consisted of a single list of ten synthetic sentences, seven words each, representing a third-order approximation to actual English sentences. The patient was seated before a console containing a list of the ten sentences and a corresponding column of push buttons. After each sentence had been presented, the patient identified the sentence he heard from the list in front of him and pushed the appropriate button. Different random presentations of the same ten sentences were used throughout the test session. Sentences were presented at an intensity level yielding 100% correct performance in both ears. For most patients, this level was 50 dB SPL. However, a few patients required louder presentation levels to achieve a criterion of 100% in both ears. The SSI task was made difficult by a competing speech message concerning the life of a Texas pioneer (Davy Crockett). Performance was measured at several message-to-competition ratios (MCR's) for both a contralateral competing message (CCM) and an ipsilateral competing message (ICM). For the CCM condition (sentences to the test ear and competition to the opposite ear) MCR's were varied in 20 dB steps over the range from 0 dB to −40 dB. For the ICM condition (sentences and competition to the same ear) MCR's were varied in 10 dB steps over the range from +10 dB to −20 dB.

Staggered Spondaic Word (SSW) test.   The SSW test (Katz, 1962) was composed of 40 pairs of partially overlapping spondaic words. The time sequence for an illustrative word pair (*upstairs* and *downtown*) consisted of the patient hearing *up* in one ear, then *stairs* and *down* simultaneously in both ears, then *town* in the opposite ear. We called the first monosyllable the *leading* condition, the simultaneous monosyllables the *competing* condition, and the last monosyllable the *lagging* condition. The 40 spondaic pairs were alternated between ears so that each ear received the leading monosyllable one-half of the time. The patient was instructed to repeat all the words he heard in either ear. The presentation level was the intensity yeilding maximum performance on PI–PB testing. The percent correct scores for the leading, competing and lagging conditions were obtained for each ear. The leading and lagging conditions were averaged in some groups to obtain one *non-competing* score. Results for each group were also scored according to the method recommended by Katz (1968).

Instrumentation and test materials

Pure-tone audiograms were obtained with either a manual audiometer (Beltone, model 10D) or a Békésy audiometer (Grason-Stadler, model E800). Impedance audiometry was carried out with an electroacoustic impedance bridge (Madsen, type ZO-70) and an associated pure-tone audiometer (Beltone, model 10D). Speech materials consisted of six PB-50 word lists (Egan, 1948), one list of ten synthetic sentences (Jerger et al., 1968), and one SSW list of 40 spondaic pairs (Katz, 1962). All materials were prerecorded on magnetic tape by the same male talker. The tape playback system (Ampex, AG440) was routed through a speech audiometer (Grason-Stadler, type 162) to earphones (Telephonic, type TDH-39) housed in CZW-6 cushions. Speech level was defined as the SPL of a 1000 Hz signal recorded at the average level of frequent peaks of the speech as monitored on a VU meter.

Procedure

Patients were tested in a single session of two to three hours duration. The entire test battery was attempted on all patients, but it was not possible to obtain all procedures on both ears of every subject. Patients

TABLE 1.
Number of Patients in Each Group with Successful Results On Both Ears for Each of the Seven Test Procedures

Test procedure	Groups							Total (N = 70)
	Normal	VIIIth nerve	Brain stem	Temporal lobe	Aphasic	Non-auditory CNS	ALS	
Pure-tone sensitivity	10	10	10	10	10	10	10	70
Békésy audiogram	10	10	8	4	7	8	3	50
Acoustic reflex	10	6	9	5	5	6	10	51
PI–PB	10	10	10	10	5	10	7	62
SSI–ICM	10	10	10	10	7	10	8	65
SSI–CCM	10	10	10	10	8	10	8	66
SSW	10	1	3	6	3	4	5	32

that did not complete the entire test battery either were unusually ill, were young children, or had other tests (i.e., radiograms) scheduled and could not stay for the entire session. Table 1 presents the number of patients in each group with successful results on both ears for each of the seven tests. All 70 patients completed pure tone sensitivity testing on both ears. At least 62 of the 70 patients had complete results for PI–PB functions, SSI–ICM, and SSI–CCM. Békésy audiometry and acoustic reflex measures were obtained in both ears in approximately 50 patients. The SSW test was successfully completed in 32 of the 70 patients.

Results

Illustrative cases

Patient A.   Figure 1 summarizes auditory findings for a 37-year-old female with a non-auditory CNS lesion on the left. Surgical exploration revealed a well circumscribed glioblastoma in the left temporoparietal region underlying the gyrus posterior to the junction of the occipital and temporal lobes and lower parietal region. The audiogram showed essentially normal sensitivity on both ears. Békésy audiograms were type I on both ears. The PI–PB functions were normal on both ears. The maximum PB (PB_{max}) scores were 100% on the right ear and 96% on the left ear. SSI–ICM scores were within the normal range, as indicated by the stippled area, on both ears. SSI–CCM scores remained at 100% on both ears at all MCR's. All diagnostic test results were negative. There was no evidence of eighth nerve or central auditory pathway involvement on either ear.

Patient B.   Figure 2 shows results for a 45-year-old female with an eighth nerve disorder on the right. An acoustic neurilemoma was removed at surgery. The audiogram showed normal sensitivity on the left ear and a mild sensori-neural loss on the right ear. Impedance audiometry showed normal, typeA, tympanograms and normal static compliance in both ears. However, acoustic reflexes were absent at all frequencies with sound in the right ear. With sound in the left ear, reflexes were present at normal HL's at 500, 1000, and 2000 Hz, but absent at 4000 Hz. The absence of acoustic reflexes at 4000 Hz only in the left ear probably has no diagnostic significance. Békésy audiograms were type IV in the right ear and type I in the left ear. The PI–PB function was normal on the left ear but showed substantial rollover on the right ear. PB_{max} scores were 96% correct on both ears. SSI–ICM scores showed unusually poor performance on the right ear only. SSI–CCM performance was unimpaired on either ear. Note that auditory deficits—sensitivity loss, abnormal adaptation on Bekesy audiometry, substantial PI–PB rollover, and SSI–ICM loss—were observed on the right ear only, the ear showing the radiographic abnormality.

Patient C.   Figure 3 presents results for a 48-year-old female with an intra-axial brain stem disorder primarily on the left side. Left vertebral angiography revealed a large intra-axial neoplasm extending from the caudal pons to the upper cervical cord and centered at the medulla oblongata with infiltration into the left cerebellar hemisphere. A shunt was performed to relieve increased ventricular pressure.

FIGURE 1. ━━━━━━━━━━━━━━━━━━━━━━━━━━
Summary of diagnostic test results for a 37-year-old female with a non-auditory CNS lesion on the left. Stippled area represents the normal range for SSI–ICM.

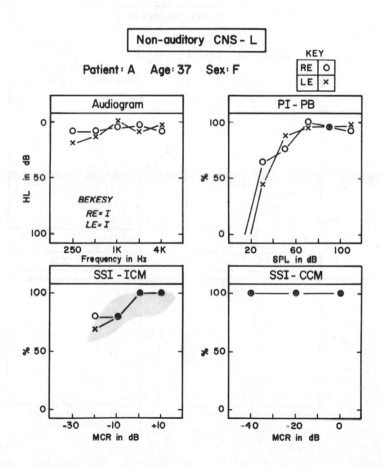

Surgery confirmed the presence of a brain stem glioma. The audiogram showed a moderate high frequency loss in both ears. Acoustic reflexes were present at normal HL's for all test frequencies on both ears. Békésy audiograms were type I on both ears. PI–PB functions showed slightly reduced maximum performance on the right ear and a mild rollover effect on the left ear. PB_{max} scores were 96% on the left ear and 84% on the right ear. SSI–ICM performance showed a deficit on the right ear only. SSI–CCM scores remained at 100% on both ears.

FIGURE 2. ━━━━━━━━━━━━━━━━━━━━━━━━━

Summary of diagnostic test results for a 45-year-old female with an eighth nerve disorder on the right. The stippled area represents the normal range for SSI–ICM.

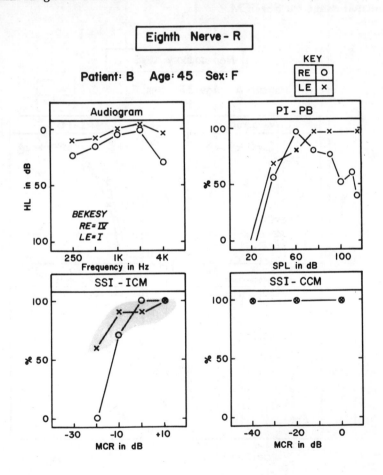

Development of the Staggered Spondaic Word Test

FIGURE 3.

Summary of diagnostic test results for a 48-year-old female with an intra-axial brain stem disorder primarily on the left side. Stippled area represents the normal range for SSI-ICM.

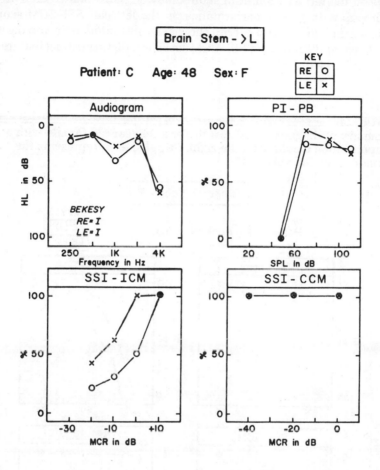

Substantial SSI–ICM losses in the presence of normal or near normal SSI–CCM performance is a distinguishing characteristic of brain stem disorder. Note that speech intelligibility deficits are observed on the right ear, the ear opposite the affected side of the brain stem.

Patient D.   Figure 4 shows results for a 24-year-old female with a temporal lobe disorder on the right. Angiography showed an ischemic area in the right temporal area with extensions into the frontal and parietal areas accompanied by cerebral edema and hydrocephalus. The audiogram showed normal sensitivity in both ears. Acoustic reflexes were observed at normal HL's for all test frequencies on both ears. The PI–PB functions showed normal maximum scores and insignificant rollover, but the left ear showed an unusually slow rise to maximum performance. PB_{max} scores were 96% on the right ear and 88% on the left ear. SSI–ICM scores showed performance deficits on both ears with poorer performance on the left ear. SSI–CCM scores were normal on the right ear but showed a substantial deficit on the left ear. Marked difficulty on SSI–CCM tasks is a distinguishing feature of temporal lobe disorder.

FIGURE 4.
Summary of diagnostic test results for a 24-year-old female with a temporal lobe disorder on the right. Stippled area represents the normal range for SSI-ICM.

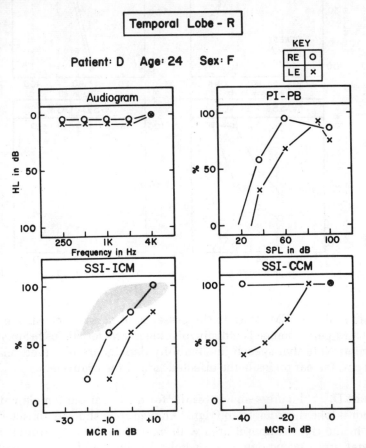

Development of the Staggered Spondaic Word Test

FIGURE 5. ▬▬▬▬▬▬▬▬▬▬▬▬▬▬▬▬▬▬▬▬▬

Summary of diagnostic test results for a 54-year-old male with aphasia. PI–PB performance could not be established (CNE) due to the patient's limited expressive ability. Stippled area represents the normal range for SSI–ICM.

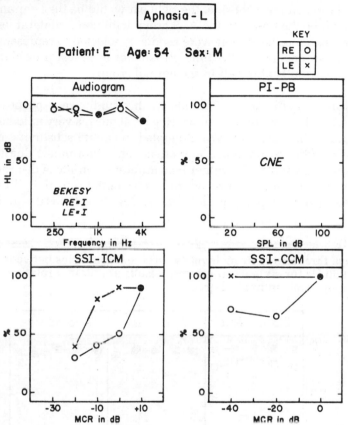

Patient E. Figure 5 presents test results for a 54-year-old male with aphasia. The patient sustained a cerebrovascular accident approximately one year prior to audiometric evaluation. The audiogram showed normal sensitivity in both ears. Acoustic reflexes were present at HL's within the normal range for all test frequencies on both ears. Békésy audiograms were type I in both ears. PI–PB functions could not be obtained (CNE) due to the patient's limited expressive ability. SSI–ICM and SSI–CCM (which require only a manual response) were within the normal range on the left ear and showed moderate impairment on the right ear. The aphasic patient usually shows a general deficit in speech intelligibility that is apparent for both monotic and dichotic listening tasks.

Distribution of auditory findings

Audiometric group data are presented in terms of the ear ipsilateral (I) and contralateral (C) to the site of disorder. For example, in a patient with a lesion on the right side, the right ear would be the I ear and left ear would be the C ear. In the ALS group with non-unilateral lesions, the right ear and the left ear were randomly selected to represent the I or the C ear one-half of the time. Results for each test procedure are referred to results obtained in the normal group.

Pure-tone sensitivity   Patients in this study were purposefully selected on the basis of normal hearing or, at most, a very mild hearing impairment in either ear. We attempted to equate sensitivity among groups in order to minimize any effects on performance due to differences in threshold HL's rather than differences in site of disorder. As a result of this selection procedure, a substantial sensitivity loss was unlikely in any group. Fig. 6 shows the average threshold HL's at octave

FIGURE 6. ▬▬▬▬▬▬▬▬▬▬▬▬▬▬▬▬▬▬▬▬▬▬▬▬▬▬▬▬

Average threshold hearing levels at octave frequencies between 500 and 4000 Hz for six patient groups. Results are plotted relative to sensitivity levels in normal group.

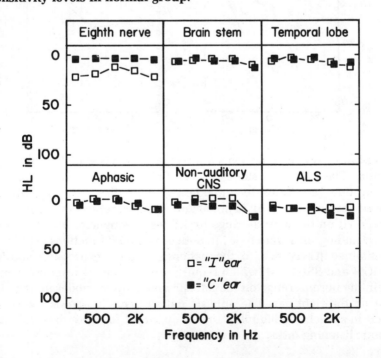

intervals between 500 and 4000 Hz for the six groups. All HL's are plotted relative to average sensitivity levels in the normal group. With the exception of the eighth nerve group, average sensitivity levels for all groups were within the normal range on both ears at all frequencies. The eighth nerve group showed an average mild loss, approximately 10 to 20 dB, on the I ear and normal sensitivity on the C ear.

Békésy audiometry   Figure 7 summarizes Békésy tracings on the I and C ears of patients in the six groups. Tracings for the normal group were type I on both ears of all patients and are not shown. Type I and II patterns are consistent with normal hearing or a cochlear site; type III and IV tracings are consistent with a retrocochlear disorder (Jerger, 1960b). Type I or II Békésy audiograms characterized both ears of all patients in the temporal lobe, aphasic, non-auditory CNS, and ALS groups. None of these patients showed a retrocochlear pattern on either ear.

Seven of eight brain stem patients showed normal, type I, tracings on both ear. This finding is consistent with the observations of Jerger (1960a) and Owens (1964, 1971). However, one patient, a 35-year-old

FIGURE 7. ━━━━━━━━
Type of Bekesy audiogram found on I and C ears of patients in each group.

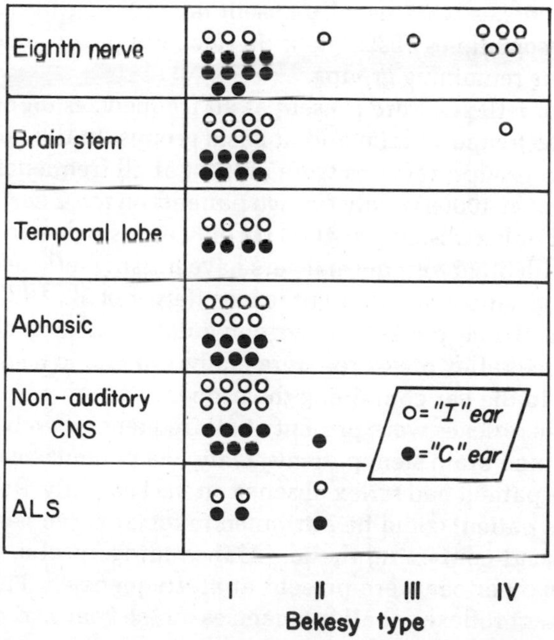

	I	II	III	IV

male, had a type I tracing on the C ear and a type IV pattern on the I ear. Pure-tone sensitivity in this patient showed a bilaterally symmetrical loss with a pure-tone average (PTA) at 500, 1000, and 2000 Hz of 17 dB on each ear. Surgical findings revealed a pontomesencephalic glioma with an exophytic extension to the right (I) side which may have indirectly involved the eighth nerve fibers.

Six of the 10 eighth nerve patients showed a type III or IV pattern on the I ear. This finding is consistent with the results of Johnson (1968), Owens (1971), and Jerger (1973). Conversely, four eighth nerve patients had a type I or II tracing on the I ear. However, two of these four patients with normal Békésy tracings showed positive, retrocochlear, results for modified Békésy audiometry. One patient had a significant discrepancy between continuous-forward versus continuous-backward sweep frequency tracings (Palva et a., 1970; Jerger et al., 1972b). The other patient had a positive (retrocochlear) pattern on Békésy comfortable loudness (BCL) audiometry (Jerger & Jerger,1974b). In short, Békésy audiometry was consistent with a retrocochlear site in eight of the 10 eighth nerve patients when the conventional procedure was supplemented by either continuous-forward versus continuous-backward tracings or BCL tracings. All eighth nerve patients had normal, type I, tracings on the C ear.

Acoustic reflex.   Figure 8 shows acoustic reflex results for the I and C ears of all patients in the six groups. Reflexes for the normal group were present at all frequencies on both ears and are not presented. Reflexes were usually absent (at 110 dB HL) in the eighth nerve group, sometimes absent in brain stem group, and generally present in the four remaining groups.

Acoustic reflexes were present at all frequencies on both ears of patients in the temporal lobe and aphasic groups. In the non-auditory CNS and ALS groups, reflexes were present at all frequencies on the I ear, but absent at 4000 Hz only for two patients on the C ear. Generally, we disregard reflex absence at 4000 Hz only on a single ear. About 4% of patients with otherwise normal ears have missing reflexes at this frequency on one ear for no apparent reason (Jerger et al., 1972a). Results for the I ear of one patient in the non-auditory CNS group are not presented since reflex measures were equivocal due to a slight middle ear disorder in the ear containing the probe.

Acoustic reflexes were present at all frequencies on both ears for seven of the nine brain stem patients. Only two patients had abnormal reflexes. One patient had reflex absence on the I ear only. Reflex abnormality in this patient could be attributed to facial nerve paresis on the side of the head containing the impedance bridge probe. Reflexes in this patient's other ear were present at all frequencies. The other patient had absent reflexes at all frequencies on the I ear and at 2000 and

Development of the Staggered Spondaic Word Test

FIGURE 8. ▬▬▬▬▬▬▬▬▬▬▬▬▬

Pattern of acoustic reflexes for the I and C ears of patients in each group.

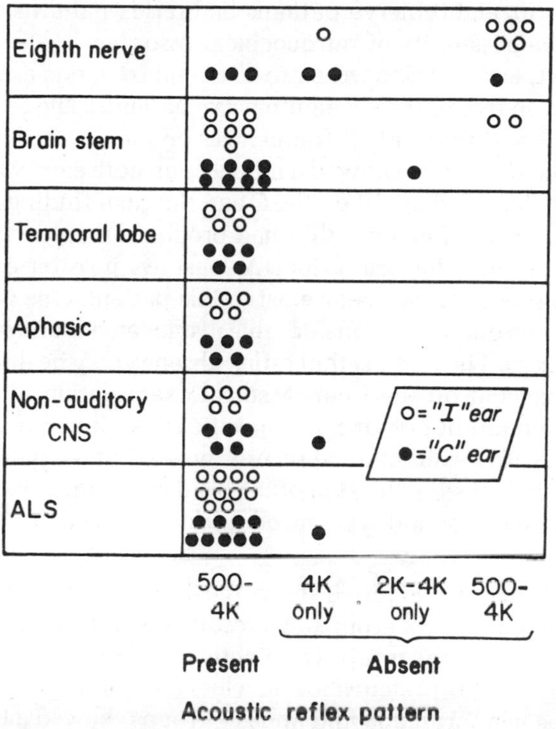

Acoustic reflex pattern

4000 Hz on the C ear. Reflexes were observed at 500 and 1000 Hz on the C ear, but threshold HL's were 110 dB and 100 dB respectively, levels at the high end of the normal range. Pure-tone sensitivity showed at moderate, bilaterally symmetrical, high frequency loss with a PTA of 9 dB on the I ear and 11 dB on the C ear. Radiographic studies revealed a pontomesencephalic glioma with an exophytic extension to the right (I) side. In short, only one of the nine brain stem patients had reflex absence that could not be explained on a peripheral basis (middle ear or motor-neuron disorder). Normal acoustic reflexes in most of the present brain stem patients is in contrast to previous studies (Greisen & Rasmussen, 1970; Lehnhardt, 1973) stressing abnormal reflex measures.

Reflexes were absent on the I ear at all frequencies in five of the six eighth nerve patients. This finding is consistent with several previous studies (Anderson et al., 1969; Sheehy, 1974; Jerger et al., 1974). The one patient with acoustic reflexes on the I ear had reflex absence at 4000 Hz and elevated reflex HL's (110 dB) at 2000 Hz. Absent reflexes at 4000 Hz only are considered equivocal, but the elevated reflex HL at 2000 Hz in conjunction with the missing reflex at 4000 Hz is unusual enough to be suspicious in our experience. According to this criterion, all six eighth nerve patients had reflex patterns on the I ear suggesting the possibility of retrocochlear disorder.

On the C ear, reflexes were present at all frequencies or absent at 4000 Hz only in five of the six eighth nerve patients. The remaining patient had reflex absence at all frequencies on the C ear as well as the I ear. Pure-tone sensitivity showed a mild loss on both ears, with a PTA of 34 dB on the I ear and 26 dB on the C ear. Surgical findings revealed a 35-mm angular neurilemoma that had produced displacement, deformity, and rotation of the brain stem. At least two possible explanations for reflex absence on the C ear exist in this patient. One is that reflex absence may be due to the considerable displacement of the brain stem noted at surgery. The other is that reflex absence may be due to seventh nerve involvement on the I ear. Medical examination at the time of hospitalization did not record any specific seventh nerve abnormality on either side. However, clinical records noted that the patient's mouth "drooped" on the I side, the side of the head containing the impedance bridge probe when sound was introduced to the C ear.

PI–PB functions. Figure 9 shows the average PB_{max} losses for each ear of patients in the six groups. All results are plotted relative to performance in the normal group. The eighth nerve group showed a loss on the I ear only; the brain stem showed a loss on both ears, but greater on the C ear; the temporal lobe and aphasic groups showed a loss on the C ear only; and the non-auditory CNS and ALS groups showed normal scores on both ears.

The largest PB_{max} deficit was observed for patients with eighth nerve disorder. Even though the average hearing loss on the impaired ear was only 18 dB, the PB_{max} score for this group was approximately 30% poorer than normal performance. Unusually poor performance for PB word tests has long been recognized as a distinguishing characteristic of eighth nerve site (Goodman, 1957; Flower & Viehweg, 1961; Johnson, 1970; Katz, 1970).

The brain stem group had a PB_{max} deficit of 17% on the C ear and 7% on the I ear even though sensitivity measures were within the normal range on both ears. Bilateral speech intelligibility deficits, with greatest impairment on the C ear, have been reported previously in patients with intra-axial brain stem lesions. (Parker et al., 1962, 1968; Calearo & Antonelli, 1968; Antonelli, 1970). However, PB_{max} deficits in the present group reflect, at most, only a mild impairment on either ear for this repetition task.

FIGURE 9. ━━━━━━━━━━━━━━━━━━━━━━━━━━━━━━━━━

Average PB$_{max}$ loss for the I and C ears of patients in each group. Results are plotted relative to performance in the normal group.

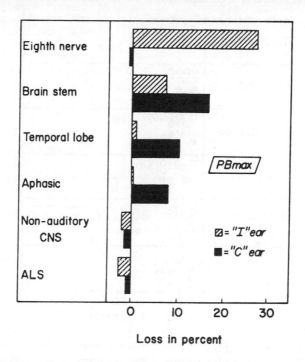

Loss in percent

Performance scores on the C ear of the temporal lobe group and the aphasic patients who could perform the task approximately 10% poorer than normal performance. PB$_{max}$ scores on the I ear were unimpaired in both groups. The observation of slight PB$_{max}$ deficits, on the C ear only, agrees with the findings of some previous investigators (Jerger, 1964, 1973; Berlin et al., 1965; Korsan-Bengsten, 1970, 1973). However, in the past, PB$_{max}$ performance in temporal lobe patients has generally been considered normal (Antonelli et al., 1963; Lynn & Gilroy, 1972; Liden & Korsan-Bengsten, 1973). Maximum scores on both ears have been within the "normal" range and slight ear differences, if present, have been presumed to be within the range of normal variability. However, our experience suggests that a very real, although slight, deficit is present on the C ear. In this project, we carefully constructed PI–PB functions across many intensity levels and found consistently poorer performance on the C ear although pure-tone sensitivity was the same on both ears. Furthermore, the performance deficit was frequently more pronounced at very low and very high intensities.

FIGURE 10. ▬▬▬▬▬▬▬

Distribution of PI–PB rollover indices for I and C ears of patients in
each group. Results are plotted relative to performance in normal
group. The stippled area represents the normal range.

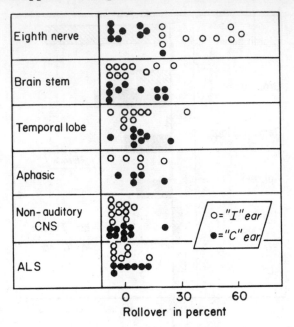

Rollover in percent

PI–PB rollover.   Figure 10 shows the distribution of rollover indices for both ears of all patients in the six groups. Rollover indices are plotted relative to performance in the normal group. Degree of rollover was defined by the difference between the maximum (PB_{max}) and minimum (PB_{min}) scores. For this purpose, PB_{min} was defined as the lowest percent correct score at any speech level above that level yielding PB_{max}. The stippled area in Figure 10 represents the range of normal performance.

The rollover phenomenon differed among the six groups. Abnormal rollover occurred on the I ear of all eighth nerve patients. This finding is consistent with previous reports (Jerger & Jerger, 1971; Igarashi et al., 1974). The amount of abnormal rollover in these patients varied from approximately 20% to 60% more than the normal group. And, indeed, only the eighth nerve group had rollover effects of more than 35%. Only one eighth nerve patient had abnormal rollover on the C ear also. Surgical reports on this patient noted an angular meningioma, 35 mm by 25 mm, that had produced displacement, deformity, and rotation of the brain stem. Bilateral rollover in this patient may have reflected the extensive amount of brain stem involvement noted at surgery.

Abnormal rollover occurred in four of the 10 brain stem patients. Two patients had abnormal rollover on both ears and two patients had abnormal rollover on the C ear only. The amount of rollover was approximately 20% on both the I and C ears of all four patients.

Rollover effects were generally within normal limits for the temporal lobe, aphasic, non-auditory CNS and ALS groups. Abnormal rollover effects occurred in only two temporal lobe patients, on the I ear only and on the C ear only; in one aphasic patient on both ears; and in one non-auditory CNS patient on the C ear only.

SSI functions (SSI-ICM and SSI-CCM). Figure 11 shows the average loss on each ear for the six groups on the ICM task. Performance was averaged across MCR's of 0, −10, and −20 dB. All results are plotted relative to performance in the normal group. The stippled area represents the range of normal findings. ICM results were within normal limits on both ears of the non-auditory CNS and ALS groups.

FIGURE 11.
Average SSI-CCM loss on the I and C ears of patients in each group. Performance was averaged across message-to-competition ratios of 0, −10, and −20 dB. Results are plotted relative to performance in the normal group. The stippled area represents the range of normal findings.

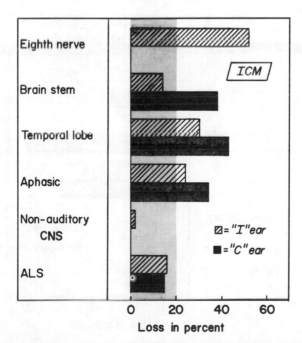

The eighth nerve and brain stem groups had performance deficits on one ear only. However, the ear reflecting the ICM loss differed in the two groups. The eighth nerve group had a loss of approximately 50% on the I ear only; the brain stem group had a loss of about 40% on the C ear only.

The temporal lobe and aphasic groups had a loss on both ears, but greater on the C ear. Average performance deficits in the temporal lobe group were approximately 30% on the I ear and 40% on the C ear. Average losses in the aphasic group were about 25% on the I ear and 35% on the C ear.

Figure 12 summarizes the average loss for each ear on the CCM task. Performance was averaged across MCR's of 0, −20, and −40 dB. All scores are plotted relative to results in the normal group. The stippled area presents the range of normal findings. CCM results were within normal limits for both ears of the brain stem, non-auditory CNS, and ALS groups. The eighth nerve group had a loss, on the I ear only, of approximately 18%. The temporal lobe group had a performance

FIGURE 12. ======================================

Average SSI-CCM loss on the I and C ears of patients in each group. Performance was averaged across message-to-competition ratios of 0, −20, and −40 dB. Results are plotted relative to performance in the normal group. The stippled area represents the range of normal findings.

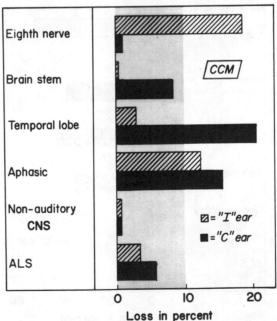

Development of the Staggered Spondaic Word Test

deficit on the C ear only of approximately 20%. The aphasic group showed poor performance on both ears, with a loss of 12% on the I ear and 16% on the C ear.

For SSI performance, diagnostic information is provided by two indices: (1) the relative configuration of results for ICM and CCM tasks and (2) the ear reflecting the performance deficits. For eighth nerve patients, the SSI procedure is characterized by poor performance on both ICM and CCM tasks. All deficits are confined to the I ear only. For brain stem patients, the SSI procedure shows poor performance for ICM and relatively good performance for CCM. The ICM deficits are observed on the C ear only and CCM performance is within normal limits on both ears. Although this "brain stem" pattern is observed in most brain stem patients, a few patients may present slightly different results. In these later patients there may be ICM deficits on both ears, instead of the C ear only, and/or a relatively mild CCM deficit on the C ear only, instead of normal performance on both ears. However, the observation of relatively more difficulty on ICM tasks than on CCM tasks holds for all brain stem patients in our experience.

For temporal lobe patients, the SSI procedure yields poor performance on both ICM and CCM. The ICM deficits are observed on both ears and the CCM deficit is observed on the C ear only. The exceptions to the expected "temporal lobe" pattern are that some temporal lobe patients may have an ICM deficit on the C ear only or normal ICM performance on both ears. The overriding principle in these patients is relatively more difficulty for CCM tasks than for ICM tasks.

For aphasic patients, SSI performance deficits did not seem to be more obvious on CCM tasks than on ICM tasks. The overriding principle for the present patients seemed to be a general speech intelligibility deficit that characterized both monotic and dichotic listening paradigms. Abnormally poor SSI scores occurred on both ears, usually with slightly greater deficits observed on the C ear than on the I ear.

SSW test.   Tables 2 and 3 show the average loss for the leading, competing, and lagging SSW conditions in the ALS, non-auditory CNS, aphasic, brain stem, and temporal lobe groups. The average PB word loss for the patients completing the SSW test is also shown. All results are presented relative to performance in the normal group. Results for the eighth nerve group are not included since only one patient completed the test.

As shown in Table 2, the ALS and non-auditory CNS groups had ear deficits of less than 10% on all three SSW conditions. The difference between ears for the competing monosyllables was small, approximately 3%, in both groups. The aphasic group had performance deficits of less than 10% on the leading and lagging conditions. On the competing condition, the C ear was essentially normal but the I ear showed a 15% loss. An ear difference of 10% was observed for competing and lagging conditions although no ear difference was observed for PB words.

In our experience, results for these three groups are essentially negative and do not suggest the presence of central auditory disorder. SSW results for the three groups scored according to Katz's method (1968) were in the range between normal (upper limit of 5) and mildly abnormal (upper limit of 15). Katz's total corrected SSW scores were 7 for the ALS group, 11 for the non-auditory CNS patients, and 14 for the aphasics. This finding of "mildly abnormal" SSW results agrees with Katz's observations (1968) on "central non-auditory" patients, but

TABLE 2. ▰▰▰▰▰▰▰▰▰▰▰▰▰▰▰▰▰▰▰▰▰▰▰
Loss in Percent Relative to Normal Group for SSW Test and PB Word Test in Both Ears of Three Control Groups

Group	Ear	SSW Lead	SSW Compete	SSW Lag	PB
ALS	C	—	3	−2	1
	I	2	7	0	−1
Ear difference			4		
Non-auditory	C	−1	7	5	−3
CNS	I	2	5	−4	−2
Ear difference			2		1
Aphasic	C	8	6	−2	0
	I	3	15	8	0
Ear difference			9		0

TABLE 3. ▰▰▰▰▰▰▰▰▰▰▰▰▰▰▰▰▰▰▰▰▰▰▰
Loss in Percent Relative to Normal Group for SSW Test and PB Word Test on Both Ears of Experimental Groups

Group	Ear	SSW Lead	SSW Compete	SSW Lag	PB
Brain	C	22	44	26	44
Stem	I	7	16	3	21
Ear difference			28		23
Temporal	C	36	65	30	14
Lobe	I	6	10	8	5
Ear difference			55		9

disagrees with Balas' (1971) comments. The latter investigator reported completely normal scores in all of his patients with non-auditory lesions involving either the frontal, parietal, or occipital lobes.

Table 3 shows the SSW results and the PB_{max} deficits for the brain stem and temporal lobe groups. The brain stem group showed a performance deficit for the leading, competing, and lagging conditions on the C ear. On the I ear, depressed performance was observed for the competing condition only. A difference between ears of approximately 15% to 25% was observed for competing and non-competing words. However, this ear difference was observed on traditional PB word tests as well as the SSW test. PB_{max} deficits were 44% on the C ear and 21% on the I ear. If we correct for PB_{max} deficits as suggested by Katz (1968), the corrected SSW scores for "condition," "ear," and "total" measures are well within Katz's normal range. For example, the "total" corrected SSW score was − 5 for the brain stem group. The negative value reflects a slightly greater loss for PB words than for SSW monosyllables. Poorer performance for PB words than for SSW conditions also characterized some of the patients studied by Lynn and his colleagues (1972). This performance difference suggests that PB monosyllables presented in isolation may be a more difficult listening task for some patients than SSW monosyllables presented in spondaic units. To us, the present difference is not unreasonable in view of the constraints on syllabic sequence imposed on monosyllables presented in the SSW paradigm.

SSW results for the temporal lobe group were essentially normal on the I ear, but showed large deficits for the non-competing and competing conditions on the C ear. The loss on the C ear was approximately 33% for the non-competing conditions and 65% for the competing condition. Pb_{max} deficits were within normal limits, 5%, on the I ear and showed only a very slight loss, 14%, on the C ear. Katz's corrected "ear" scores were 11 (normal) on the I ear and 39 (moderately abnormal) on the C ear. Abnormal performance on the C ear only for temporal lobe patients has been previously reported by Katz (1968), Balas (1971), Berlin & Lowe (1972), Lynn and his colleagues (1972) and Gilroy & Lynn (1974).

In short, only the temporal lobe group showed significant SSW performance deficits according to Katz's criterion. The other four groups had essentially negative results when PB_{max} losses were subtracted from the SSW deficits.

Comment

Auditory findings in these six patient groups varied considerably on any one individual test of auditory function. For example, one of the present intra-axial brain stem patients had an abnormal, type IV,

Békésy audiogram. This pattern would be expected in a patient with peripheral eighth nerve disorder, but is not expected in a patient with a brain stem site. On the other hand, two of the present eighth nerve patients had type I or II conventional Békésy audiograms and no abnormalities on either of the modified Békésy procedures. This result is expected in patients with brain stem disorder, but is a false-negative result for eighth nerve site. Acoustic reflex results also produced confusing findings in a few isolated patients. For example, one eighth nerve patient in this series had abnormal reflexes on both ears, instead of the I ear only. This pattern is more typical of an intra-axial brain stem site than of a peripheral eighth nerve disorder.

In spite of these inconsistencies on individual test procedures, the overall battery of test results seemed to produce a pattern unique to each of the six groups. Figure 13 summarizes the overall pattern characterizing the three groups with specific auditory disorders: either eighth nerve, brain stem, or temporal lobe. The overall pattern of results differed significantly among these gorups. The eighth nerve group was usually characterized by abnormal Békésy audiograms, absent or decaying acoustic reflexes, relatively poor PB_{max} scores, substantial PI–PB rollover, SSI–ICM loss, SSI–CCM loss, and auditory symptoms on the ipsilateral ear only. The eighth nerve control group contrasted sharply with the intra-axial brain stem group. The latter group

FIGURE 13.

Overall pattern of diagnostic test results on seven indices for the eighth nerve, brain stem, and temporal lobe groups.

Tests	VIII th Nerve	Brain Stem	Temporal Lobe
Bekesy Audiogram	●	○	○
Acoustic Reflexes	●	○	○
PB max	●	⊘	⊘
Rollover	●	⊘	○
SSI-ICM	●	●	●
SSI-CCM	●	⊘	●
SSW	—	⊘	●
Ear symptoms observed on	Ipsi only	Both or contra only	Both or contra only

(Legend: ○ Normal, ⊘ Questionable, ● Abnormal — Experimental Groups)

was generally characterized by normal Békésy audiograms; normal acoustic reflexes; mild, if any, PB_{max} deficits; mild, if any, PI–PB rollover; substantial SSI–ICM deficits; relatively normal SSI–CCM performance; relatively normal SSW results; and auditory symptoms on both ears or the contralateral ear only. In distinction to the above two groups, the temporal lobe group was usually characterized by normal Békésy audiograms, normal acoustic reflexes; mild, if any PB_{max} loss; no PI–PB rollover; SSI–ICM deficits; SSI–CCM deficits; abnormal SSW results; and auditory symptoms on both ears or on the contralateral ear only. The unique difference between the brain stem and temporal lobe groups was that the brain stem group had more difficulty with degraded monotic signals and the temporal lobe group had more difficulty with dichotic signals.

At the present time, we are not suggesting that the test procedures shown in Figure 13 comprise the perfect test battery. However, the combination of the SSI procedure and the SSW test did seem to offer an unusually effective diagnostic tool for differentiating brain stem and temporal lobe sites. In the present study, the SSW test offered unique assistance in differentiating temporal lobe disorders, but did not consistently identify patients with brain stem disorders. Conversely, the SSI procedure provided unique assistance in differentiating brain stem site, but did not consistently identify temporal lobe site. For example, the temporal lobe patients usually showed substantial SSW deficits, but the SSI–CCM deficits varied considerably. Some temporal lobe patients had clearcut SSI–CCM losses; other patients performed better than we expected. On the other hand, the brain stem patients consistently showed striking SSI–ICM deficits, but SSW results varied considerably. Some brain stem patients had no SSW deficits; others had unusually poor SSW performance. Also the relation between PB_{max} scores and SSW scores varied in the brain stem patients. Sometimes SSW scores could be corrected by PB_{max} deficits to within the normal range; at other times, however, SSW deficits remained, even when corrected; and still other times the PB_{max} deficits were so much more severe than SSW deficits that a negative corrected SSW score appeared. The overriding principle that characterized the combination of the two procedures was that the brain stem patients consistently showed SSI–ICM deficits whereas temporal lobe patients consistently showed SSW deficits.

Conclusions

1. Does the physical discomfort characterizing patients with central nervous system disease produce abnormal test results on a central auditory test battery? *Probably not.* For example, findings in the present ALS control group were consistently within normal limits, although these patients were typically extremely ill and uncomfortable.

2. Does *any* central nervous system disorder produce abnormal auditory test results even though there is no direct involvement of the auditory pathways, per se? *Probably not.* For example, findings in the present non-auditory CNS control group were consistently within the normal range.

3. Does the presence of aphasia in patients with temporal lobe disorder compromise the diagnostic value of degraded speech audiometry? *To some extent.* The present aphasic patients usually showed a performance deficit on both ears for difficult speech tasks, rather than the expected deficit only on the ear contralateral to the affected side of the brain. Further, performance deficits seemed just as pronounced for monotic listening conditions as for dichotic conditions.

4. Can auditory test results differentiate brain stem disorders from eighth nerve disorders? *Yes, fairly well.* In the present eighth nerve and brain stem groups, there were no patients in whom secondary symptoms masked the primary site of disorder when results for the entire test battery were considered. However, isolated test procedures showed some overlap between the two groups. Whenever individual patients showed both eighth nerve and brain stem auditory symptomatology, surgical and/or radiographic findings usually noted either (1) eighth nerve neoplasms rotating, distorting, and/or compressing the brain stem, or (2) brain stem neoplasms critically invading the cerebellopontine angle.

Acknowledgements

This project was supported by Public Health Service Research grants NB-08542 and NS-10940 from the National Institute of Neurological Diseases and Stroke.

References

Anderson, H., Barr, B. & Wedenberg, E. 1969. Intra-aural reflexes in retrocochlear lesions. In *Nobel symposium 10: Disorders of the skull base region* (ed. C. Hamberger & J. Wersall), p.49. Almqvist & Wiksell, Stockholm.

Antonelli, A. 1970. Sensitized speech tests: Results in lesions of the brain. In *Speech audiometry* (ed. C. Røjskjær), p. 176, Second Danavox Symposium, Odense, Denmark.

Antonelli, A., Calearo, C. & De-Metri, T. 1963. On the auditory function in brain stem diseases. *Int. Audiol* 2, 55.

Balas, R. 1971. Staggered spondaic word test: Support. *Ann Otol 80*, 1.

Berlin, C. & Lowe, S. 1972. Temporal and dichotic factors in central auditory testing. In *Handbook of clinical audiology* (ed. J. Katz), p. 280. The Williams & Wilkins Co., Baltimore.

Berlin, C., Chase, R., Dill, A. & Hagepanos, T. 1965. Auditory findings in patients with temporal lobectomies. *Amer Speech Hearing Assoc 7*, 386.

Calearo, C. & Antonelli, A. 1968. Audiometric findings in brain stem lesions. *Acta Otolaryngol* (Stockholm) 66, 305.

Egan, J. 1948. Articulation testing methods. *Laryngoscope 58*, 955.

Flower, R. & Viehweg, R. 1961. A review of audiologic findings among patients with cerebellopontine angle tumors. *Laryngoscope 71*, 1105.

Gilroy, J. & Lynn, G. 1974. Reversibility of abnormal auditory findings in cerebral hemisphere lesions. *J Neurol Sci 21*, 117.

Goodman, A. 1957. Some relations between auditory function and intracranial lesions with particular reference to lesions of the cerebellopontine angle. *Laryngoscope 67*, 987.

Greisen, O. & Rasmussen, P. 1970. Stapedius muscle reflexes and otoneurological examinations in brain stem tumors. *Acta Otolaryngol* (Stockholm) *70*, 366.

Igarashi, M., Jerger, J., Alford, B. & Stasney, R. 1974. Functional and histological findings of bilateral acoustic tumor. *Arch Otolaryngol* (Chicago) *99*, 379.

Jerger, J. 1960a. Audiological manifestations of lesions in the auditory nervous system. *Laryngoscope 70*, 417.

—1960b. Békésy audiometry in the analysis of auditory disorders. *J Speech Hearing Res 3*, 275.

—1964. Auditory tests for disorders of the central auditory mechanism. In *Neurological aspects of auditory and vestibular disorders* (ed. W. Fields & B. Alford), p. 77. Charles C. Thomas, Springfield, Ill.

—1973. Diagnostic audiometry. In *Modern developments in audiology* 2nd ed. (ed. J. Jerger), p. 75. Academic Press, New York.

Jerger, J. & Jerger, S. 1971. Diagnostic significance of PB word functions. *Arch Otolaryngol* (Chicago) *93*, 573.

—1974a. Auditory findings in brain stem disorders. *Arch Otolaryngol* (Chicago) *99*, 342.

—1974b. Diagnostic value of Békésy comfortable loudness tracings. *Arch Otolaryngol* (Chicago) *99*, 351.

Jerger, J., Jerger, S. & Mauldin, L. 1972a. Studies in impedance audiometry. I. Normal and sensori-neural ears. *Arch Otolaryngol* (Chicago) *96*, 513.

—1972b. The forward-backward discrepancy in Békésy audiometry. *Arch Otolaryngol* (Chicago) *96*, 400.

Jerger, J., Speaks, C. & Trammell, J. 1968. A new approach to speech audiometry. *J Speech Hearing Dis 33*, 318.

Jerger, J., Harford, E., Clemis, J. & Alford, B. 1974. The acoustic reflex in eighth nerve disorders. *Arch Otolaryngol* (Chicago) *99*, 409.

Johnson, E. 1968. Auditory findings in 200 cases of acoustic neuromas. *Arch Otolaryngol* (Chicago) *88*, 598.

—1970. Auditory test results in 268 cases of confirmed retrocochlear lesions. *Audiology 9*, 15.

Katz, J. 1962. The use of staggered spondaic words for assessing the integrity of the central auditory nervous system. *J Aud Res 2*, 327.

—1968. The SSW test: An interim report. *J Speech Hearing Dis 33*, 318.

—1970. Audiologic diagnosis: Cochlea to cortex. *Menorah Med Jour 1*, 25.

Korsan-Bengsten, M. 1970. Some comparisons between ordinary and sensitized speech tests in patients with central hearing loss. In *Speech audiometry* (ed. C. Røjskjær), p. 123. Second Danavox Symposium, Odense, Denmark.

—1973. Distorted speech audiometry. *Acta Otolaryngol* (Stockholm) Suppl. *310*, 34.

Lehnhardt, E. 1973. Audiometric localization of brain stem lesions. *Z Laryng Rhinol Otol 52*, 11.

Liden, G. & Korsan-Bengtsen, M. 1973. Audiometric manifestations of retrocochlear lesions. *Scand Audiol 2*, 29.

Lynn, G. & Gilroy, J. 1972. Neuroaudiological abnormalities in patients with temporal lobe tumors. *J Neurol Sci 17*, 167.

Lynn G., Benitez, J., Eisenbrey, A., Gilroy, J. & Welner, H. 1972. Neuroaudiological correlates in cerebral hemisphere lesions. Temporal and parietal lobe tumors. *Audiology 2*, 115.

Owens, E. 1964. Békésy tracings and site of lesion. *J Speech Hearing Dis 29*, 456.

—1971. Audiologic evaluation in cochlear versus retrocochlear lesions. *Acta Otolaryngol* (Stockholm) Supp. *283*, 1.

Palva, T., Karja, J. & Palva, A. 1970. Forward vs. reversed Békésy tracings. *Arch Otolaryngol* (Chicago) *91*, 449.

Parker, W., Decker, R. & Garner, W. 1962. Auditory function and intracranial lesions. *Arch Otolaryngol* (Chicago) *76*, 425.

Parker, W., Decker, R. & Richards, N. 1968. Auditory function and lesions of the pons. *Arch Otolaryngol* (Chicago) *87*, 228.

Sheehy, J. 1974. Impedance audiometry in otologic practice. Cited in Jerger, J.: 2nd International Symposium on Impedance Measurement, Houston, Texas. *Audiology 13*, 271.

Wolfgram, F. & Meyers, L. 1973. Amyotrophic lateral sclerosis: Effect of serum on anterior horn cells in tissue culture. *Science 179*, 579.

Errors on the Staggered Spondaic Word (SSW) Test in a Group of Adult Normal Listeners

Dennis J. Arnst

The Staggered Spondaic Word (SSW) Test was developed as a means to assess central auditory function. In the present study, the SSW Test was administered to a group of normal-hearing young adults (N = 86) with no history of central auditory problems in an attempt to evaluate previous normative data and the types of errors made by this group. Mean number of errors for corrected (C-SSW) scores were consistent with the "normal" category established by Katz. Response bias (ear effects, order effects, and reversals) was not prevalent in this population. Although two subjects obtained a significant number of reversals, it seemed that changes in listening strategy rather than auditory dysfunction was accountable for this finding.

In 1968, Katz (9) published an "interim" report in which he detailed the construction, rationale, procedures, and preliminary validation of the Staggered Spondaic Word (SSW) Test. The SSW Test was developed to evaluate the central auditory nervous system by means of a dichotic listening task in which 2 spondaic words are presented

Ear and Hearing, 2, 112–116, 1981.

simultaneously to opposite ears in a partially overlapped manner. Performance patterns in competing and noncompeting conditions for both ears have been related to areas of auditory dysfunction from the cochlea to the cortex (8, 10, 15, 18, 20). Also, error categories have been established (9) which serve as a basis for classifying these results on a continuum from normal to severe dysfunction.

Katz (10–12), Katz and Pack (18), Balas (1), Lynn and Gilroy (19), Jerger and Jerger (8), and Winkelaar and Lewis (20) have reported clinical data describing the ability of the SSW Test to differentiate auditory from nonauditory reception area dysfunction as well as brainstem, VIIIth nerve, and cochlear problems. It seems that the dichotic task and the complex presentation method of the SSW Test challenges the central auditory pathway in such a way that specific areas of dysfunction can be identified. Individuals with normal brain and brainstem function have little difficulty with the task (4, 10). In fact, they are often not aware that the stimuli are overlapped in time (4).

Several normative studies have been reported using various versions of the SSW Test (3, 7, 15, 17). Researchers have indicated that subjects with normal central auditory function between the ages of 11 and 60 years make few errors. Average total SSW scores (percentage correct) range between 97.0 and 98.8% (4). The variability within the data has been small, indicating that the SSW Test has good internal consistency. Also, few errors have been reported for subjects demonstrating pure conductive and sensorineural types of hearing loss (9, 10). This fact strengthens the interpretation of SSW Test results because the absence of central dysfunction is clearly categorized.

When the central auditory pathway is intact, individuals make few errors on the SSW Test and usually obtain a corrected SSW (C-SSW) (percentage of error) score within the normal range. Individuals with lesions outside Heschl's gyrus usually score in the normal or mild categories, but demonstrate significant response bias additionally (11, 13, 14, 18). Individuals with auditory reception area lesions tend to make many errors in the competing listening condition presented to the ear opposite the involved hemisphere. Significantly different patterns of results have also been associated with VIIIth nerve, low brainstem, and high brainstem problems (11, 13, 14, 18).

Only minor modifications have been made in the interpretation and scoring of the test since Katz' original discussion (13, 14). An "over-corrected" category has been added which has been shown to be associated with cochlear, VIIIth nerve, and low brain stem type problems. The over-corrected score occurs when SSW performance is good, but the word discrimination scores are depressed. The computation of the C-SSW score results in a negative number which suggests that the errors reflect a peripheral problem and do not involve a central (cortical) component (11, 12).

The second modification in interpretation involves response bias, the type of errors the individual makes on the SSW Test. These patterns of response were originally thought to be an artifact of the test (9), but more recently have been demonstrated to provide diagnostic information concerning the location of the dysfunction within a hemisphere in cases of lesions outside Heschl's gyrus (11).

Response Bias refers collectively to ear effects, order effects, and reversals. Each category represents a qualitative analysis of the listener's responses.

Ear effects represent a greater number of errors occurring when the stimulus set is begun in the right ear or the left ear. Significant ear effects are associated with dysfunction involving the anterior temporal or parietal areas of the cortex. Order effects represent more errors made on the first versus the second spondaic word. Significant order effects have been related to frontal lobe and/or temporoparietal lobe dysfunction. Reversals are changes in the sequence of the stimulus words made by the listener. This type of error has been most closely associated with dysfunction located in the central fissure are (10–14, 18).

The present study was undertaken to (1) evaluate the performance on the SSW Test by listeners with normal hearing sensitivity and no history of central auditory problems, and (2) consider the types of errors (i.e., response bias) made by this population.

Procedures

Eighty-six subjects (26 males; 60 females) were evaluated in the present study. Their ages ranged from 18 to 26 years with a mean age of 22 years. Each subject reported no history of hearing loss or central nervous system impairments. All subjects were required to have normal hearing and middle ear function based on pure-tone air conduction thresholds, speech audiometry, and impedance audiometry. Word discrimination scores (i.e., CID W-22 lists presented at 40 dB-SL re: speech reception threshold) were 90 to 100%. All subjects had type A tympanograms with acoustic reflex thresholds obtained between 75 and 100 dB HL. Pure-tone sensitivity for all subjects was symmetrical bilaterally, and interaural thresholds did not differ by more than 10 dB. Mean audiometric data for the entire population are reported in Table 1.

TABLE 1. ▬▬▬▬▬▬▬▬▬▬▬▬▬▬▬▬▬▬▬
**Mean Audiometric Data for Subjects
Participating in the Present Study (N = 86)**

	Speech Average		Word Discrimination Score		Acoustic Reflex Threshold	
	Right	Left	Right	Left	Right	Left
Mean	2.3	2.0	98.6	98.8	87.5	86.7
S.D.	2.8	2.7	2.6	2.4	6.6	6.5
Range	0-10	0-13	92-100	92-100	82-110	78-100

All test data were obtained using Maico 24-B or Tracor RE-115 dual-channel clinical audiometers. Impedance results were obtained using either an American Electromedics Impedance Meter (model AE83) or a Peters portable Impedance Meter (model AP61A). To facilitate acoustic reflex threshold measurement with the Peters Impedance Meter, the unit was coupled with a Beltone model 10-D portable audiometer. The equipment was calibrated just before the study and was monitored daily throughout the collection of the data. Subjects were seated in a single-walled, sound-treated room (1AC-400) throughout the entire test session.

After the basic hearing test battery, the SSW Test was administered to each subject and scored using the procedures described by Katz (11–14). The SSW Test was admininstered in its complete form. All 40 items from a commercially prepared 2-channel tape recording of List EC (12) were presented to each listener at 50 dB SL (re: pure-tone average at 500, 1000, and 2000 Hz) (2, 11–14). The test stimuli were routed through separate speech circuits of the dual-channel clinical audiometers from a Sony dual-channel tape recorder. All subjects were tested with the stimulus set beginning in the right ear first (REF).

Results and Discussion

Total Errors

None of the subjects reported having difficulty with the dichotic task. All subjects were able to repeat the stimuli after simple instructions. No subject scored more than 8 errors on the test. The total number of errors for all subjects and the total errors made for each listening condition are reported in Table 2. The mean total number of errors was 1.45 with a standard deviation of 1.72. This result compares favorably with Brunt and Goetzinger (6) who reported a mean total error score of 1.25 (SD = 1.2) for their population of 16 normal listeners.

The mean correct score for all subjects was 98.4% which is similar to other normative studies summarized by Brunt (4) (see Table 3). The present results support previous observations that the SSW test is quite easy for normal-hearing listeners with no history of central auditory dysfunction.

The mean number of errors obtained for the right ear was 0.96 (SD = 0.56), and for the left ear, it was 1.11 (SD = 0.89) (see Table 2). The difference between these scores was calculated to be 0.15, suggesting little difference in ear performance. Analysis of the right and left ear errors produced a nonsignificant t-test result of 1.88 ($p > 0.01$).

Brunt and Goetzinger (6) reported mean right ear errors of 0.3 (SD = 0.05) and mean left ear errors of 1.0 (SD = 0.6). These authors found that the obtained between-ear performance difference of 0.7 was statistically significant at the 0.02 level of confidence using the Wilcoxon Matched-Pairs Sign-Ranks Test: However, the small ear differences observed by Brunt and Goetzinger (6) and also by Katz and Fishman (16) were considered to be insignificant clinically.

Because the differences noted in earlier research on smaller populations were slight, the large number of subjects in the present study may have obliterated small individual differences. Moreover, Brunt (4) reported that dichotic tasks do not always show ear laterality effects when stimuli are familiar, highly associated, and not overlapped completely. Consequently, the lack of sensitivity to ear laterality effects at a clinical level for normal-hearing adults may be inherent to the design of the SSW Test. When significant ear differences are obtained,

---

TABLE 2

Summary of Errors Made on the SSW Test by Normal-Hearing Young Adults ($N = 86$)

		Ear		Condition			
	Total	Right	Left	RNC[a]	RC	LC	LNC
Total errors	125	48	77	9	39	64	13
Mean no. of errors	1.45	0.96	1.11	0.05	0.22	0.37	0.08
S.D.	1.72	0.56	0.89	0.27	0.54	0.68	0.28
% correct	98.4	98.8	98.6	99.4	98.6	98.3	99.3

[a]RNC, right noncompeting; RC, right competing; LC, left competing; LNC, left noncompeting.

TABLE 3

Comparison of Total R-SSW and Total C-SSW Scores [after Brunt (4)]

Study	Mean Age	Total R-SSW	Total C-SSW	S.D. C-SSW
Katz, Basil and Smith (15)	20	98.8	−0.4	1.5
Katz and Fishman (16)	22	98.3	−0.8	1.9
Goldman and Katz (7)	24	98.3	−0.3	2.2
Katz and Myrick (17)	23	97.8	−1.3	2.2
Present study (1980)	22	98.4	−0.3	2.2

deviance from normal function is suggested rather than the influence of ear laterality. The minimum amount of ear difference which can be used as a clinical sign for auditory dysfunction should be determined.

From Table 2, it can be noted that a total of 103 errors (i.e., 82.4% of total errors) were made in the competing conditions of the test. This result is similar to that reported by Brunt and Goetzinger (6). When comparing overall performance (i.e., percentage correct) under competing and noncompeting listening conditions, an approximate 1% difference exists. As a result, performance of normal listeners does not seem to be affected by the type of listening condition (i.e., competing versus noncompeting).

Percentage of Error Scores

Results on the SSW Test are interpreted based on percentage of error scores. The total number of errors in each of the listening conditions (i.e., competing and noncompeting conditions for the right and left ears) is multiplied by 2.5, and the product is the raw SSW score (R-SSW). The R-SSW represents the total percentage of error and has been shown to reflect errors due to central impairments as well as peripheral distortion (11, 12). Therefore, a C-SSW is calculated by subtracting the Word Discrimination Score (WDS) (percentage of error) from the R-SSW. Katz (11, 12) has indicated that this computation is effective in neutralizing the influence of peripheral distortion. Consequently, the C-SSW represents errors related primarily to central impairment.

Development of the Staggered Spondaic Word Test

TABLE 4
TABLE 4
**Mean (S.D.) R-SSW and C-SSW Scores Obtained for a Group (N = 86)
of Normal-Hearing Young Adults**

	RNC[a]		RC		LC		LNC	
R-SSW								
Condition	0.22	(0.92)	1.10	(1.98)	1.70	(2.49)	0.18	(0.58)
Ear	0.71	(1.18)					1.00	(1.35)
Total			0.93	(1.10)				
C-SSW								
Condition	−1.02	(2.66)	−0.28	(3.09)	0.56	(3.27)	−0.90	(2.26)
Ear	−.56	(2.77)					−0.16	(2.54)
Total			−0.33	(2.21)				

[a]RNC, right noncompeting; RC, right competing; LC, left competing; LNC, left noncompeting.

The mean (SD) R-SSW and C-SSW results obtained in the present study are shown in Table 4. As can be seen, the R-SSW shows minimal percentage of error (i.e., <2%). An analysis of the C-SSW scores based on performance ranges established by Katz (9, 11) revealed mean scores (i.e., total, ear, and condition scores) within the "normal" range. Similar scores for each subject were in the normal range; no other performance category was obtained. It should be evident that the normal listener with no peripheral hearing impairment and no history of central auditory nervous system dysfunction performs very well on the SSW Test. Moreover, the small standard deviations found in the present study and those reported in the 1960's (see Table 1) show the consistency of performance within the normal-hearing population on this test.

Response Bias

Response bias (i.e., ear effects, order effects, and reversals) represents a qualitative aspect of the SSW Test which assists in designating the location of dysfunction (10–12). Significant ear effects are shown when errors on the REF and left-ear-first (LEF) overlapped word pairs differ by 5 or more. Significant order effects are shown when errors on the first spondee and second spondee differ by 5 or more. Significant differences are designated by either "low/high" or "high/low" to reflect the condition with the greatest number of errors (e.g., ear 12/4 = ear high/low). Reversals represent any change in the sequence of the test stimuli reported by the subject. Ear and order effects obtained in the present study are summarized in Table 5. The number of reversals is shown in Table 6.

TABLE 5 ▰▰▰▰▰▰▰▰

**Ear and Order Effects Obtained on the SSW Test
in Normal-Hearing Young Adults** ($N = 86$)

	Ear Effect	Order Effect
Nonsignificant	84 (97.8)[a]	85 (98.8)
High/low	1	0
Low/high	1	1

[a]Numbers in parentheses, percentage.

TABLE 6 ▰▰▰▰▰▰▰▰

**Reversals Obtained on the SSW Test
in Normal-Hearing Young Adults** ($N = 86$)

No. of Reversals	No. of Subjects
0	73 (85)[a]
1	8 (10)
2	2 (2)
3	1 (1)
13	1 (1)
26	1 (1)
Mean = 0.62	

[a]Numbers in parentheses, percentage.

Ear and Order Effects

Ninety-eight percent of the subjects showed no significant ear or order effects. On the average, normal hearing individuals with no history of central dysfunction seem to lack either ear and/or order effects. A total of 3 subjects demonstrated response bias: 2 subjects had signficant ear effects; one subject had a significant order effect. All 3 subjects made all of their errors on one aspect of the test: on the second spondee (one subject with order low/high (0/5)); on the REF condition (one subject with ear high/low (5/0)); on the LEF condition (one subject with ear low/high (0/5)). The effect of the subjects' error pattern produced the significant response bias. However, those subjects with the same overall number of errors, but distributed fairly equally across all listening conditions, had no significant response bias.

Although approximately 2% of this population showed significant ear or order effects, the fact the C-SSW results were normal suggests it would be inappropriate to conclude that a central problem existed. Katz and Pack (18) and Brunt (5) have indicated that caution should be used when ear or order effects are significant and C-SSW scores are normal. In the 3 cases noted in the present study, it seemed that the pattern of error responses created the significance and if interpreted out of context, would lead the clinician to an inappropriate conclusion.

Reversals

The mean number of reversals observed in the present study averaged less than one (see Table 6). Eighty-five percent of the subjects did not change the stimulus order in any way. Katz and Pack (18) have correlated the presence of 2 or more reversals with lesions involving the pre- and postcentral gyri as well as the anterior temporal lobe. This area was subsequently labeled the "reversal strip." Of the 17 cases reported with damage to the motor and sensory strips along the central fissure, 9 (53%) evidenced reversals ranging from 1 to 28 (mean = 11 reversals). Seventy-six percent of the cases had 4 or more reversals.

In the present study, 84 (98%) of the subjects showed less than 4 reversals as compared with 24% of the cases with damage to the reversal strip as observed by Katz and Pack (18). The fact that almost all the subjects in the present study did not change the stimulus sequence is consistent with previous conclusions indicating that reversals are evident when there is damage to the central fissure area.

Two subjects in the present study made an unusually large number of reversals (i.e., 13 and 26 reversals). These are notable in a normal-hearing population because they probably represent a shift in listening strategy by the individual. When both subjects were reinstructed and asked to report the stimuli in the order in which they were presented on the tape, reversals were eliminated.

Because the SSW Test is a very easy task for normal hearing individuals, a change in listening strategy may occur in which stimuli are reported in random order. Clinically, it may be necessary to check the accuracy of inordinately large numbers of reversals. It has been observed that when reversals are indeed related to a specific area of dysfunction (i.e., the central fissure area), simple precautionary comments or reinstruction will not change the manner in which the stimuli are reported. Katz (11) has indicated that it is not advisable to stress or even mention order/sequence when giving the instructions. It is better to note the patient's natural style before intervening. Whenever reversals persist after reinstruction of the patient, changes in stimulus order can be accepted with confidence because they are manifestations of damage to the reversal strip.

Conclusions

It can be concluded that if the SSW Test is presented according to the prescribed procedure (11, 12) results indicating normal performance can be accpted with confidence and that the central auditory nervous system is intact. A certain amount of performance variability is acceptable, but has been reflected in the range of scores defined as normal. This is evident from the fact that all subjects in the present study fell within the normal category defined by Katz (9, 11, 12). It should be evident that normal central auditory function is rather precisely defined by the norms published previously.

Secondly, response bias results which are used to locate the area of dysfunction (i.e., particularly in nonauditory reception area dysfunction) are not prevalent in the normal popultion. Whenever signficant results do occur, a careful assessment of other supporting clinical findings needs to be made. Reversals, one particularly important indicator, should be cautiously interpreted in the light of other normal results (e.g., C-SSW). Because of the easy task presented for the normal listener, changes in listening strategy may create a false-positive finding. Reinstructing the patient to report the stimuli in the order heard will safeguard against misinterpretation because true changes in stimulus word will not be affected.

Acknowledgements

The author wishes to acknowledge the following persons for their assistance with this project: Jon Bryant, David Hicks, Dan Kallaus, Laura Mastick, Marion Meyerson, Lynn Price, Steven Rawiszer, Michael Shrinian, Marti Todebush, and Lynn Williams.

References

1. Balas, R. F. 1971. Staggered spondaic word test. Support. Ann. Otol. Rhinol. Laryngol. 80, 134–139.

2. Balas, R. F. and G. R. Simon. 1965. The articulation function of a staggered spondaic word list for a normal hearing population. J. Aud. Res. 4, 285–289.

3. Brunt, M. A. 1969. *Auditory Sequelae of Diabetes.* Doctoral dissertation, University of Kansas.

4. Brunt, M. A. 1972. The staggered spondaic word test. pp. 334–356, in J. Katz, ed. *Handbook of Clinical Audiology.* (Ed. 1). The Williams & Wilkins Co., Baltimore.

5. Brunt, M. A. 1978. The staggered spondaic word test. pp. 262–275, in J. Katz, ed. *Handbook of Clinical Audiology.* (Ed. 2). The Williams & Wilkins Co., Baltimore.

6. Brunt, M. A. and C. P. Goetzinger. 1968. A study of three tests of central function with normal hearing subjects. Cortex 288–297.

7. Goldman, S., and J. Katz. 1966. A comparison of the performance of normal hearing subjects on the staggered spondaic word test given under four conditions—dichotic, diotic, monaural (domininant ear), and monaural (nondominant ear). Paper presented at American Speech and Hearing Association Convention. Chicago.

8. Jerger, J., and S. Jerger. 1975. Clinical validity of central auditory tests. Scand. Aud. 4, 147–163.

9. Katz, J. 1968. The SSW Test—an interim report. J. Speech Hear. Disord. 33, 132–146.

10. Katz, J. 1970. Audiologic diagnosis: cochlea to cortex. Menorah Med. J. 1, 25–38.

11. Katz, J. 1977. The staggered spondaic word test, pp: 103–128, in Central Auditory Dysfunction, ed. R. W. Keith, Grune & Stratton, New York.

12. Katz, J. 1977. The SSW Test Manual. Auditec of St. Louis, Brentwood, MO.

13. Katz, J. 1978. SSW workshop—Basic. Santa Barbara, CA. January 9–11.

14. Katz, J. 1978. SSW workshop—Advanced. San Mateo, CA. July 17–18.

15. Katz, J., R. A. Basil, and J. M. Smith, 1963. A staggered spondaic word test for detecting central auditory lesions. Ann. Otol. Rhinol. Laryngol. 72, 908–918.

16. Katz, J., and P. Fishman. 1978. The use of the staggered spondaic word test as a means of detecting differences between age groups. Unpublished study, 1964, cited in M. A. Brunt.

17. Katz, J., and D. K. Myrick. 1965. A normative study to assess performance of children, aged seven through eleven, on the staggered spondaic word (SSW) test. Unpublished study, cited in M. A. Brunt (1978).

18. Katz, J., and G. Pack. 1975. New developments in differential diagnosis using the SSW test. pp. 85–107, in M. Sullivan, ed. Central Auditory Processing Disorders. University of Nebraska Press. Omaha, NE.

19. Lynn, G. E. and J. Gilroy, 1972. Neuro-audiological abnormalities in patients with temporal lobe tumors. J. Neurol Sci. 17, 167–184.

20. Winkelaar, R. G., and T. K. Lewis. 1977. Audiological tests for evaluation of central auditory disorders. J. Otolaryngol. 6, 127–134.

Related Readings

M. Brunt. The Staggered Spondaic Word Test. The Handbook of Clinical Audiology. J. Katz (ed) 1st edition (1972), Chapter 18, 334–356; 2nd edition, 1978, Chapter 23, 262–275. Baltimore: Williams & Wilkins.

This section contains papers dealing with acoustics, psychoacoustics, and other factors associated with the SSW Test. Overlapping words on the test are the subject of the first four papers. Since the words are spoken in a normal manner, the durations of the words differ from word to word. There is still no "proper criterion" for overlapping the words even after one has decided on a given measure. The papers bring into question whether perceptual or acoustic methods would be best. In the perceptual procedures the words sound overlapped and in the acoustic method there is a certain speech–energy relationship between the competing signals. With the acoustic method, one would need to determine whether to match up the initial portion, the final portion, the peak of energy, or to center the energy of the shorter word on the longer one.

While the discussion of the test parameters in the first four papers is interesting and might someday lead to refinements in the procedure, it is solely of academic interest at this time. The important point from a clinical stance is that the procedure is highly effective for evaluating central auditory function. This is true because of or despite the criteria and methods that were used to align the competing words.

The next paper (Goldman and Katz) offers variations in the standard dichotic presentation of the SSW. This method of study helps to shed light on the test material and how different routings of the signal may be dealt with by the auditory system. In the next paper Katz and Goldman compared the data for left- and right-handed subjects. There are Important Implications to be derived from these results which could provide further diagnostic implications. Unfortunately, there have been no published reports of the same type of work in non-normal populations.

The paper by Katz and Arndt deals with the split-half reliability of the SSW Test (List EC). The study shows that in a large group of individuals with various problems the first half ofthe test is a good predictor of performance

3

Acoustic and Psychoacoustic Factors

for the second half. This is true for the C-SSW score. We presume that the SSW has good test–retest features as well, but there are no published data to back this up. A study should be carried out on a stable, pathologic population in order to provide more information.

The last three papers contain information on performance intensity curves for the SSW Test. Balas and Simon contributed the first study of this type in 1965. Doyle recently repeated the study using current materials and found that the performance intensity function was steeper than the one reported earlier. This difference may be due in part to the scoring procedure and materials used by Balas and Simon. Conant extended the consideration to include a high-intensity presentation of the SSW in normal listeners.

Lead and Lag Effects Associated With the Staggered Spondaic Word Test

Barry A. Freeman and Daniel S. Beasley

This study was designed to determine to what extent onset times of overlapping spondaic words were controlled in the development of the Staggered Spondaic Word Test (SSW) (List EC), a measure which is used to detect central auditory dysfunction. The results showed that the SSW (List EC) was not well controlled relative to onset times. Further, the scores of 10 normal-hearing listeners who were administered the SSW were found not to suffer when the onset times were closely matched. The results were related to the effects that leading and lagging onset times have on the perception of dichotically presented stimuli.

The Staggered Spondaic Word Test was introduced by Katz (1962) and has been found to be useful in the differential diagnosis of perceptual processing problems associated with central nervous system auditory pathways (Katz, Basil and Smith, 1963; Katz, 1968; Balas, 1971). There are several possible sources of variability, however, inherent in dichotic listening tasks, including the amount of temporal delay between the onset times of competing stimulus items. Studdert-Kennedy, Shankweiler, and Schulman (1970) and Berlin et al. (1973)

Journal of Speech and Hearing Research, 19, 572–577, 1976.

showed that a temporal delay of 15 to 30 msec in onset time between competing CV stimuli resulted in a decrease in the recall accuracy of the leading stimuli. Onset time differences greater than 60 msec resulted in improved recall accuracy of both the leading and lagging stimulus items. Katz,[1] however, expressed concern that the dichotic listening task on the SSW may be too difficult for even normal-hearing subjects if the competing stimuli were too closely matched in time. Nevertheless, adequate control of the temporal characteristics of auditory stimuli may provide information pertaining to the systematic confusions which occur with various types of stimuli (for example, CVs vs. words). The purpose of the present study was to measure the onset times of the competing stimuli on the SSW, and further to determine if onset time delays differentially affected perceptual accuracy.

Method

The present investigation was composed of two parts. In Part 1, the SSW (List EC) was presented to a group of normal hearing persons. In Part 2, the onset times of the two overlapping syllables for each word pair of the SSW (List EC) were measured.

Subjects

Ten normal-hearing young adults served as listeners in the study. Each subject was required to pass a pure-tone audiometric screening examination at 10 dB HTL (ANSI, 1969) for the octave frequencies from 250 through 8000 Hz. All of the subjects showed a normal SRT as determined through standard administration of the CID W-1 word list.

Listener Presentation

The 40 word pairs of the SSW test (List EC) (see Table 1) were administered to each of the 10 listeners individually at a 50-dB sensation level (re: SRT) in the manner described by Katz (1968). The presentation of the SSW was performed with the subject seated in a prefabricated double-walled test suite (IAC, 1200 Series) and the experimenter seated in an adjacent single-walled control room. The SSW tapes were presented via a high-quality tape recorder (Sony ESP Model 770) coupled to a speech audiometer. (Grason-Stadler Model 162) through a stereo headset (TDH-39 mounted in MX 41/AR cushions). Equipment used for speech and pure-tone audiometric measurements was calibrated before and after each experimental session in accordance with ANSI (1969) recommendations.

---

[1] J. Katz, personal communication, 1974.

TABLE 1 ▬▬▬▬

Stimulus Items from the SSW
(List EC) and the Onset Time Differences (in msec).

Stimulus Item	Lead	Lag	Stimulus Item	Lead	Lag	Stimulus Item	Lead	Lag
Upstairs downtown	–	65	Whitewall doghouse	–	12	Cornstarch soap flakes	–	50
Outside in-law	–	175	Back door playground	60	–	Birthday first place	–	70
Daylight lunchtime	150	–	Schoolboy church bell	–	10	Daybreak lamplight	50	–
Washtub blackboard	25	–	Snow white football	100	–	Doorknob cowbell	–	36
Cornbread oatmeal	–	40	Band saw first aid	–	90	Bird cage crow's nest	–	30
Bedspread mushroom	–	25	Bluejay blackbird	–	52	Weekend workday	–	70
Floodgate flashlight	–	25	Iceland sweet cream	35	–	Bookshelf drugstore	–	25
Seashore outside	–	145	Hair net toothbrush	–	48	Woodwork beach craft	50	–
Meat sauce baseball	–	65	Fruit juice cupcake	40	–	Handball milk shake	–	80
Blackboard airmail	–	48	Ash tray tin can	32	–	Fishnet skyline	4	–
Housefly woodwork		30	Night-light yardstick	–	12	Forgive milkman	–	27
Green bean homeland	8	–	Key chain suitcase	50	–	Sheepskin bulldog	–	70
Sunday shoeshine	18	–	Playground batboy	–	75	Racehorse streetcar	60	–
						Greenhouse string bean	74	–

Lead **means the onset of the second syllable of the first word precedes the onset of the first syllable of the second word.** *Lag* **means the onset of the second syllable of the first word follows the onset of the first syllable of the second word.**

Lead and Lag Effect Measurements

The onset times of the second syllable of the first spondee and first syllable of the second spondee for each of the items on the SSW was measured, using a high-quality tape recorder (Ampex Model AG 440B) coupled to a dual-channel storage oscilloscope (Tektronix Model 564B). The SSW recording was monitored by the experimenters using the stereo headset coupled to the tape recorder. To measure the onset times of each item on the test, the experimenters triggered the oscilloscope at the termination of the first syllable of the first spondee, thereby allowing the oscilloscope to trace and store the second syllable of the first spondee and the first syllable of the second spondee. The onset times of the traced syllables for each of the test items were then measured using a procedure suggested by Speaks[2]. Onset time was defined as any output which exceeded a baseline noise level preceding the syllable (see Figure 1). The onset time measurements were repeated on randomly chosen test items by the experimenters. The agreement between the first and second set of measurements of the experimenters as well as the agreement between the experimenters were found to average ±2 msec.

Results

Listener Results

There were a possible 160 errors associated with a single presentation of the SSW (List EC). That is, there were 40 spondee words on the test, and each spondee was presented under a competing and a non-competing condition, resulting in a total of 80 stimulus items. When scoring the SSW, the two single-syllable words per spondee were scored separately, thereby allowing for two possible errors per spondee, and a possible total of 160 errors per listener.

The 10 listeners in the study committed a total of only seven errors out of a possible total of 1600. Of these seven errors, only one was made on a spondee pair matched within 4 to 30 msec.

Lead and Lag Effects

The onset times of the spondees for the 40 stimulus pairs of competing items on the SSW (List EC) were found to be highly variable (see Figure 1 and Table 2). The onset of the second syllable of the first spondee was found to lead the onset of the first syllable of the second spondee in 15 (38%) of the stimulus pairs (range = 4 msec to 150 msec, mean = 50.4 msec, standard deviation = 36.01 msec). The onset of the second syllable of the first spondee was found to lag behind the onset of the

---

[2] C. Speaks, personal communication, 1974.

Acoustic and Psychoacoustic Factors

first syllable of the second spondee in 25 (62%) of the stimulus pairs (range = 10 msec to 175 msec, mean = 55 msec, standard deviation = 38.36 msec).

FIGURE 1. ══════════════════════════

Sample tracing of a competing stimulus item from the SSW test, including the points at which the onset-time measurements were made (arrows). Top tracing represents the second syllable of the word and lower tracing represents the first syllable of the word. Each division equals 40 msec.

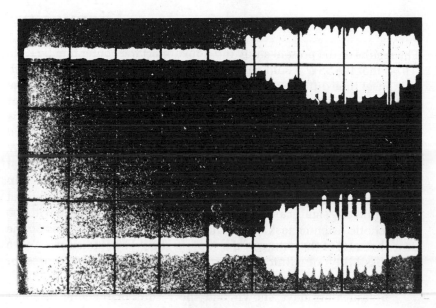

TABLE 2.

The number and percentage (in parentheses) of items and mean onset time differences, ranges, and standard deviations (in msec) for the items on the SSW that showed a lead effect and those that showed a lag effect. The results are depicted according to the three onset time difference categories employed.

Onset Time Difference Categories (in msec)	Lead				Lag			
	No. of items	Mean	Range	SD	No. of items	Mean	Range	SD
0-30	4 (10%)	13.8	4-25	–	9 (22%)	21.8	10- 30	–
31-50	6 (15%)	42.8	35-50	–	5 (13%)	44.4	36- 50	–
51 +	5 (13%)	88.8	60-150	–	11 (28%)	87.0	52-175	–
Total	15 (38%)	50.4	4-150	36.0	25 (62%)	55.0	10-175	38.4

Discussion

The results of the present study did not support the contention by Katz (1974) that the SSW would be too difficult for normal listeners if word-pair onset time differences were controlled. The spondaic words of the SSW are characterized by significantly more phonetic and spectral redundancy than the CV stimuli used in earlier investigations (Studdert-Kennedy et al., 1970; Berlin et al., 1973). The increased redundancy likely enhances the perceptual processing of the SSW words compared to the CV stimuli, thereby minimizing for normal listeners the deleterious effects associated with variable onset times. In turn, Berlin et al. (1974) found neurologically impaired listeners did not show clinically significant lead and lag effects when presented with the CV dichotic listening task. Nevertheless, onset time differences on the SSW, because of the nature of the stimuli, should be studied relative to the possibility of clinically significant effects on the scores of neurologically impaired listeners.

Investigators have shown that the results of dichotic listening tasks can vary depending upon the signal-to-noise ratios which are employed (Speaks, 1974; Berlin et al., 1973), the type of signals employed (Speaks et al., 1973), and intensity levels of the respective competing stimuli (Speaks and Bisonette, 1974; Cullin et al., 1973; Roeser, Johns, and Price, 1972). The SSW, a dichotic listening task, has been used in the differential diagnosis of auditory processing problems, and its use may be improved as the effects of these and other variables become apparent and are applied in a controlled and systematic manner.

Acoustic and Psychoacoustic Factors

Acknowledgement

This study was supported in part by an All-University Research Grant No. 8813 (Project No. 11-6893), awarded to the second author. The authors wish to express their gratitude to Charles Speaks of the University of Minnesota and Jack Katz of the University of Buffalo for their suggestions and comments. Requests for reprints should be directed to Daniel S. Beasley, Department of Audiology and Speech Pathology, Memphis State University, Speech and Hearing Center, 807 West Jefferson Avenue, Memphis, Tennessee 38105.

References

American National Standards Institute, *Specifications for Audiometers*. ANSI S3.6 1969. New York: American National Standards Institute (1969).

Balas, R., Staggered Spondaic Word Test: Support. *Ann. Otol. Rhinol. Laryng.*, 80, 132–134 (1971).

Berlin, C., Cullen, J., Lowe-Bell, S., and Berlin, H., Speech perception after hemispherectomy and temporal lobectomy. Paper presented at the Speech Communication Seminar, Stockholm (1974).

Berlin, C., Lowe-Bell, S., Cullen, J., Thompson, C., and Loovis, F., Dichotic speech perception: An interpretation of right ear advantage and temporal offset effects. *J. acoust. Soc. Am.*, 53, 699–709 (1973).

Cullen, J., Thompson, C., Samson, D., and Hughes, L., The effects of monaural and binaural masking on a dichotic speech task. Paper presented at the Annual Convention of the American Speech and Hearing Association, San Francisco (1973).

Katz, J., The SSW Test: An interim report. *J. Speech Hearing Dis.*, 33, 132–146 (1968).

Katz, J., The use of staggered spondaic words for assessing the integrity of the central auditory system. *J. aud. Res.*, 2, 327–337 (1962).

Katz, J., Basil, R., and Smith, J., A staggered spondaic word test for detecting central auditory lesions. *Ann. Otol. Rhinol. Laryng.*, 72, 908–917 (1963).

Roeser, R., Johns, D., and Price, L., Effects of intensity on dichotically presented digits. *J. aud. Res.*, 12, 184–186 (1972).

Speaks, C., Dichotic listening: A clinical or research tool? Paper presented at the Conference on Central Auditory Processing Disorders, Univ. Nebraska Medical Center, Omaha (1974).

Speaks, C., and Bissonette, L., Inter-aural-intensive differences and dichotic listening. Paper presented at the 88th Meeting of the Acoustical Society of America, St. Louis (November 1974).

Speaks, C., Kuhl, P., Trooien, T., Marth, S., Rubens, A., and Podraza, B., Interference by speech and nonspeech signals. Paper presented at the 85th Meeting of the Acoustical Society of America, Boston (April 1973).

Studdert-Kennedy, M., Shankweiler, D., and Schulman, S., Opposed effects of a delayed channel on perception of dichotically and monotically presented CV syllables. *J. acoust. Soc. Am.*, 48, 599–602 (1970).

Lead/Lag Analysis of SSW Test Items*

J. Katz, N. K. Harder, and P. R.Lohnes

The SSW Test is a procedure which is used for locating dysfunction in the brain and brainstem. Over the past 16 years a considerable amount of data has been collected on normal and non-normal subjects. Many investigators and clinicians have found the test to be effective in locating lesions in various parts of the central nervous system. The test is now being used widely in the United States and elsewhere.

The SSW Test is a procedure in which one spondaic word is presented to each ear. The spondees are partially overlapped in time as shown in Figure 1. We will begin with the word, *upstairs* presented to the right ear. The word *downtown* trails and is presented to the left ear. The words *stairs* and *down* (which we will refer to as 2a and 2b, respectively) arrive at the same time. This paper will deal with the temporal relationships between the two competing words of the SSW items. It should be noted that the items begin alternately in the right and left ears.

In 1976 Freeman and Beasley reported on the the temporal relationships of the competing words on the SSW Test. They tried to determine whether the pairs that were more closely overlapped were also the more difficult ones. They divided the 40 items from the SSW (EC List) into those they called "leading" and those they called "lagging." A

ASHA Convention, Chicago, Illinois, 1977.

Acoustic and Psychoacoustic Factors

leading item was one in which the competing word of the leading spondee (2a) preceded the competing word of the trailing spondee (2b). A leading item is shown in the upper diagram of Figure 2. The opposite situation constitutes a lagging item. This is shown in the lower diagram in which the trailing spondee (2b) begins before the competing word of the first spondee (2a).

Freeman and Beasley found that 15 of the items were leading and 25 were lagging. They indicated that the onset differences varied from 4 to 175 msec. They tested 10 young, normal-hearing college students to determine whether there was a difference in performance as a result of the onset differences. The subjects made a total of only seven errors. Since only one error was on an item that was closely matched, they concluded that onset time was not a critical feature for normal listeners on the SSW Test.

The present study attempted to replicate the work of Freeman and Beasley with a larger sample of subjects, including a more typical normal population. The SSW records of 174 subjects were studied. Forty control subjects from Brunt's 1968 study comprised the normal group.

FIGURE 1. ▬▬▬▬▬▬▬▬▬▬▬▬▬▬▬▬▬▬▬▬▬▬▬▬▬▬▬▬▬▬

An SSW item showing the time sequence of the words. The competing words are labeled 2a and 2b.

	Time Sequence		
	1	2	3
		(a)	
First spondee	UP	STAIRS	
		(b)	
Second spondee		DOWN	TOWN

FIGURE 2. ▬▬▬▬▬▬▬▬▬▬▬▬▬▬▬▬▬▬▬▬▬▬▬▬▬▬▬▬▬▬

Onset lead is shown as being the competing word 2a beginning before the competing word 2b (upper curve). The onset lag is shown to be the initiation of 2b before 2a.

	Onset Lead		
First spondee	UP	STAIRS	
Second spondee		DOWN	TOWN

	Onset Lag		
First spondee	UP	STAIRS	
Second spondee		DOWN	TOWN

These subjects ranged from 16–61 years of age and represented a wide socioeconomic population. Both blacks and whites, men and women were employed in the sample.

The other groups represented—elderly, cochlear, retrocochlear, cerebral auditory reception (i.e., having lesions involving Heschl's gyrus), cerebral nonauditory reception (i.e., brain lesions not involving Heschl's gyrus), mentally retarded, and learning disabled. On the handout you will see the mean ages, number of subjects, and correlations with Freeman and Beasley's lead/lag data.

Pearson product–moment correlations were computed between the number of errors on each item and their respective onset time differences. In order to replicate the work more closely, we used the onset time data which were reported by Freeman and Beasley. For the normal group and each of the other seven groups there was a consistent but small negative correlation. That is, there was a tendency in each group for the items with the closest onset times to have the most errors. The multiple R was .54, which was statistically significant the .05 level of confidence.

Since the primary purpose of the SSW Test is to differentiate auditory reception from nonauditory reception disorders (Katz, 1968), we were particularly interested in these two groups as well as the normals. Berlin et al. (1973) indicate that certain patients with brain lesions require 500 msec between dichotically presented monosyllables in order for them to correctly identify both of the words. Since the maximum onset time differences reported by Freeman and Beasley was only 175 msec on the SSW items, we would predict that such differences would have a negligible benefit for the AR subjects. This was indeed the case. The AR group had the smallest correlation of any group ($-.06$). As one might expect, when Heschl's gyrus is damaged, the contralateral competing word is missed, regardless of the minor onset time discrepancies.

On the other hand, the cases with cerebral involvement sparing Heschl's gyrus (as well as each of the other groups in the study) had more errors on the items that were more precisely aligned. The correlation for the NAR group was $-.36$ (which is significant at the .05 level of confidence).

The purpose of the quantitative analysis on the SSW Test is to differentiate the performance of the AR cases from the NAR cases. By closer alignment of the competing words on the SSW Test there should be a tendency to reduce the difference between these two groups, thus weakening the test.

We studied the correlations for the lead and lag items to see how they corresponded to the number of errors in the normal group. There was a signficant correlation for the 25 lag items ($r = -.39$). The correlation for the 15 lead items was not statistically signficant. It appears that while onset time differences play a part in determining the difficulty level of an item, there are many other factors that also influence the results. This latter point was properly made by Freeman and Beasley.

Recently, Rudmin and Harder studied the discriminability of the recorded words on the SSW tape. They found the highest correlation to exist for the *normal subjects* who were more likely to say *ice bland* for *ice land* because of the acoustic characteristics on the tape rather than any onset time differences. This no doubt explains the Freeman and Beasley results when dealing with their supra-normal population.

The lag effect was first reported by Studdert-Kennedy *et al.* in 1970. Their findings were supported by Berlin *et al.* (1973). They noted that when two monosyllables were delivered to opposite ears, the one that lagged slightly behind the other was more frequently identified. A delay of 30 to 90 msec seemed to benefit the lagging member. Studdert-Kennedy *et al.* suggest that this is due to incomplete processing of the first word before shifting attention to the second word.

All of our groups except the AR group made more errors on the words that were most closely matched in onset. The AR group apparently could not take advantage of the lead or lag time because of the overriding influence of the pathology effect, in which the competing word in the contralateral ear was extinguished.

One more word of caution seems appropriate for those who would be included to "tighten up" the SSW onset times. Berlin *et al.* noted that lag difference of less than 30 msec produced a right ear advantage. If the onset times were more closely aligned this could introduce an undesirable source of variability into the procedure. The SSW Test is surprisingly free from the influence of dominance and can only be weakened by this added variable factor.

In the present study we were unable to confirm the assumption of Freeman and Beasley that onset time differences did not alter SSW test performance. Since the purpose of the test is to identify and categorize auditory pathologies and since it does an effective job, there seems little reason for adjusting the onsets of the competing words at this time.

Author's Note

Rudmin and Katz replicated the measurements of Freeman and Beasley. Rudmin and Katz used the standard SSW EC tape, which, apparently; Freeman and Beasley also used. Numerous discrepancies were noted. The most important problem that was noted in the data by Freeman and Beasley is that most of the items were reversed (i.e., *lead* was incorrectly shown as *lag* and vice versa, but not in all cases).

Lead/Lag Analysis of SSW Test Items
Correlations between competing-word errors and Lead/Lag temporal difference data of Freeman and Beasley, 1976.

Group	N	Mean Age	Pearson r
Normals	40	45	−.25
Elderly	8	66	−.34*
Cochlear	35	45	−.14
Retrocochlear	13	43	−.24
Cerebral Auditory Reception	7	49	−.06
Cerebral Nonauditory Reception	13	37	−.36*
Mentally Retarded	37	31	−.12
Learning Disabled	23	9	−.26
Multiple R			.54*

J. Katz, B. K. Harder, and P. R. Lohnes

*significant at .05 level

Normal Adult Performance on a Temporally Modified Staggered Spondaic Word Task

Melanie L. Matthies and D. C. Garstecki

Competing syllables in the Staggered Spondaic Word (SSW) test exhibit considerable variation in alignment. These alignment variations have shown discrepant effects on selected subject populations. Since Berlin et al. (1973) found that dichotic presentation of temporally off-set CV syllables may result in improved intelligibility of the trailing syllable, the same lag effect would be expected to influence performance on a staggered spondaic word identification task. The purpose of this study was to examine the effect of temporal alignment of competing syllables in a staggered spondaic word identification task. Forty-eight adults having no prior experience with or knowledge of the SSW test and no history of speech, language, hearing or reading disorders participated in the study. Each subject was administered two recorded versions of the SSW test. One recording contained items as presented on the commercially available test. The second recording contained SSW test items in which competing monosyllables were temporally aligned. Results revealed no significant difference in performance between the two alignment conditions. In addition, no significant ear effect was demonstrated. Variables which may influence subject performance are described.

Scand Audiol 9:89–92, 1980

Introduction

The Staggered Spondaic Word (SSW) test (Katz, 1962) is one of few commercially available dichotic listening tests of central auditory system function. In this test, each item consists of a pair of spondaic words. The pairs of words are presented dichotically with the second syllable of the first word overlapping with the first syllable of the second word. Thus, the initial syllable of the first spondee is received without competition, the second syllable of the first spondee competes with the first syllable of the spondee presented to the opposite ear, and the final monosyllable of the second spondee is also received without competition.

Since depressed ear performance on the SSW test may be indicative of dysfunction in the opposite hemisphere (Katz, 1976), it would seem that a significant right ear advantage could confound the results. Various studies using the SSW test have demonstrated statistically significant laterality effects (Goldman & Katz, 1966; Brunt & Goetzinger, 1968; Katz & Fishman, 1972). However, these findings were not considered to be clinically significant.

In the construction of the commercially available SSW test, precise alignment of overlapping syllables was not achieved. For example, Freeman & Beasley (1976) examined the alignment of SSW test item syllabic overlap and found that the onset of the second syllable of the first word was misaligned from the onset of the first syllable of the second word by as much as 175 milliseconds. Freeman & Beasley also provided item error analyses based on the responses of ten normal subjects to SSW test recordings. These subjects made a small number of errors, which were not correlated with onset alignment precision. Katz et al. (1977) reported a study in which SSW test performance of 174 peripherally and/or centrally hearing-impaired subjects was compared with that of a control group comprised of 40 normal subjects. They found that onset time did influence SSW test performance. Further investigation is warranted to examine the seeming discrepancies between these two studies. The purpose of this study was to re-assess the effect of alignment of the onset of competing SSW test syllables on the performance of normal adults in an effort to better understand factors which may influence performance on a diagnostic test of this type.

Method

Subjects

Forty-eight female university students ranging in age from 20 to 32 years of age (mean age, 22.2 years) served as subjects in this study. Selection criteria for these subjects required that each have no prior experience with or knowledge of the SSW test along the no history of speech, language, hearing or reading disorders. A homogeneous group of subjects was selected in order to minimize the influence of individual subject variables on the results of the experiment. Each subject passed a hearing screening at 20 dB HL (ANSI, 1969) at octave frequencies from 500 to 4000 Hz bilaterally.

Experimental Tape Preparation

Initially, it was necessary to measure the magnitude of alignment discrepancy within each of the 40 SSW test items. Measurements were made with a Crown (Model 700) audio tape playback unit used in conjunction with a two-channel storage oscilloscope (Tektronix, Model 1501) equipped with a camera (Tektronix, Model C-12). As competing syllable pairs were displayed on the two-channel oscilloscope, a high-speed black and white Polaroid photograph was taken of the speech signal and superimposed measuring grid. Figure 1 (upper) is a graphic sketched from a photograph to represent the temporal characteristics of the monosyllables 'break' (upper) and 'lamp' (lower) in the spondaic word pairs 'daybreak' and 'lamplight' as recorded on the commercially available SSW test tape. Onset alignment discrepancy values recorded on each photograph were measured with a millimeter rule. Our measurements were within 5 msec of the alignment discrepancy values reported by Freeman & Beasley (1976). Having determined competing syllable onset differences, onset times of competing SSW test stimuli were aligned by computer. The spondaic word pairs of the SSW test were used as input into a PDP-8L laboratory computer using an Ampex (Model 350) audiotape playback unit. Competing syllable lead or lag time difference for each pair of spondaic words was calculated as an octal number and its binary representations was toggled into the PDP-8L computer, Using a specifically designed assembly language program (DLAY), the two channel signal input was samples, digitized and stored in the core memory of the computer with one channel being programmed to delay the input signal by a predetermined amount of time. By delaying input from one channel, lead or lag time differences were resolved and competing syllable onset times were aligned.

Following alignment, the comuter line output was displayed on the Tektronix (Model 1501) storage oscilloscope and competing syllable pairs were photographed (Tektronix, Model C-12) for measurement of onset alignment. Figure 1 (lower) is a graphic sketch of the monosyllables 'break' (upper) and 'light' (lower) after syllabic onset alignment. The mean post-alignment discrepancy between competing syllables was 5.65 msec (SD = 3.8; range = 2–15 msec). Mean pre-alignment discrepancy was 52.95 msec (SD = 37.2; range = 5–175

FIGURE 1. ▬▬▬▬▬▬▬

Graphics sketched from photographs to represent the temporal characteristics of the unaligned and aligned experimental stimuli at output from Channel 1 and Channel 2.

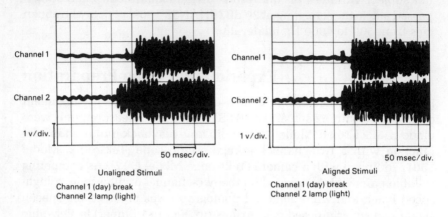

Unaligned Stimuli

Channel 1 (day) break
Channel 2 lamp (light)

Aligned Stimuli

Channel 1 (day) break
Channel 2 lamp (light)

msec). To control for any change in tape quality which might be attributable to computer processing, the original SSW test tape was also sampled and digitized. The computer output was recorded on an Ampex (Model 700) reel-to-reel tape recorder. Recordings of the unaligned and aligned item computer processed tapes were band-pass filtered (Krohn-Lite, Model 3550) from 150 to 8000 Hz. Filtered tapes were re-recorded on cassette tape using a Pioneer (Model CT-5151) stereo tape recording deck. Half-lists were recorded in alternate presentation order to provide two experimental test tapes each containing aligned and unaligned test items.

Experimental Design and Procedure

Test stimuli were presented using an Advent (Model 202) tape player in conjunction with a Maico (Model MA-24) diagnostic audiometer. The speech signal was transduced through TDH-39 headphones set in MX 41/AR cushions and presented at 50 dB SL re: spondee threshold. Subjects were seated in a double walled audiologic testing room and instructed to listen to recorded instructions. Subjects were presented with four practice items which are normally included as the introduction to the standard SSW test. They were then presented with a test tape, receiving the first 20 items in either the aligned or unaligned condition, with the second 20 items presented in the alternate alignment condition. Thus, each subject received both aligned and unaligned test items. Subject responses were recorded and categorized as to ear and alignment condition. Each subject obtained four scores, one score for each ear under each alignment condition.

Acoustic and Psychoacoustic Factors

Results

Since two experimental tapes were used in this study, it was necessary to determine their equivalency. Comparison of scores obtained for each ear under each alignment condition for each tape revealed essentially similar results. Student's t-test distribution scores obtained using the means for all ear-alignment conditions indicated no significant difference in performance among subjects on the two experimental tapes ($t = 1.96$; $p < 0.01$).

The effect of alignment of competing syllable onset time is summarized in Table 1. Subjects made relatively few errors under any condition. The mean overall number of errors was 2.21. No significant differences in subject performance were found for ear or alignment conditions using a two-way analysis of variance (Winer, 1971; Nie et al., 1975).

Discussion

The performance of normal adults on an aligned and unaligned staggered spondaic word task was compared. No significant difference was found between the magnitude of errors made on the aligned versus unaligned test items. There was also no significant interaction between ear and alignment conditions. The results of this study support earlier research demonstrating that alignment of competing syllabic onsets does not influence normal adult performance on an SSW identification task (Freeman & Beasley, 1976). Both Katz et al. (1977) and Freeman & Beasley (1976) used an item analysis technique to ascertain possible effects of alignment on SSW test performance. A more direct test of the effects of alignment on test performance was undertaken in this study, e.g., we directly manipulated syllabic onset alignment.

The findings of the present investigation were interpreted to suggest that factors other than the alignment characteristics of competing

TABLE 1 ▬▬▬▬▬▬▬▬▬▬▬▬▬▬▬▬▬▬▬▬▬▬▬▬▬▬▬▬▬▬▬▬▬▬

Mean standard deviation (SD) and variance data for each ear and alignment condition for all subjects (n = 48) expressed in percent incorrect.

Ear	Aligned Items			Unaligned Items		
	Mean	SD	Variance	Mean	SD	Variance
Right	1.92	2.53	6.44	2.60	2.47	6.11
Left	2.03	2.28	5.22	2.34	2.95	8.61

syllables contributed to the variability in performance of normal listeners to the experimental task. Factors worthy of consideration include semantic variability present among SSW test items. Consideration of word familiarity and the role of semantics has only recently been recognized as an important factor in test item selection (Kalikow et al., 1977). For example, some of the items used in the SSW test included familiar bi-syllabic words such as 'baseball' and 'hotdog', while others seem less common, i.e. 'bandsaw' and 'beachcraft'. Differences in semantic content may influence subject performance and require further study.

A second factor that may influence test performance which has not been addressed by other investigators is concerned with the fact that new spondee stimuli may, in some cases, be formed by combining the second syllable of the first word with the first syllable of the second word, i.e. 'outside' and 'inlaw' can be recombined to form 'inside'. For most test items, such recombinations are not possible, i.e. 'meatsauce' and 'baseball'. During the conduct of the present investigation, several subjects reported greater difficulty in responding to the task when recombinable items were presented. The degree in which this factor influences test performance has not been systematically appraised.

There are two additional factors which merit consideration. First, wide variability is present in the silent time between the monosyllables of the spondaic words. Although it was not the intent of this study to measure the variability in silent interval, we were impressed with the degree of variation apparent in our oscilloscopic records of the stimuli. The degree to which this factor influences the competing nature of the SSW test stimuli merits more careful observation. Finally there is the issue of a potential masking effect of the background noise on the competing stimuli. The true nature of this masking effect may be particularly important for test items with sibilant and fricative consonant content (Miller & Nicely, 1955).

In conclusion, examination of the competing syllabic onsets of SSW test items has led to further questions concerning the use of this test as a diagnostic instrument. Use of a staggered spondaic word paradigm to evaluate central auditory system processing must also take into consideration other, potentially critical factors. Possible factors may include test word familiarity, semantic cues, recombinability of monosyllables to form spondees and masking effects. Further evaluation of these variables may serve to increase the clinical utility of the SSW test and similar central auditory test procedures.

Acknowledgements

This article is based on a master's thesis completed by Melanie L. Matthies in the Department of Audiology and Speech Sciences, Purdue University. The authors wish to express their appreciation to Yoshiyuki Horii for use of his DLAY computer program and to William A. Cooper and Bernd Weinberg for their critical review of earlier versions of the manuscript.

References

ANSI S3.6 1969. *Specification for Audiometers.* Acoustical Society of America, New York.

Berlin, C., Lowe-Bell, S., Cullen, J., Thompson, C. & Loovis, F. 1973. Dichotic speech perception: An interpretation of right ear advantage and temporal offset effects. *J Acoust Soc Am 53*, 699.

Brunt, M. & Goetzinger, C. 1968. A study of three tests of central function with normal hearing subjects. *Cortex 4*, 288.

Freeman, B. & Beasley, D. 1976. Lead and lag effects associated with the Staggered Spondaic Word Test. *J Speech Hear Res 19*, 572.

Goldman, S. & Katz, J. 1966. A comparison of the performance of normal hearing subjects on the Staggered Spondaic Word Test given under four conditions—dichotic, diotic, monaural (dominant ear) and monaural (non-dominant ear). Paper presented at the Annual Meeting of the American Speech and Hearing Association, Chicago, Illinois.

Kalikow, D., Stevens, K. & Elliot, L. 1977. Development of a test of speech intelligibility in noise using sentence materials with controlled word predictability. *J Acoust Soc Am 61*, 1337.

Katz, J., Harder, B. & Lohnes, P. 1977. Lead/lag analysis of SSW test items. Paper presented at the Annual Meeting of the American Speech and Hearing Association, Chicago, Illinois.

Miller, G. & Nicely, P. 1955. Analysis of perceptual confusions among some English consonants. *J Acoust Soc Am 27*, 388.

Nie, N., Hull, C., Jenkins, J., Steinbrenner, K. & Bent, D. 1975. *SPSS—Statistical Package for the Social Sciences.* McGraw-Hill, New York.

Winer, B. 1971. *Statistical Principles in Experimental Design.* McGraw-Hill, New York.

Katz, J. 1962. The use of the Staggered Spondaic Word Test for assessing the integrity of the central auditory nervous system. *J Aud Res 2*, 327.

Katz, J. 1976. *The SSW Test Manual —A Brief Explanation.* Auditec of St. Louis, St. Louis, Mo.

Katz, J. & Fishman, P. 1972. The use of the Staggered Spondaic Word Test as a means of detecting differences between age groups. Unpublished study in *Handbook of Clinical Audiology.* (ed. J. Katz) Williams & Wilkins, Baltimore.

Dichotic Onset and Offset Parameters on the SSW Test

Floyd Rudmin and Jack Katz

The alignment of the competing words of the SSW Test (EC recording) was analyzed using an auditory-manual method. Oscilloscopic tracings were also made. Word onsets and offsets were marked directly on the recording tape. In addition, sonorancy onsets and offsets were noted. Time differences between the competing words were calculated and displayed. Information for each item is shown. Alignment differences were calculated for six acoustic reference points: word onsets, word offsets, word centers, sonorancy onsets, sonorancy offsets, and sonorancy centers. Word center and sonorancy onset alignment differences were smallest and least variable. The word onset measures of this study were compared to those of a similar oscilloscopic study by Freeman and Beasley (1976). Some important differences were noted between the studies indicating limitations with the purely oscilloscopic study.

Broadly defined, dichotic speech testing refers to the simultaneous or overlapping presentation of different messages to each ear, such that the messages compete for the subject's processing capacities. Cherry introduced the dichotic speech paradigm in 1953. Since then the procedure has been developed for a wide variety of experimental and clinical purposes. Feldmann (1960) first described a dichotic speech test for central auditory testing. The Feldman Test (in German) consists of dichotic presentations of numbers, such as *twenty-five* to one ear and *forty-three* to the other. Kimura (1961) employed dichotic digits for similar purposes. In this test, three digits are presented simultaneously to each ear. In 1962, Katz introduced the Staggered Spondaic Word (SSW) Test as a clinical measure of central auditory dysfunction. Other dichotic central auditory tests include the

Acoustic and Psychoacoustic Factors

Synthetic Sentences Index with a contralateral competing message [SSI–CCM] (Jerger and Jerger, 1974), the Competing Sentences Test (Willeford, 1976), and Berlin's (1976) simultaneous and time-staggered CV syllables.

The SSW Test is a modified dichotic speech procedure in which each ear is presented a different spondaic word in a partially overlapping manner. First, one monosyllable is presented to one ear. Then, while the second monosyllable from the first spondee is being presented, the second spondee is started in the other ear. For example, the first SSW item is *upstairs, downtown.* The word *up* is presented monaurally to the first ear, followed by *stairs* and *down* dichotically, and then *town* monaurally to the second ear. The two monosyllables presented to each ear are semantically linked as a single spondee.

A number of SSW test lists and tapes have been produced. For some of them, dichotic alignment was based on word onset adjustment. However, in preparing the EC tape, the competing monosyllables were not aligned on the criterion of simultaneous word onset. Rather, two monophonic tapes were played and replayed, making small time adjustments until the competing words sounded overlapped in time. This was checked dichotically and monaurally. Using this listening method, no one acoustic, phonetic, physiologic, or psychological criterion was considered paramount. The human auditory perceptual system was allowed to weigh and balance the many factors involved in dichotic simultaneity for each of the 40 test items. The overlap as also checked by drawing the tape slowly across the playback heads. This ensured that there were no gross discrepancies between the competing words. Perceptual simultaneity has been discussed in the psychological literature as an appropriate, reliable, and perhaps preferred procedure for preparing dichotic speech materials (Morton, Marcus, and Frankish, 1976). In retrospect, the procedure used to align the SSW EC tape might be labelled *two-channel P-center alignment* to differentiate it from the alignment of monaurally determined P-centers described by Morton et al. (1976).

Of the SSW tapes produced, the EC tape has proven to be a broadly applicable and clinically efficient procedure. It is used by approximately half of the audiologists responding to a recent survey (Martin and Forbis, 1978). The EC tape's clinical strength results in part from two characteristics. First, laterality effects due to hemispheric dominance for speech are clinically insignificant on the EC recording (Brunt, 1978). On simultaneous dichotic tests, right ear advantage precludes ready comparisons of ear scores (Kimura, 1961). Berlin et al. (1973) review evidence that right ear effects are maximized by word onset alignment and are reduced by boundary alignment (i.e., sonorancy onset alignment).

Secondly, with the EC recording, a correction factor may be used to offset the effects of poor speech discrimination. Miltenberger, Dawson, and Raica (1978) found that cochlear hearing loss disrupts a number of central auditory speech tests. However, when SSW scores are corrected, the resulting C-SSW scores are excellent for both normal hearing and peripheral hearing loss cases (Brunt, 1978). This ability to estimate and discount the portion of a depressed SSW score that is due to peripheral effects is possible because of the close relationship between raw SSW scores and W-22 scores for normals (Balas and Simon, 1964) and for cochlear cases (Katz, 1977). In this last study using subjects with cochlear pathology, raw SSW scores and percent error on the W-22 test were found to have nearly identical means and standard deviations, and to correlate with an r of .86. Reported correlations of total raw SSW scores and PB error are .92 and .93 (Katz, Basil, and Smith, 1963; Katz, 1968). It is not known whether or not dichotic alignment is one of the factors that allows a half-dichotic spondee to have approximately the same difficulty as a PB monosyllable.

The ultimate validity of the SSW Test design, including dichotic alignment, is that it is differentially sensitive to lesions at various levels of the central auditory nervous system (CANS). These include the cerebral auditory reception area (Jerger and Jerger, 1975; Balas, 1971; Katz, 1968), cerebral nonauditory reception areas (Katz, 1978; Winkelaar and Lewis, 1977; Katz and Pack, 1975; Balas, 1971), and upper and lower brainstem areas (Katz, 1970). The test has also been effective in the evaluation of learning disabled children (Dempsey, 1977; White, 1977; Stubblefield and Young, 1975; Katz and Illmer, 1972).

In 1976, Freeman and Beasley reported on a study of one parameter of SSW dichotic alignment. Using a two-channel oscilloscope, they examined the alignments of the word onsets of the competing monosyllables of the EC recording. They found that competing monosyllables did not, as a rule, have simultaneous word onsets, and that 10 normal subjects missed 7 of the 1600 monosyllables presented. They concluded that the EC recording was not well controlled relative to onset times and that normal listeners were not disrupted when onset times were closely aligned. The purpose of the present study was to replicate the word onset measurements of Freeman and Beasley, using an auditory-manual technique rather than an oscilloscope. However, oscilloscopic tracings were made for illustrative purposes. In addition to word onsets, dichotic alignment was examined at five other acoustic reference points: word offsets, word centers, sonorancy onsets, sonorancy offsets, and sonorancy centers. Finally, intraspondee silence durations, competing monosyllable durations and duration differences, and the amount of unoverlapped time were quantified.

Method

Using the principles of a dichotic alignment technique described by Rubino (1972), the commercially available SSW EC tape was re-recorded at double the normal speed. At the new recording speed of 38 cm/sec, one mm of tape equals 2.63 msec. This permits a time resolution of about 3 msec. This tape was threaded through a tape recorder so as to bypass the capstan, allowing the tape to be pulled across the playback head by hand in either direction. The output was amplified and played through soundfield speakers. Two experimenters made independent measures on separate occasions. The tape was manipulated and listened to one channel at a time. Onsets and offsets were marked directly onto the tape with color-coded pens. Measurements on which the experimenters' judgments differed by more than 1 cm were re-examined by each experimenter. Final measurements were the midpoints between the two experimenters' final judgments. Two-channel oscilloscopic tracings of each item were made and photographed to provide visual illustrations of word onset alignments.

Results

There was a high degree of consistency between the judgments of the two experimenters. Of the 160 word onsets and offsets measured, re-examination was required eight times. The absolute mean difference of the final judgments was 2.6 msec (SD = 3.02) for word onsets and 5.4 msec (SD = 5.38) for word offsets. Maximum differences were 10 msec and 24 msec, respectively. Word onsets were easier to judge than were word offsets. Differences in the judgments of the two experimenters were significantly smaller for the onset condition ($t = 8.55$; $p < .001$).

An illustration of the final measurements of the dichotic alignments of the 40 test items is shown in Figure 1. Very clearly, the competing items do not have simultaneous word onsets. On only three occasions did word onsets coincide, ±13 msec. Using this range of measurement error, word offsets were aligned on four items, word centers five times, sonorancy onsets eight times, sonorancy offsets twice, and sonorancy centers six times. Visual inspection shows a general tendency for word centering, with word duration differences divided between onset lead and offset lag. Since none of the competing pairs have equal word durations, there is a given amount of unoverlapped time for each item. Word centering would therefore tend to minimize onset and offset differences.

The spondaic words were not recorded as continuous speech. Rather, there is an intraspondee silence duration. The average competing monosyllable was 549 msec (SD = 110) in duration, and was

FIGURE 1.

Competing monosyllables for the 40 SSW items, EC recording. The thick lines represent sonorancy and the thin lines represent nonsonorancy. The initial onset begins on the left side. The competing monosyllable of the leading spondee is always on top. The time scale is presented for 200 msec.

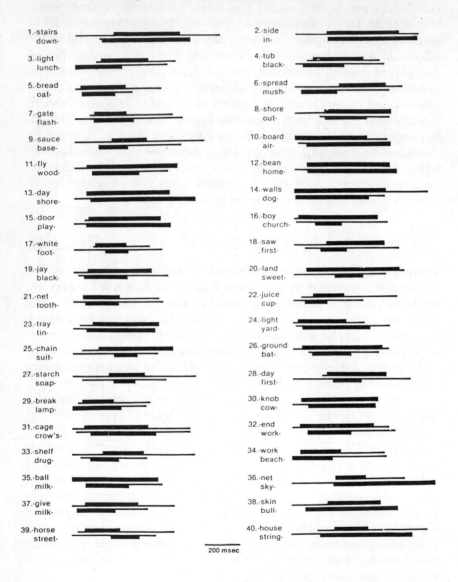

1.-stairs down-
2.-side in-
3.-light lunch-
4.-tub black-
5.-bread oat-
6.-spread mush-
7.-gate flash-
8.-shore out-
9.-sauce base-
10.-board air-
11.-fly wood-
12.-bean home-
13.-day shore-
14.-walls dog-
15.-door play-
16.-boy church-
17.-white foot-
18.-saw first-
19.-jay black-
20.-land sweet-
21.-net tooth-
22.-juice cup-
23.-tray tin-
24.-light yard-
25.-chain suit-
26.-ground bat-
27.-starch soap-
28.-day first-
29.-break lamp-
30.-knob cow-
31.-cage crow's-
32.-end work-
33.-shelf drug-
34.-work beach-
35.-ball milk-
36.-net sky-
37.-give milk-
38.-skin bull-
39.-horse street-
40.-house string-

200 msec

separated from its other half-spondee by 371 msec (SD = 36). Both competing word durations and intraspondee gaps showed considerable ranges. On an average, one of the competing monosyllables was 135 msec, or 20% longer in duration than the other. Thus, with any alignment criterion, 100% simultaneous dichotic presentations would not be possible. As aligned by its author, the EC tape's mean unoverlapped time was 168 msec, or 26% of the total duration of the competing condition. These figures do not include the considerable durations of the noncompeting monosyllables.

Dichotic alignment simultaneity was measured at six acoustic reference points along the competing condition: word onsets, word offsets, word centers, sonorancy onsets, sonorancy offsets, and sonorancy centers. Word center and sonorancy onset alignment differences were smallest and least variable. Mean absolute differences were 51 msec (SD = 37) and 56 msec (SD = 51), respectively. Sonorancy offset and word offset alignment differences were largest and most variable.

Discussion

Considering the original alignment procedure of the SSW EC tape, it was expected that no one acoustic parameter would stand out as the alignment criterion. A factor analysis study in progress may reveal significant interactions of acoustic parameters. Considering the 40 test items as a homogeneous set and disregarding nonacoustic parameters, it may be hypothesized that word centering and sonorancy onset alignment were more heavily weighted on the EC tape than were word onsets. With monaurally determined P-centers, Morton et al. (1976) report that P-centers did not correspond to word onsets, stressed vowel onsets, or peak vowel intensities, and that they are not a result of a simple energy integration. They suggest that it may be fruitful to consider phonologic, semantic, and syntactic variables in P-center allocations. Assuming that there are similarities between monaural P-centering and the method of SSW alignment, it may not be valid to evaluate SSW alignment solely on acoustic parameters. In any case, the presence of two simultaneous channels, of noncompeting monosyllables, and of semantic linkage will make SSW alignment analysis more complex than the analysis of monaural P-center allocation.

This study does support the finding of Freeman and Beasley (1976) that competing monosyllables on the EC recording do not uniformly exhibit simultaneous word onsets. However, it does not replicate their word onset measurements. Table 1 presents a tabulation of the data, comparing the Freemn and Beasley oscilloscopic study and the present investigation. The positive (+) signs indicate that the competing word of the leading spondee begins before the competing word in the other ear. The negative (−) signs indicate that the competing word of the leading spondee trails the competing word in the other ear. It is obvious that a major discrepancy between the two studies is a difference in signs, and not always the measurements *per se*. The reversal of this data is demonstrated clearly in Figure 2, an oscilloscopic display of the dichotic onsets of the competing words of item 8. *Shore* is in the upper trace and *out* is in the lower. The traces should be read left to right, with arrows pointing to the approximate onsets of the two words. Freeman and Beasley report that *out* precedes *shore*. However, it is clear from the figure that the reverse is true. On 40% of the items, the absolute values of the measurements of the two studies are within 10 msec, but all of the signs are reversed. On only one item (item 21) is there relative agreement on both measurement and sign.

TABLE 1. ▬▬▬▬▬
Word onset alignments of the competing SSW monosyllables are shown for the Freeman and Beasley (1976) study (column F&B) and for the present investigation (column R&K). Units are milliseconds. A " + " indicates that the competing monosyllable of the leading spondee begins before the competing monosyllable of the second spondee. A " − " indicates that the competing monosyllable of the leading spondee begins after the competing monosyllable of the lagging spondee.

ITEM	R&K	F&B	ITEM	R&K	F&B
1. stairs/down	+142	− 65	2. side/in	+189	−175
3. light/lunch	−123	+150	4. tub/black	− 66	+ 25
5. bread/oat	+ 34	− 40	6. spread/mush	+ 31	− 25
7. gate/flash	− 87	− 25	8. shore/out	+136	−145
9. sauce/base	+136	− 65	10. board/air	+ 10	− 48
11. fly/wood	+102	− 30	12. bean/home	− 73	+ 8
13. day/shoe	− 76	+ 18	14. walls/dog	+ 3	− 12
15. door/play	− 63	+ 60	16. boy/church	+ 10	− 10
17. white/foot	−123	+100	18. saw/first	+ 63	− 90
19. jay/black	+ 24	− 52	20. land/sweet	− 73	+ 35
21. net/tooth	− 55	− 48	22. juice/cup	− 42	+ 40
23. tray/tin	− 34	+ 32	24. light/yard	+ 16	− 12
25. chain/suit	− 50	+ 50	26. ground/bat	+ 97	− 75
27. starch/soap	+ 55	− 50	28. day/first	−168	− 70
29. break/lamp	− 31	+ 50	30. knob/cow	− 54	− 36
31. cage/crow's	+ 24	− 30	32. end/work	+ 87	− 70
33. shelf/drug	+ 50	− 25	34. work/beach	− 47	+ 50
35. ball/milk	+ 81	− 80	36. net/sky	−255	+ 4
37. give/milk	+ 26	− 27	38. skin/bull	+ 89	− 70
39. horse/street	− 31	+ 60	40. house/string	−150	+ 74

FIGURE 2.

Oscillographic display of the onsets of the competing monosyllables of SSW item 8.

Shore **onset is in the upper trace, and** *out* **onset is in the lower. The traces read left to right. Arrows indicate approximate word onsets. One grid unit equals 25 msec. Note that** *shore* **onset precedes** *out* **onset. There is glottal frication preceding sonorancy onset in** *out*. **Sonorancy is shown by the large, quasi-periodic amplitudes on the right.**

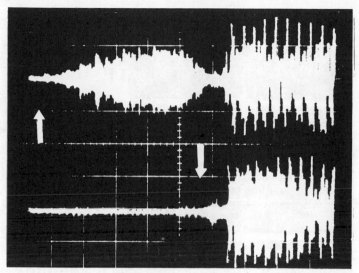

A second area of discrepancy between the two studies shows a limitation on the purely oscilloscopic study. Since an oscilloscope technique is based on identifying word onsets by rises in amplitude on the trace, there is an apparent tendency to focus on sonorancy onsets and to overlook some of the low amplitude presonorancy speech sounds. This is most dramatically exemplified in item 36. Even when this item is played at normal speed, it is easy to hear that *sky* starts before *net*. The near-simultaneous word onsets reported by the oscilloscopic study probably refer to the near-simultaneous sonorancy onsets. Another example is item 7. Assuming an overall reversal of data, the oscilloscope study reports that *gate* precedes flash by 25 msec. Figure 3 shows the onset of *flash* in the upper trace and *gate* in the lower. It can be seen that *gate* word onset precedes sonorancy onset in *flash* by about 25 msec. This may represent the data reported by Freeman and Beasley. However, this would fail to account for the low intensity /fl/ friction which precedes sonorancy. This type of problem is not limited to initial frication only. Figure 4 shows an oscilloscopic tracing of item 30. *Knob* is in the upper trace and *cow* is in the lower. It can be seen that *knob* word onset precedes *cow* sonorancy onset by

FIGURE 3.

Oscillographic display of the onsets of the competing monosyllables of SSW 7.
Flash onset is in the upper trace and *gate* onset is in the lower. The traces read left to right. Arrows indicate approximate word onsets. One grid unit equals 25 msec. Note /fl/ frication preceding sonorancy onset in *flash*. Sonorancy is shown by the large, quasi-periodic amplitude on the right.

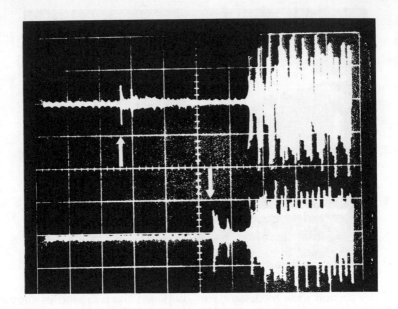

about 35 msec. Again assuming a reversal of data, this may represent the information reported by Freeman and Beasley. If so, it would omit the considerable duration of /k/ release and aspiration.

Excluding sign differences, measurement differences on at least 55% of the SSW items can be accounted for by omission of some or all of the presonorancy speech sounds by the oscilloscopic technique. This apparent risk with a purely oscilloscopic method has important implications for its use in preparing and evaluating dichotic speech tapes. It is particularly relevant to experimenters attempting very precise alignments of speech signal onsets and offsets.

Primarily, however, this study recommends that visual oscilloscopic measurements of speech be cross-checked with auditory listening measurements for greater validity. The oscilloscopic technique transforms the transient, auditory, linguistic event of speech into the static, visual, nonlinguistic abstraction of a time–amplitude trace. This apparently results in tendencies to overlook low amplitude

FIGURE 4.

Oscillographic display of the onsets of the competing monosyllables of SSW item 30.
Knob onset is in the upper trace and *cow* onset is in the lower. The traces read left to right. Arrows indicate approximate word onsets. One grid unit equals 25 msec. Note /k/ release and aspiration preceding sonorancy onset in *cow*. Sonorancy is shown by the large, quasi-periodic amplitude on the right.

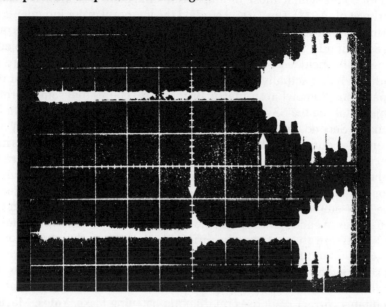

presonorancy speech sounds and to become disoriented as to the identities of the items, resulting in the reversal of the data. The listening technique, on the other hand, requires only a time transformation (i.e., a slowing) of the real speech event. But the event is still transient and difficult to measure precisely. In short, the oscilloscopic method may risk validity as the price for precision and the listening method risks precision as the price for validity. But an acoustic signal is speech only by human perception. As a problem for science in general, the preference for abstract precision over perceptual concreteness has been discussed by Whitehead (1967).

Based on the present experience, it is not possible to recommend either technique alone as superior. Measures from both procedures are highly correlated ($r = -.99$) when the words begin with sonorancy. With presonorancy speech sounds, however, the two techniques result in different findings. For example, in item 7 this study reports that *flash* begins 87 msec before *gate*. The oscilloscopic display in Figure 3 shows a 70 msec lead. Possible sources of error with the auditory-manual method occur during the perceptual judgments of speech onsets, during the manual markings on the tape, and during the measurements of the tape.

As Freeman and Beasley hypothesized, normal listeners are probably not disrupted by simultaneous word onsets on the SSW Test for a number of reasons. First, the SSW Test uses real words and not CV syllables, on which most of the onset alingment research is based (Berlin *et al.*, 1973). Day (1970) studied the temporal order judgments of normal subjects on a dichotic speech task using phonologically normal speech stimuli. She found that in certain conditions some subjects (those she concluded were "language bound") would report a word as leading when it actually lagged by as long as 100 msec, the limits of the experiment. Somewhat similarly, Brunt (1972) claims that some normal subjects taking the SSW Test fail to realize that the items are partially dichotic. Second, because the competing monosyllables of the SSW are of unequal durations, there is always some nonsimultaneous information presented to at least one of the ears. Third, the SSW incorporates higher language perceptual parameters that may override purely acoustic parameters, such as word onsets, at least for normal subjects. The SSW employs a monaural-dichotic semantic linkage between the two halves of each spondee. Considering item 1, the words *up, upstairs,* and *stairs* are three distinctly different semantic units as are *down, downtown,* and *town.* There is possibly a critical language perception tension perceiving monosyllables versus spondees. Experiments by Kadesh, Riese, and Anisfeld (1976) show that semantic association facilitates correct responses on dichotic listening tasks. Yates, Martin, and DiLollo (1970) report that facilitation due to semantic categorization tends to override rate, ear, and order factors. Clinical observations by the authors suggest that an SSW item is perceived as an easy two-word task by normals, but as a difficult four-word task by subjects with CANS involvement. Semantic linkage on the SSW Test probably facilitates correct responses for normals.

Acknowledgement

The authors wish to express their appreciation to Henry Ilecki of McGill University for his suggestions and comments, and to Victor Moser of McGill University and Steven Perlow of the University of Buffalo for their technical assistance.

References

Balas, R. F. Staggered spondaic word test: support. *Ann. Otol. Rhinol. Laryngol.* 80, 132–134 (1971).

Balas, R. F. and Simon, G. R. The articulation function of a staggered spondaic word list for a normal hearing population. *J. Aud. Res.*, 4, 285–289 (1964).

Berlin, C. I. New developments in evaluating central auditory mechanisms. *Ann. Otol. Rhinol. Laryngol.*, 85, 833–841 (1976).

Berlin, C., Lowe-Bell, S., Cullen, J., and Thompson, C. Dichotic speech perception: an interpretation of right ear advantage and temporal offset effects. *J. Acoust. Soc. Am.*, 53, 699–709 (1973).

Brunt, M. A. The staggered spondaic word test. In J. Katz (ed.), *The Handbook of Clinical Audiology.* Baltimore: William & Wilkins (1972).

Brunt, M. A. The staggered spondaic word test. In J. Katz (ed.(, *The Handbook of Clinical Audiology,* 2nd edition. Baltimore: William & Wilkins (1970).

Cherry, E. C. Some experiments on the recognition of speech with one and with two ears. *J. Acoust. Soc. Am.*, 25, 975–979 (1953).

Day, R. S. Temporal order judgments: are individuals language bound or stimulus bound? *Haskins Lab. Status Report on Speech Res.,* SR-2/22, 71–87 (1970).

Dempsey, C. Some thoughts concerning alternate explanations of central auditory test results. In R. Keith (ed.), *Central Auditory Dysfunction.* New York: Grune & Stratton (1977).

Feldmann, H. Untersuchungen zur diskrimination differenter schallbilder bei simultaner, monauraler under binauraler darbietung. *Arch. Ohr. usw. Heilk. u. Z. Hals-usw. Heilk.*, 176, 600–605 (1960).

Freeman, B. A. and Beasley, D. S. Lead and lag effects associated with the staggered spondaic word test. *J. Speech Hear. Res.*, 19, 572–577 (1976)

Jerger, J. and Jerger, S. Audiological findings in brainstem disorders.*Arch. Otololaryngol.*, 99, 342–350 (1974).

Jerger, J. and Jerger, S. Clinical validity of central auditory tests. *Scand. Audiol.* 4, 147–163 (1975).

Kadesh, I., Reise, M., and Anisfield, M. Dichotic listening in study of semantic relationships. *J. Verbal Learn. Verbal Behav.*, 15, 213–225 (1976).

Katz, J. The use of staggered spondaic words for assessing the integrity of the central auditory nervous system. *J. Aud. Res.*, 2, 327–337 (1962).

Katz, J. The SSW Test: an interim report. *J. Speech Hear. Dis.*, 33, 132–146 (1968).

Katz, J. Audiologic diagnosis: cochlea to cortex. *Menorah Med. J.*, 1, 25–36 (1970).

Katz, J. The staggered spondaic word test. In R. Keith (ed.) *Central Auditory Dysfunction.* New York: Grune & Stratton (1977).

Katz, J., Basil, R. A., and Smith, J. M. A staggered spondaic word test for detecting central auditory lesions. *Ann. Otol. Rhinol. Laryngol.*, 72, 908–918 (1963).

Katz, J., and Illmer, R. Auditory perception in children with learning disabilities. In J. Katz (ed.), *The Handbook of Clinical Audiology.* Baltimore: Williams & Wilkins (1972).

Katz, J., and Pack, G. New developments in differential diagnosis using the SSW test. In M. Sullivan (ed.), *Central Auditory Processing Disorders.* Omaha: University of Nebraska Press (1975).

Katz, J., Harder, B., and Lohnes, P. R. Lead/lag analysis of the SSW test items. Presented at ASHA Convention, Chicago, IL (1977).

Kimura, D. Some effects of temporal lobe damage on auditory perception. *Can. J. Psychol.*, 15, 156–165 (1961).

Martin, R., and Forbis, N. The present status of audiometric practice: a follow-up study. *ASHA*, 20, 531–541 (1978).

Miltenberger, G., Dawson, G., and Raica, A. Central auditory testing with perhipheral hearing loss. *Arch. Otolaryngol.*, 104, 11–15 (1978).

Morton, J., Marcus, S., and Frankish, C. Theoretical note: Perceptual centers (P-centers). *Psychol.Rev.*, 83, 405–408 (1976).

Rubino, C. A. A simple procedure for constructing dichotic listening tapes. *Cortex*, 8, 335–338 (1972).

Stubblefield, J. and Young, C. Central auditory dysfunction in learning disabled children. *J. Learn. Disabil.*, 8, 89–94 (1975).

White, E. Children's performance on the SSW test and the Willeford battery. In R. Keith (ed.), *Central Auditory Dysfunction*. New York: Grune & Stratton (1977).

Whitehead, A., *Science and the Modern World*. New York: Free Press (1967).

Willeford, J. A. Central auditory function in children with learning disabilities. *J. Audiol. Hear. Educ.*, 2, 12–20 (1976).

Winkelaar, R. and Lewis, T. Audiologic tests for evaluation of central auditory disorders. *J. Otolaryngol.*, 6, 127–134 (1977).

Yates, A., Martin, M., and Di Lollo, V. Retrieval strategy in dichotic listening as a function of presentation rate and structure of material. *J. Exp. Psychol.*, 86, 26–31 (1970).

THE SSW TEST: DICHOTIC, DIOTIC, AND MONAURAL

Sheila Goldman and Jack Katz

Recently, there has been more and more interest in our field in the assessment of central auditory disorders. Katz *et al.* recently investigated the Staggered Spondaic Word (SSW) Test, a measure of central integrity. This test has been administered to over 500 pathologic and normal subjects. Central auditory dysfunction is revealed by deteriorated performance in the ear contralateral to the affected hemisphere. The SSW Test (outlined below) is a competing message task that is presented to both ears.

BINAURAL (DICHOTIC)

	Time Sequence				
	1		2		3
Right Ear	up	–	stairs		
Left Ear			down	–	town

DIOTIC

	Time Sequence				
	1		2		3
Right ear	up	–	stairs		
			down	–	town
Left ear	up	–	stairs		
			down	–	town

ASHA Convention, Chicago, Illinois 1965

MONAURAL

	Time Sequence			
	1		2	3
Either ear	up	–	stairs	
			down	– town

We felt that the contribution of an instrument that could unilaterally and bilaterally measure central hearing loss would be considerable. Therefore, 24 right-handed normal hearing subjects with no history of neurologic impairment were given the SSW Test under four conditions in a counterbalanced order. The order in which each subject reported the monosyllables was not considered in scoring the test.

Test Conditions

Binaural Condition. This is the standard presentation of the test. The output was switched in this condition so that the ear receiving the first word was alternated. As can be seen, we have a dichotic stimulus with one monosyllable arriving simultaneously at the right with another monosyllable at the left ear. Two noncompeting monosyllables also were presented to each ear. The two monosyllables presented to each ear form a spondaic word. In addition, the two noncompeting monosyllables arriving in separate ears form another spondaic word.

Diotic Condition. All four monosyllables are presented to both ears in the staggered fashion described above. Instead of concentrating on a simple stimulus (spondee) in one ear first and then in the other, the subject concentrates on a complex stimulus (two spondees with two simultaneous monosyllables on each side). The diotic aspect of hearing has not been studied sufficiently to see how the central auditory system handles this type of information. We were interested in seeing whether the system operates on an additive basis or whether one side provided supplementary information for the other side, thus resulting in better scores than those achieved in the separate monaural conditions.

Monaural Right-Ear Condition. All four monosyllables are presented to the right ear in staggered fashion.

Monaural Left-Ear Condition. All four overlapped monosyllables are presented to the left ear. Studies have not demonstrated dominant ear superiority with monaural stimuli. We were interested in seeing whether the dominance effect would show up.

172   Acoustic and Psychoacoustic Factors

Results

The results of this study indicated that the standard binaural condition yielded the greatest number of correct responses. The diotic and monaural right-ear conditions proved more difficult, while the poorest performance was on the monaural left-ear condition. In Figure 1 we have plotted the number of errors along the ordinate; along the abscissa we have the four conditions. The standard deviation is indicated by the dashes. Statistical analysis revealed that the binaural condition was signficantly better than each of the other three conditions. The diotic and monaural right-ear conditions were not significantly different; however, both had better mean scores than the left-ear condition. Therefore, we can consider the four means to be divisible into three groups. The highest ranking (or lowest error condition) is the binaural condition, the poorest ranking (or highest error condition) is the left-ear condition, and the middle group comprises both the diotic and monaural right-ear conditions. This portion of the study clearly indicates that binaural competition is far simpler for the central nervous system to handle than if the identical stimuli were presented in one or both ears.

FIGURE 1. ▬▬▬▬▬▬▬▬▬▬▬▬▬▬▬▬▬▬▬▬▬▬▬▬▬▬▬▬▬▬▬
Mean number of errors and standard deviations for right-handed subjects on four SSW tasks.

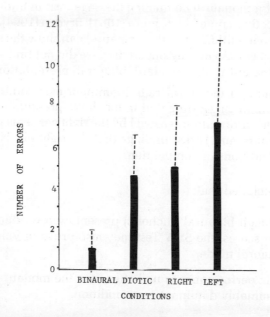

Discussion

The mean number of errors for the binaural condition was .88, resulting in a 2.19 percentage of errors. The percentage of error replicated the normative data obtained by Katz, Balas, and Fishman (unpublished) for the SSW Test with other young, normal adult subjects.

The findings of the SSW Test in the monaural conditions demonstrates the possibility of using it as a unilateral tool. The rather small standard deviations in the two monaural conditions suggest that we might set up a baseline for performance of normal listeners and expect relatively little deviation. Verification of the SSW Test as a unilateral measure would require the evaluation of test performances by peripheral sensory-neural patients and CNS disorder patients, in addition to normal control subjects.

It is particularly interesting to note the superiority of the right ear over the left ear in the present study. All of the subjects employed for this study were right-handed and were assumed to be left-hemisphere dominant for language. Goodglass and Quadfasel (1942), Kimura (1961; 1963), Palmer (1963; 1964), and Penfield and Roberts (1959) have found that right-handers are almost invariably left-dominant for language, but that either the right or left hemisphere may mediate language functions in the left-handed. Our finding of right-ear superiority demonstrates that right and left ears can be differentiated on the basis of a monaural competing message task in addition to the binaural competition noted by Kimura (1961), Bryden (1964), and Dirks (1964). Thus, competition other than binaural can show the superiority of the dominant ear. As in previous studies, we did not find any laterality effects on the test in the standard (binaural) presentation.

The diotic and monaural right (dominant ear) conditions were remarkably similar, suggesting that in the diotic presentation the subject relies on the information received by the right ear. This would tend to support Kimura and Dirks' findings that the right ear is more efficient under conditions of competition.

It is concluded that:

1. Although binaural (dichotic) presentation produced optimal scores, the SSW Test may also prove of value in a monaural mode.

2. Diotic performance is no better than the monaural right (presumably dominant ear) condition.

Acoustic and Psychoacoustic Factors

3. Right-ear proficiency is greater than left. This demonstrates that ear dominance is discernible not only under certain conditions of binaural competition (as shown by other investigators), but also under some conditions of monaural competition.

References

Bryden, N. P. Order of Report in Dichotic Listening. *Canadian Journal of Psychology,* 16, 291–199, 1962.

Dirks, D. Perception of Dichotic and Monaural Verbal Material and Cerebral Dominance for Speech. *Acta Otolaryngolica,* 58, 73–80, 1964.

Goodglass, H. and Quadfasel, F. A. Language Laterality in Left-Handed Aphasics. *Brain,* 65, 205–219, 1942.

Kimura, D. Cerebral Dominance and the Perception of Verbal Stimuli. *Canadian Journal of Psychology,* 15, 166–171, 1961 b.

Kimura, D. Speech Lateralization in Young Children as Determined by an Audiological Test. *Journal of Comparative and Psychological Psychology,* 56, 899–902, 1963.

Palmer, R. D. Hand Differentiation and Psychological Function. *Journal of Personality,* 31, 445–461, 1963.

Palmer, R. D. Cerebral Dominance and Auditory Asymmetry. *Journal of Psychology,* 58, 157–167, 1964.

Penfield, W. and Roberts, L. *Speech and Brain Mechanism,* Princeton, N.J. Princeton University Press, 89–102, 1959.

Author's Note:

After the Goldman and Katz study was completed we wondered if the similarity between left-monaural and diotic would be found in a group of young *left-*handed subjects. Goldman tested 12 left-handed individuals (see follow-up study below) using the same procedures as in the previous study. The results were quite interesting.

Similar performance for right- and left-handers on two of the four conditions was noted. The binaural and the left-monaural conditions were essentially the same for the two groups (see Figure 1). However, performance on the diotic and especially the right-monaural conditions seemed to favor the right-handers. If these differences are signficant, it might suggest that under these conditions, left-handers are at a disadvantage because their right ears are poorer than the right-handers and their left ears are no better than the left ears of right-handed listeners. If diotic listening is dependent on the better ear, it is not surprising that the left-handers seem to perform poorly. It is interesting that the discrepancy in right-ear performance is not reflected in the binaural condition. Is it possible that the left ear plays a major role in binaural (dichotic) listening?

SSW Performance in Left-Handers: Dichotic, Diotic, and Monaural

Jack Katz and Sheila O. Goldman

Since our previous findings suggested that languange dominance influenced the performance in the monaural conditions (right ear being better than left), it was reasonable to wonder how left-handed listeners would perform on these same conditions. Twelve young, normal left-handed individuals were evaluated in the same manner as in the first experiment. The results and the comparisons with the right-handers turned out to be quite interesting.

On two of the four conditions the right- and left-handers performed in a very similar way. Figure 1 shows that both groups had equivalent scores for the binaural and monaural left conditions. Thus, for the standard administration of the SSW Test the right- and left-handers had the same level of accuracy. They had identical left performance as well. However, in this study the monaural right and left conditions were not significantly different.

The right- and left-handers differed significantly (at the .05 level) on the diotic and monaural right conditions. In both cases the right-handers demonstrated better scores. This might imply that under monaural competing conditions, right-handed individuals tend to have

Acoustic and Psychoacoustic Factors

FIGURE 1.
Mean number of errors for right- (black bar) and left- (white bar) handed subjects on the four SSW tasks.

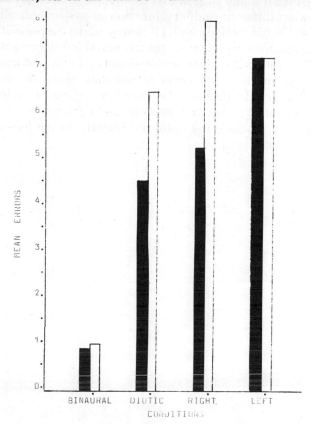

an advantage. They are no worse off than the left-handers in the left ear, but they are better than the left-handers in the right.

One would think that the advantage of the right-handers over the left-handers would show up in the diotic condition as well. This would be logical, since the first experiment showed that diotic was about the same as the better ear (the right ear for the right-handers). However, the same type of relationship was noted for the left-handers. The diotic versus monaural right for the right-handers and the diotic versus monaural left for the left-handers was about the same and less than one error apart.

One could also assume that the right-handers would have an advantage in the binaural condition because they were better in the right and no poorer in the left. However, this does not appear to be the case, as the performance for both groups is extremely close. If significant differences cannot be found under more adverse binaural conditions (e.g., at 15 dB SL), then it would suggest that the monaural procedure is tapping a somewhat different auditory function or system. An alternate hypothesis is that binaural (dichotic) listening, under the present conditions, is more highly dependent on the monaural left than right.

The SSW Test, when given under dichotic, diotic, and monaural conditions, appears to offer useful information about the auditory system. It could help to answer some questions regarding the learning disabled, those with conductive losses and unilateral problems. A first step would be to replicate the data, particularly on the left-handers because of the small sample.

A Split-Half Evaluation of the SSW Test

Jack Katz and William B. Arndt

Unfortunately, many audiologic tests require considerable clinical time, which reduces their practical value. Word discrimination procedures (Elpern, 1961) and the SISI test (Griffing, 1963) have been studied with a view toward saving time and maximizing their diagnostic value. The present study was undertaken to determine if the first half of the Staggered Spondaic Word (SSW) Test provides a reasonable estimate of the full 40 item test.

The SSW test is a measure of central auditory function (Katz, 1962). Its primary focus is to identify lesions in various parts of the cerebrum and brainstem. The test requires about 15 minutes to administer. However, with aphasic patients or others who are difficult to test, the testing time might be protracted. In other cases patients might be feeling ill or extremely agitated because of their inability to handle the task. Under such circumstances it has been necessary to administer only half of the items.

In this project we studied 4 parameters using 120 pathological cases. The parameters were the number of errors, reversals, ear effects and order effects on the first half of the test versus the second. The data were analyzed separately and combined into the following subgroups: conductive ($n = 18$), unilateral cochlear ($n = 20$), bilateral cochlear ($n = 22$), and retrocochlear hearing loss groups ($n = 17$), as well as central auditory reception [damage to Heschl's gyrus] ($n = 20$) and central nonauditory reception [cerebral damage sparing Heschl's gyrus] ($n = 23$).

ASHA Convention, Las Vegas, Nevada, 1974.

FIGURE 1.
SSW Split-Half Analysis

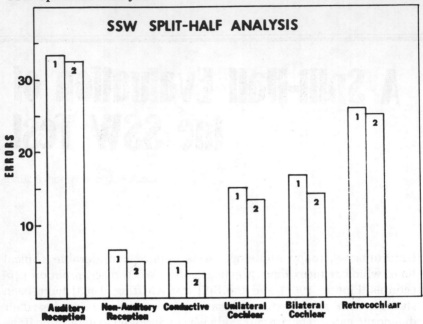

As a group, the subjects had 1.5 fewer errors on the second half than the first half ($M_1 = 16.9$; $M_2 = 15.4$). In addition the correlation between them was $r = .96$, which was significant at less than the .01 level of confidence. (See Figure 1 for the performance of the individual groups on the two halves of the test. The errors on the first half are designated by "1" and on the second half by "2."

Despite the close relationship between the two halves of the SSW test when looking at the number of errors, this was not true for the other parameters. The three types of response bias that we studied were reversals, ear effects, and order effects. These are used to refine the SSW diagnosis, especially in the central nonauditory reception areas. Response bias refers to a consistent peculiarity in the patient's verbal answer.

As expected, a relatively small number of subjects had reversals in some of the subgroups. A reversal refers to an item in which the words are repeated out of order and in which there is no error or just one error. Only central nonauditory, conductive, and unilateral cochlear subgroups had 10 or more reversal cases. For the subjects in these subgroups that reversed, the mean on the first half was 3.0 and on the second half 4.0. The $r = .76$ was significant, but was due mainly to the central nonauditory subgroup ($r = .74$). The peripheral hearing loss

FIGURE 2.

Number of Reversals Scored by Subjects.

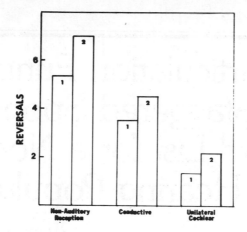

subgroups did not have significant correlations. (See Figure 2 for the number of reversals on the first and second halves of the SSW Test for each of the three groups.)

All groups were studied for ear and order effects. The number of significant effects were counted on the first half versus the total test and submitted to x^2 analysis. None of the subgroups nor the total group had statistically significant correspondence.

In order to make use of the valuable response bias, the SSW test should be given in its entirety; however, if it is necessary to give only half of the items, the total C-SSW score can be relied upon with confidence to tell if there is a reception dysfunction or not. If there is no hearing loss and there is a probable central lesions, it would be possible to double the number of reversals to get a gross estimate of the total test results.

The Articulation Function of a Staggered Spondaic Word List for a Normal Hearing Population

Robert F. Balas * and George R. Simon

During the past ten years, a number of investigators have reported techniques to demonstrate the hearing performance of subjects with central auditory impairment (Bocca et al., 1955; Bocca, 1961; Walsh and Goodman, 1955; Matzker, 1959; Katz, 1962). The rationale for these procedures is reviewed by Bocca and Calearo (1963).

Katz (1962) proposed a competing message technique using bilateral, partially overlapped spondaic words. Balas (1962), Katz, Basil and Smith (1963) report results of a staggered spondaic word list on a limited number of normal and various impaired hearing populations. These pilot studies tend to indicate the potential use of the proposed procedure as a clinical tool. However, before a staggered spondaic word list can be of clinical value, rigid standardization is imperative. The performance of a substantial number of normal hearing and various impaired hearing subjects must be objectively determined before clinical interpretation of such a methodology can be considered valid.

The purpose of this study was to establish an articulation curve for a staggered spondaic word list with a normal hearing, young adult population.

* This study is part of a preliminary investigation for a dissertation at the University of Denver.

J. Auditory Res. 4, 285–289, 1965.

Acoustic and Psychoacoustic Factors

Subjects

The subjects consisted of 27 male and 45 female college students with no history of hearing loss or central nervous system impairment. The age range of the subjects was from 17 to 30, with a mean age of 21 years. The mean pure tone average threshold for the subjects was -6 dB HL. None of the subjects had prior experience in listening to the test material.

Apparatus and Procedure

A list of 40 pairs of spondaic words was prepared. For each pair of spondaic words, the initial syllable of the first spondaic word if combined with the second syllable of the second spondaic word formed a third familiar spondaic word in American English.

This list of 40 paired spondaic words was recorded using an Ampex PR-10-2 Magnetic Tape Recorder/Reproducer with an MX-10/MX-35 Mixer Assembly in an I.A.C. Series 400 sound suite. The recording of each item (spondaic word pair) was made so that the first word was recorded in one channel with the second syllable of the first word and the first syllable of the second word recorded simultaneously as in the procedure reported by Katz (1962). The following illustrates the recording procedure:

Channel	Ear		Time	
I	Right (or left)	day	light	
II	Left (or right)		lunch	time

In order for the syllables in the competing condition (simultaneous recording) to be at the same level, the initial recorded list was re-recorded using a 1 dB step attenuator (Hewlett-Packard, Model 350 BR) between the outputs of a tape reproducer and the inputs of a tape recorder to correct for level errors in the original recording.

A pure tone air conduction threshold was measured for each subject using conventional pure tone audiometry. The subjects were randomly assigned to six groups. The staggered spondaic word list was presented to each group through a two channel speech audiometer (Grason-Stadler, E-664) at a determined sensation level. The sensation levels were 0, 10, 20, 30, 40, and 50 dB. The sensation level of presentation for each subject within each group was relative to the average pure tone threshold of each ear for the frequencies 500, 1000, and 2000 Hz. For each word pair then, the first syllable of the first word and the second syllable of the second word was alone and in opposite ears while the second syllable of the first word and first syllable of the second word were heard simultaneously but in opposite ears.

Each subject was required to repeat all the words heard, and his responses were recorded by the examiner. Testing time was approximately 10 minutes.

Results and Discussion

Table 1 summarizes the performance of the six groups. The mean incorrect responses of monosyllables indicate that the subjects had progressively more difficulty in the competing syllable conditions at the lower sensation levels. Errors in both competing and non-competing conditions diminished when the list was presented at the higher sensation levels.

In determining the articulation curve a test item (spondaic word pair) was counted wrong if the subjects' responses were only partially correct. The slightest alteration of a phoneme, e.g., [bæd] for [bæt], within any one of the four monosyllables made the response incorrect. As in articulation curves for other word lists, score performance (percentage of correct responses) increased as a function of sensation level. A maximum score was obtained at 50 dB SL. Figure 1 shows the articulation curve and standard deviations for each sensation level. Inspection of the curve shows an initial rapid increase of the slope with 50% correct obtained at approximately 13 dB SL. The average slope between 20% and 80% is about 3%/dB. This representation of heterogeneity of the words, similar to that of PB words, indicates that this type of word list may provide the difficult sitmuli for evaluating higher auditory performance.

On the basis of the above data it seems plausible to administer a staggered spondaic word list at different sensation levels. That is, errors at 30 and 40 dB SL in both competing and non-competing conditions are minimal. This factor renders the technique clinically flexible, particularly when certain hearing problems would not permit presentation of the list at 50 dB SL. Sharply sloping audiograms may require the reference level for the list presentation to be relative to the SRT which was used in the pilot studies cited.

Summary

An articulation curve was established for a list of 40 pairs of staggered spondaic words. The subjects consisted of 72 normal hearing young adults. The level of maximum performance was 50 dB SL. The results

Acoustic and Psychoacoustic Factors

TABLE 1
Summary of Performance to Monosyllables and Complete (Spondaic Word Pair) Stimulus Conditions

| | Mean Incorrect of Monosyllables | | Complete Stimulus | |
Group (SL)	Noncompeting	Competing	Mean Incorrect	Mean Correct (%)
0	–	–	39.83	0.42
10	15.75	23.08	23.00	42.50
20	4.33	10.91	9.08	77.30
30	1.50	3.16	4.25	89.38
40	0.33	1.83	1.83	95.42
50	0.00	0.42	0.42	98.96

FIGURE 1.
Articulation function of a staggered spondaic word list for a normal hearing population. The standard deviation for each sensation level is represented by the vertical lines.

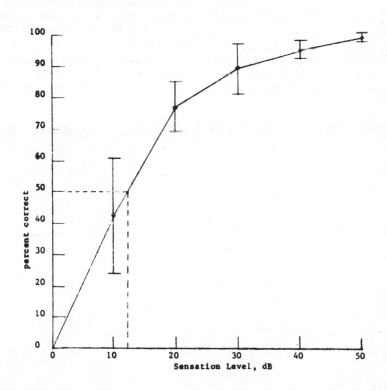

indicate that the paired spondaic words may be presented at lower sensation levels when particular hearing problems indicate so. The articulation curve represents a relative lack of homogeneity of the words, indicating that this list may provide the difficult stimuli necessary in evaluating the performance of higher auditory function.

References

1. Balas, R. F. Results of the staggered spondaic word test with an old age population. Unpublished M.A. thesis, Northern Illinois University, 1962.

2. Bocca, E., Calearo, C., Cassinari, V., and Migliavacca, F. Testing "cortical" hearing in temporal lobe tumours. *Acta Oto-laryngol.*, 1955, 45, 289–304.

3. Bocca, E. Factors influencing binaural integration of periodically switched messages. *Acta Oto-laryngol.*, 1961, 53, 142–144.

4. Bocca, E., and Calearo, C. Central hearing processes. Chap. 9, *Modern Developments in Audiology*. Jerger, J. (Ed.) New York: Academic Press, Inc., 1963.

5. Katz, J. The use of staggered spondaic words for assessing the integrity of the central auditory nervous system. *J. Aud. Res.*, 1962, 2, 327–337.

6. Katz, J., Basil, R., and Smith, J. A staggered spondaic word test for determining central auditory lesions. *Ann. Otol., Rhinol., Laryngol.*, 1963, 72, 908–917.

7. Matzker, J. Two new methods for the assessment of central auditory functions in cases of brain disease. *Ann. Otol., Rhinol., Laryngol.*, 1959, 68, 1185–1197.

8. Walsh, T., and Goodman, A. Speech discrimination in central auditory lesions. *Laryngoscope*, 1955, 65, 1–8.

Performance–Intensity Functions for a Normal Hearing Population on the Staggered Spondaic Word (SSW) Test

Philip C. Doyle

Introduction

The use of the Staggered Spondaic Word (SSW) Test for assessing the integrity of the central auditory nervous system (CANS) was first developed and presented by Jack Katz in 1962. The SSW Test is a dichotic speech task which requires the listener to identify two spondaic words which are presented in a partially overlapped manner. As can be seen in Figure 1, an overlap occurs between the second syllable of the first spondee, "stairs," and the first syllable "down," of the second spondee. As a result of this partial overlap, noncompeting and competing listening conditions for both ears are accomplished (RNC = right noncompeting; RC = right competing; LC = left competing; and LNC = left noncompeting).

The entire test is comprised of 40 test items or, spondaic word pairs. For example, the spondaic words "upstairs" and "downtown"

Presented at the 29th Annual Conference of the California Speech-Language-Hearing Association, April 10–12, 1981, San Francisco, California

FIGURE 1.

Example of SSW test items showing presentation (temporal) sequence of stimulus words and the reversal of the leading ear.

	Time Sequence of SSW Test Item		
T1	1	2	3
Item 1 (REF)	RNC up	RC stairs	
		down LC	town LNC
Item 2 (LEF)	LNC out	LC side	
		in RC	law RNC

comprise an entire test item (see Figure 1). Further, each individual test item consists of four elements. That is, four monosyllables, "up," "stairs," "down," and "town," each representing either a non-competing or competing presentation condition for the right or left ear. The 40 test items are preceeded by four practice items not used in the final scoring of the test.

Standard procedures require that the test is presented at 50 dB-sensation level (SL), referencing the pure-tone average (PTA) of 500, 1000, and 2000 Hz for the respective ear. A number of studies have indicated that normal subjects exhibit little difficulty and make few errors on the test when presented using standard procedures (Arnst, in press; Goldman and Katz, 1966; Katz and Myrick, 1963; and Katz, Basil, and Smith, 1963).

In developing the test, Katz chose spondaic words for three reasons: First, spondaic words are relatively familiar to a majority of subjects; second, spondaic words have been demonstrated to be intelligible to subjects over a wide range of intensities; and third, by using spondees, Katz proposed that errors which result from peripheral distortion could be corrected and accounted for, resulting in a more sensitive measure of central auditory function. The rationale of Katz suggests that due to the high level of redundancy found in spondaic words, they are more likely to be intelligible in difficult or degraded listening situations. Based on the high amount of redundancy found within spondaic words and the resulting high degree of their intelligibility, questions regarding the identification of spondaic words presented in a dichotic manner at intensity levels less than 50 dB-sensation level are raised.

In 1965, Balas and Simon sought to identify the intensity level at which normal hearing subjects revealed maximum performance when presented a staggered spondaic word list. In their study, 72 subjects ranging in age from 17 to 30 years (mean = 21–0) were randomly assigned to one of six sensation level presentation groups. The staggered spondaic word list used in their study *was not* the standard SSW Test List EC currently in clinical use, but rather, a precursor to it. Prior to presenting their test list, Balas and Simon evaluated each subject using pure-tone (ASA, 1951), speech reception threshold, and word discrimination tests to ensure hearing within normal limits. Following these procedures, 6 groups of 12 subjects each were presented Balas and Simon's entire 40-item staggered spondaic word list at one of six sensation levels, either 0, 10, 20, 30, 40, or 50 dB-SL. Each subject was presented the entire list at only one sensation level.

In scoring subject responses, Balas and Simon used the following method. A substitution, omission, or distortion on any part of a given test item resulted in the entire item being counted as an error. Using Balas and Simon's scoring method for the example shown in Figure 1, an error of omitting the word "stairs" in item 1 or the inability of the subject to identify any of the four monosyllables in item 2 would be scored as an equal error. As a result, each test item was scored in an "all-or-none" manner. Using this method of scoring, Balas and Simon reported the group mean percent errors and standard deviations for each of the six presentation groups shown in Table 1. Based on these findings, it can be seen that their list was virtually unintelligible for the 0 dB-SL presentation group. Intelligibility increased at 10 and 20 dB-SL, with good performance being reported at 30 dB-SL and above. Maximum intelligibility was found with the 50 dB-SL presentation group. From these findings, the articulation function shown in Figure 2 was plotted. Despite maximum intelligibility at 50 dB-SL, viewing the function it can be seen that an increase in intelligibility is exhibited from the mean performance at 40 dB-SL. When inspecting the values presented in Table 1, an increase of around 4% is found at 50 dB-SL from the 40 dB-SL presentation.

TABLE 1

Mean Error Percentages and Standard Deviations Using 40–Item Scoring (N = 12 per SL) (Balas and Simon, 1965, Balas, 1964)

	dB-Sensation Level					
	0	10	20	30	40	50
Mean	99.6	57.5	22.7	10.7	4.6	1.1
SD	.85	18.3	8.2	8.0	3.1	1.2

Although the test list developed and used by Balas and Simon appears to be similar to the standard SSW Test List EC, no comparative function for the clinical list presently used has been obtained. Results from my pilot studies with List EC indicated that the intelligibility of the Balas and Simon list might not be representative of normal performance on the current clinical list. Based on these preliminary results, it is the purpose of this study to evaluate SSW Test performance by normal listeners and thus establish an articulation or performance–intensity function on the standard SSW Test list now in use. Further, a second

FIGURE 2.
Performance–intensity function established by Balas and Simon (1965). Mean group values and standard deviations are depicted.

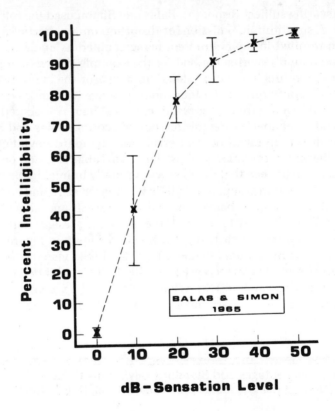

Acoustic and Psychoacoustic Factors

objective of the study is to obtain a performance–intensity function using a more sensitive scoring procedure which may better reflect performance of the normal listener.

Procedures

Sixty subjects (45 females and 15 males) between the ages of 18 and 30 years (mean age 24.2) served as subjects for this study. All subjects who participated received pure-tone air and bone conduction (ANSI, 1969) speech reception threshold (SRT), and word discrimination (WDS) testing using standard clinical methods prior to administration of the SSW Test. Due to the difference in audiometric standards used by Balas and Simon (ASA, 1951) and in the present study (ANSI, 1969), appropriate correction factors to ensure subject similarity were employed. All subjects exhibited pure-tone air conduction thresholds of 20 dB-HTL for octave frequencies 250–8000 Hz. Bone conduction thresholds for 250–4000 Hz did not exceed plus or minus 5 dB-HTL of the respective air conduction threshold. Speech reception thresholds for each ear of no more than plus or minus 5 dB-HTO of the ears PTA were exhibited. Word discrimination scores of 96% or better bilaterally were exhibited by all subjects using 50 item, W-22 word lists. Standard tape recordings for all speech audiometry tests (SRT, WDS, SSW) were used for each subject.

All subjects reported (1) no known history of hearing loss, ear disease, or neurological impairment;(2) no persistent history of headaches or dizziness; (3) English as the native spoken language; (4) no current use of stimulating or tranquilizing medications; and (5) no previous experience with or exposure to the SSW Test.

Following initial audiometric testing, subjects were randomly assigned to one of six SSW Test presentation conditions—0, 10, 20, 30, 40, and 50 dB-SL—as in the Balas and Simon study. Regardless of which presentation condition a subject was assigned to, standard SSW Test instructions and the four practice items included on the standard recording were presented at 50 dB-SL.

The resulting data were scored using two methods. The first procedure was the same as that previously described in the Balas and Simon study. That is, if any one of the four elements comprising a test item was substituted, omitted, or distorted, the entire test item was counted as an error, each of the 40 test items being scored in an "all-or-none" manner.

In contrast, the second procedure was scored by individual elements, for example, "up," "stairs," "down," and "town". Thus, the second scoring method did not penalize the listener for missing an entire test item if they missed only one, two, or three of the four elements comprising a test item (see Figure 1). The test item was completely in error *only* if all four elements were in error. Therefore, 160 items (40 test items × 4 elements) were now scored as opposed to only 40 scorable items used by Balas and Simon.

Results

Using the 40-item scoring procedure, the below mean percent error and standard deviations for each sensation level group performance were obtained (see Table 2). A mean percent error of approximately 56% was exhibited by the 0 dB-SL group, with a rapid decrease in error percentage to around 15% by the 10 dB-SL group. It is also apparent that at sensation levels of 20 dB and above, group performance was quite similar.

From these findings using List EC, the performance–intensity function seen in Figure 3 was generated. A one-way Analysis of Variance (ANOVA) revealed a statistically significant main effect ($F = 64.04$; $df = 5, 54$; $p = .01$). Use of Scheffe's post-hoc test revealed that a statistically significant difference in group performance was found only for the 0 dB-SL presentation group ($F = 3.34$; $df = 5, 54$; c. diff. = 11.69). Further, we see that the performance by groups at 20 dB-SL and above is very high with standard deviations that are quite narrow. Using the Balas and Simon criterion for scoring the data, results indicate that even with a stringent "all-or-none" procedure, SSW Test List EC is quite intelligible to normal subjects at 10 dB-SL and above.

In comparing the present findings to those reported by Balas and Simon using the same method of scoring on a similar list, the following

TABLE 2 ━━━━━━━━━━
Mean Error Percentages and Standard Deviations Using 40-Item Scoring ($N = 10$ per SL) (present study)

	dB-Sensation Level					
	0	10	20	30	40	50
Mean	56.5*	16.0	2.8	2.5	2.0	2.3
SD	18.9	7.8	2.4	2.3	1.9	1.8

*$p = 0.01$

findings were revealed. Using a two-tailed *t*-test, significantly better performance on List EC was found for the 0, 10, and 20 dB-SL groups

$$
\begin{array}{llll}
(0 \text{ dB-SL-}t = 8.08; & df = 20; & PL = 2.84; \\
10 \text{ dB-SL-}t = 6.12; & df = 20; & PL = 2.84; \\
20 \text{ dB-SL-}t = 4.56; & df = 20; & PL = 2.84; \\
30 \text{ dB-SL-}t = 1.90; & df = 20; & PL = 2.84; \\
40 \text{ dB-SL-}t = .88; & df = 20; & PL = 2.84; \\
50 \text{ dB-SL-}t = .54; & df = 20; & PL = 2.84)
\end{array}
$$

as shown in Figure 4. Further, it should be noted that a mean error percentage of less than 3% was exhibited on List EC at the 20 dB-SL presentation.

FIGURE 3.
Performance–intensity function established in present study using 40–item scoring procedure. Mean group values and standard deviations are depicted.

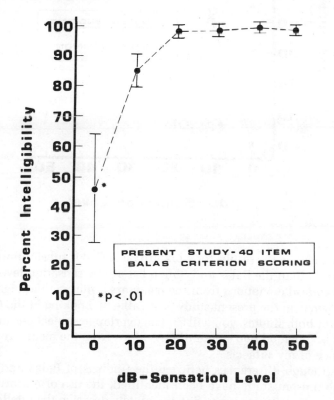

FIGURE 4.

Comparison of performance–intensity functions established by Balas and Simon (1965) and in the present study using identical scoring procedures.

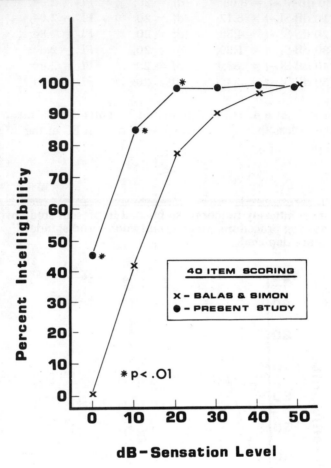

In viewing the results for standard List EC, it is substantially more intelligible than the Balas and Simon list at low sensation levels. Further, standard deviations from the mean are quite small at higher sensation levels in the present study (see Table 3). Looking at the 0 dB-SL group for both studies, you will find no overlap in subject performance even if you extend two standard deviations from the mean group performance of my subjects.

Although differences between the findings of Balas and Simon and the present study have been identified, the use of a scoring procedure such as this one may not adequately describe the intelligibility

TABLE 3

Comparison of Mean Error Percentages and Standard Deviations Using 40-Item Scoring Procedure

| | dB-Sensation Level | | | | | |
	0	10	20	30	40	50
	Balas and Simon (1965)					
Mean	99.6	57.5	22.7	10.7	4.6	1.1
SD	.85	18.3	8.2	8.0	3.1	1.2
	Present Study-List EC					
Mean	56.5*	16.0*	2.8*	2.5	2.0	2.3
SD	18.9	7.8	2.4	2.3	1.9	1.8

* $p = 0.01$

of either test list by normal listeners. Although the "all-or-none" scoring criterion is stringent, it may misrepresent the intelligibility of a word list that requires a four monosyllable response. Therefore, the second method of scoring was employed. As previously mentioned, partial credit was given if the subject identified one, two, or three monosyllables of the test item correctly.

In rescoring my data using this new method, the mean error percentages and standard deviations seen in Table 4 were obtained. It is apparent that when each element of an entire test item is scored, slightly different performance is obtained at 0 and 10 dB-SL. When viewing the performance–intensity function obtained using the more sensitive scoring procedure, SSW Test List EC appears quite intelligible to normal subjects even at low sensation levels (see Figure 5). Once again, a one-way ANOVA revealed a statistically significant main effect ($F = 32.22$; $df = 5, 54$; $p = .01$). Post-hoc analysis revealed only the performance of the 0 dB-SL group to be significantly different from other groups ($F = 3.34$; $df = 5, 54$; c. diff = 15.66).

A statistical comparison was conducted between the performances of my subjects using both scoring procedures by using a two-tailed t-test for dependent measures (see Table 5). Results of this analysis revealed a statistically different performance by groups at 0 ($t = 12.0$; $df = 20$; $PL = 2.84$), 10 ($t = 6.62$; $df = 20$; $PL = 2.84$), 20 ($t = 3.52$; $df = 20$; $PL = 2.84$), and 30 ($t = 3.20$, $df = 20$; $PL = 2.84$) and dB-SL, at a .01 level of confidence. Comparison of functions obtained by using both scoring methods is shown in Figure 6.

An overall comparison of the functions reported by Balas and Simon and in the present study using both methods of scoring is presented in Figure 7. It can be seen that normal performance is quite different on standard List EC when compared to those data presented by Balas and Simon.

TABLE 4

Mean Error Percentages and Standard Deviations Using 160-Element Scoring Procedure (present study)

| | dB-Sensation Level | | | | | |
	0	10	20	30	40	50
Mean	29.3*	5.0	.8	.7	.6	.7
SD	15.3	3.1	.8	.6	.5	.5

*p = 0.01

FIGURE 5.

Performance–intensity function established in present study using 160-item (monosyllable) scoring. Mean group values and standard deviations are depicted.

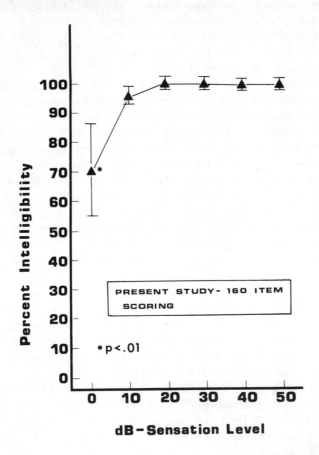

Acoustic and Psychoacoustic Factors

TABLE 5 ▬▬▬▬▬▬

Comparison of Mean Error Percentages and Standard Deviations from Present Study Using 40-Item and 160 Element Scoring Procedures

dB-Sensation Level
40-item scoring

	0	10	20	30	40	40
Mean	56.5	16.0	2.8	2.5	2.0	2.3
SD	18.9	7.8	2.4	2.3	1.9	1.8

			160-element scoring			
Mean	29.3*	5.0*	.8*	.7*	.6	.7
SD	15.3	3.1	.8	.6	.5	.5

* $p = 0.01$

Discussion

The results of the present study reveal that SSW Test List EC is highly intelligible to normal subjects at low sensation levels. In addition, there was no significant difference between group performance at the 10, 20, 30, 40, or 50 dB-SL presentation levels. Although performance findings on the Balas and Simon list and List EC are quite similar at the more intense sensation levels (40 and 50 dB-SL), the functions separate dramatically at lower levels, List EC being significantly more intelligible at levels of 30 dB-SL and below. The findings of Balas and Simon (1965) are frequently cited in the literature; however, their articulation function may not be indicative of normal performance on the standard list currently in use.

The performance differences noted appear to be primarily attributable to the lack of homogeneity between the test list used by Balas and Simon and List EC which was used in the present study. Further, the scoring procedure employed by Balas and Simon may have resulted in added misrepresentation of subject performance. That is, their method of scoring may result in a poorer intelligibility score than is actually exhibited. For this reason, an articulation or performance–intensity function that is generated using this scoring method may not be adequate. Therefore, the need for a more sensitive scoring procedure was indicated.

The second procedure for scoring subject responses used in this investigation was sensitive to performance on each element of a test item, therefore, establishing a more accurate representation of a normal performance-intensity function was possible. This second procedure followed the standard method of scoring the SSW Test, that is, each monosyllable of a spondaic word is scored individually. Using this

FIGURE 6.

Comparison of performance–intensity functions established in present study using 40–item and 160–element scoring procedures.

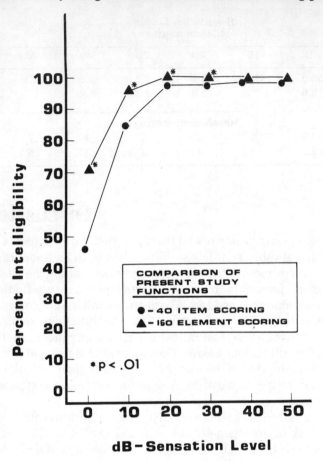

scoring method, a more precise measurement of the true function for the test, regardless of the specific subject population used, can be obtained.

The present findings of high intelligibility by normal listeners on List EC at lower than standard presentation levels appears to support previous suggestions that the SSW Test is indeed a simple task for normal subjects. In the evaluation of subjects ranging in age from 11 to 60 years, few errors are exhibited in subjects with normal central auditory function (Katz, 1977). Based on the findings of this study, it may be possible to administer the SSW Test at sensation levels lower than 50 dB-SL. This possibility may allow clients who exhibit severe hearing

Acoustic and Psychoacoustic Factors

FIGURE 7.

Overall comparison of performance-intensity functions obtained by Balas and Simon (1965), and in the present study using a 40-item and 160-element scoring procedure.

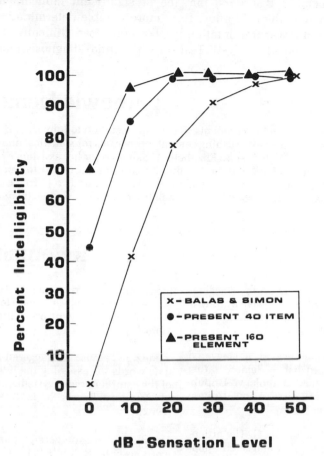

losses and/or tolerance problems to be evaluated with this test. However, rigorous standardization at lower presentations levels must first be completed prior to the clinical application of the present findings.

Future research should attempt to determine if factors related to low intensity level presentations, such as vowel–consonant masking effects, will alter performance of subjects exhibiting central auditory dysfunction. Further, research directed at conducting similar studies with younger and older normal populations, as well as investigations to determine if hearing impaired subjects exhibit parallel performance–intensity functions, are warranted. In view of the present results, additional investigations using presentation levels of 50 dB-SL and greater would determine whether presentation at more intense levels interferes with intelligibility. Results from this type of study, particularly if data is obtained from specific hearing impaired populations (sensory-neural and retrocochlear disorders) may be of significant clinical value. Research such as this will allow for a more reliable determination of whether or not lower presentation levels can be used clinically. Thus, wider application of the SSW Test for differential diagnosis may be possible.

Acknowledgement

The author would like to express his sincere appreciation to John C. Burke for invaluable assistance in establishing computer programs for statistical analysis. Appreciation is also extended to Elizabeth A. Skarakis for her assistance in the additional analysis of these data. Gratitude is further expressed to Dennis J. Arnst for his encouragement and technical assistance, and to Jeffrey L. Danhauer and Sanford E. Gerber for their helpful comments during this study.

References

Arnst, D. J. Errors on the staggered spondaic word (SSW) test in a group of adult listeners. In press, *Ear and Hearing* (1981).

Balas, R. The use of a staggered spondaic word list in demonstrating central auditory pathology. Unpublished doctoral dissertation, University of Denver (1964).

Balas, R. and Simon, G. The articulation function of a staggered spondaic word list for a normal hearing population. *Journal of Auditory Research*, 5, 285–289 (1965).

Brunt, M. The staggered spondaic word (SSW) test. In J. Katz (ed.), *Handbook of Clinical Audiology*, 2nd edition, Baltimore: Williams and Wilkins (1978), pp. 262–275.

Goldman, S. and Katz, J. A comparison of the performance of normal hearing subjects on the staggered spondaic word test given under four conditions—dichotic, diotic, monaural (dominant ear) and monaural (nondominant ear). Paper presented at the American Speech and Hearing Association Convention, Chicago, 1966.

Katz, J. The use of staggered spondaic words for assessing the integrity of the central nervous system. *Journal of Auditory Research*, 2, 327–337 (1962).

Katz, J. The staggered spondaic word test. In R. Keith (ed.), *Central Auditory Dysfunction*, New York: Grune and Statton (1977).

Katz, J., Basil, R., and Smith, J. The staggered spondaic word test for determining central auditory lesions. *Ann. Otol., Rhinol., Laryngol.*, 72, 908–917 (1963).

Katz, J. and Myrick, D. A normative study to assess performance of children aged seven through eleven, on the staggered spondaic word test. Unpublished study cited in M. Brunt.

Acoustic and Psychoacoustic Factors

Abstract

Analysis of High Intensity Performance– Intensity Function for the SSW Test in a Group of Normal Listeners

Janet L. Conant, M.A.

Traditional speech audiometry—the measurement of speech discrimination ability at a single fixed presentation level above threshold—is an extremely limited diagnostic tool. Limitations are exemplified by inadequate detection of retrocochlear pathology as well as poor differentiation between cochlear and retrocochlear lesions (Jerger, 1974).

The observation of a "rollover" phenomenon in the performance–intensity function for phonetically balanced words (PI–PB) of patients with retrocochlear disorder enhanced the diagnostic signficance of speech intelligibility measures. Jerger and Jerger (1971) described a "rollover index" which differentiated cochlear from VIIIth nerve pathology. Other nontraditional speech materials have been evaluated at high intensity levels to observe differences between pathologic and nonpathologic auditory systems (Jerger and Jerger, 1967). Again, differences in performance were obtained between individuals with normal, cochlear, and retrocochlear pathology at high intensity levels.

The SSW Test is used primarily to detect lesions of the central auditory nervous system. However, it has been noted that extremely large over-corrected SSW scores may be indicative of VIIIth nerve and low brainstem lesions (Katz, 1970). Interestingly, Katz et al. (1963) noted a high correlation between the percentage of error of the SSW and the percentage of error on the W-22 speech discrimination test on patients with peripheral hearing loss. Other studies have demonstrated the close relationship between the articulation function for the SSW Test and PB words in normal listeners (Doyle, 1981; Balas and Simon, 1964).

The purpose of the present study was to obtain normative data on the ability of normal hearing subjects to respond to items on the SSW Test at high intensity levels up to a maximum of 90 dB SL. Forty

Master's Thesis, California State Univeresity, Sacramento, 1981.

individuals served as subjects in this study. To define the performance–intensity function for this test necessitated a deviation from standard procedure. The initial presentation level was 30 dB SL (re: PTA), and following every 10 test items, the intensity level was raised 20 dB. The performance–intensity function, therefore, was examined from 30 dB SL to 90 dB SL.

Many studies have indicated that subjects with normal hearing reach a plateau on the PI–PB function and exhibit little or no decrease in performance as intensity is increased. Based on such results, it is anticipated that performance of a normal hearing, young adult population on the SSW Test will remain constant at high levels of intensity once maximum performance has been obtained.

References

Balas, R. F., and Simon, G.R., The Articulation Function of a Staggered Spondaic Word List for a Normal Hearing Population. *Journal of Auditory Research*, 4, 285–289 (1964).

Doyle, P., Performance Intensity Function for a Normal Hearing Population on the Staggered Spondaic Word Test. Unpublished Master's thesis, University of California, Santa Barbara (1981).

Jerger, J., and Jerger, S., Psychoacoustic Comparison of Cochlear and VIIIth Nerve Disorders. *Journal of Speech and Hearing Research*, 10, 659–688 (1967).

Jerger, J., and Jerger, S., Diagnostic significance of PB Word Functions. *Archives of Otolaryngology*, 93, 573–580 (1971).

Jerger, J., Diagnostic Audiometry. J. Jerger (Ed.), *Modern Developments in Audiology*, Second Edition. New York: Academic Press (1973).

Katz, J., Basil, R. A., and Smith, J. M., A Staggered Spondaic Word Test for Detecting Central Auditory Lesions. *Annals of Otology, Rhinology, and Laryngology*, 72, 908–918 (1963). Katz, J., Audiological Diagnosis: Cochlea to Cortex. *Menorah Medical Journal*, 1, 25–38 (1970).

Janet L. Conant, M.A.

Katz and Pack (a neurologist) presented a careful consideration of the reponse bias aspects of the SSW Test at a symposium in Omaha in 1975. Their study (the first article in this section) emphasized the importance of all aspects of the SSW Test in interpreting patient performance. The second paper, by the same authors and Kushner, was a poster session at the ASHA Convention in Washington, D.C. in 1975. In It the Competing Environmental Sounds (CES) Test is described and shown to be an aid to the SSW in localizing the hemisphere involved. The strong relationship between neurologic diagnosis of the problem and the SSW results is emphasized with a case study.

Audiological Diagnosis: Cochlea to Cortex relates SSW results to a full range of audiologic tests in various types of problems. It emphasizes the importance of relating SSW results to the entire audiologic test battery.

Musiek and his colleagues at the Dartmouth-Hitchcock Medical Center have presented two interesting case studies involving the SSW Test. Both point up the possibility of using the test to monitor a disease process, pre- and post-surgery performance, and possibly treatment (i.e., therapy). Winkelaar and Lewis provide detailed examples comparing three cases and central auditory tests—the SSW, competing sentences, and rapidly alternating speech.

4

Advanced Use of the Staggered Spondaic Word Test Introduction

New Developments in Differential Diagnosis Using the SSW Test

Jack Katz, Ph.D.   Gary Pack, M.D.

The title of this paper suggests that you already know what the SSW test is and are familiar with the "old developments" in differential diagnosis. This is a big assumption and we presume that in many cases a false one. For this reason, we will first describe the Staggered Spondaic Word (SSW) Test and some of the important findings from earlier research.

The SSW test was designed as a technique to identify dysfunction in auditory centers of the brain. The literature contains ample information about the purpose of the test, its administration, scoring and interpretation (Katz, 1962, Katz, Basil and Smith, 1963, Katz, 1968, Brunt, 1972). It will be briefly reviewed here.

The SSW Test

The SSW Test is a dichotic speech procedure. Each item is made up of two spondaic words which are presented in a partially overlapped fashion. Figure 1 shows an example of a test item. In this case, the first spondee "upstairs" is presented to the right ear and the second one "downtown" to the left ear.

Central Auditory Processing Disorders: Proceedings of the Conference. Omaha, Nebraska, January, 1975.

The monosyllables like "up" and "town" which arrive independently at each ear are referred to as right non-competing (RNC) and left non-competing (LNC) conditions, respectively. The items are counter-balanced so that if the odd ones are routed to the right ear first then the even items go to the left ear first. The words are recorded rather slowly on tape and presented to the patient at a comfortably loud level (50 dB SL).

Many auditory tests of central function are described in the literature (Bocca, et al., Matzker, 1959, deQuiros, 1964, Walsh and Goodman, 1955 and others). The common diagnostic sign in each of these techniques is that the ear contralateral to the disordered cerebral hemisphere is depressed. For example, a temporal lobe tumor in the left hemisphere would be revealed by a reduced score in the right ear and vice versa.

One factor on which the tests differ is their sensitivity to language dominance. The Broadbent procedure, as used by Kimura (1961), is so sensitive to language dominance that it overrides the effects due to brain pathology. The side the lesion is on must be inferred by compar-ing the relationship between the two ears.

The SSW test is essentially free of contamination due to language dominance in testing adults (Brunt, 1972). There is no evidence of a clinically significant difference between the ears in normal adults (Brunt and Goetzinger, 1968) when it is presented dichotically (Goldman and Katz, 1966). The SSW Test is most depressed when there is a lesion in the middle posterior portion of the superior temporal gyrus. The depressed score is noted in the ear contralateral to the damaged hemisphere regardless of dominance.

FIGURE 1
An illustration of an SSW item in which the first monosyllable is presented to the right ear and the second to the left ear.

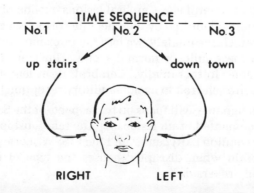

Auditory central tests differ in their sensitivity to hearing loss and word discrimination problems in patients who are being studied for cerebral disorders. Matzker (1959) pointed out that his "Binaural Test" was most effective in picking out temporal lobe tumors in the absence of peripheral hearing loss. The Rush Hughes difference test is also subject to disruption when there is a substantial hearing loss or discrimination problem (Goetzinger, 1972).

The SSW test is relatively free from the influence of peripheral hearing loss and discrimination difficulty. Three factors contribute to this. The use of spondaic words aid the person with a peripheral hearing loss since they are more easily identified than monosyllablic words. There is also a correction for lack of clarity of hearing. The percentage of error on the W-22 test or an equivalent discrimination test is subtracted to compensate the person with a discrimination problem (presumably on a peripheral basis). These are called corrected or C-SSW scores. Finally, lowered discrimination has a predictable effect on the test which is taken into consideration in the norms. An overcorrected C-SSW score is typically obtained with a sensory-neural loss. This means that any errors on the SSW test are over compensated by the correction. A moderate (or severe) score identifies the patient with a cerebral auditory reception lesion. This score is highly positive as opposed to the overcorrected score which is in the negative direction.

Most clinical procedures use a simple signal, require a simple response and are scored "correct" or "incorrect." Those types of unidimensional tests do not permit much qualitative information. We would expect various type of errors to occur with lesions in different parts of the brain. These variations could not be identified by a simple test.

The SSW test can identify or support the diagnosis of disorder in parts of the auditory system. Lesions in the peripheral centers and brainstem are shown in the ipsilateral ear (Katz, 1970). Heschl's gyrus or auditory reception (AR) center disease is identified by the defective score in the contralateral ear. Cerebral lesions outside of the reception centers are usually identified by their peculiar responses rather than by the SWW scores. Unfortunately, we lose the information about the side of lesion with these mild or normal scores. However, one can often identify the area intracranially. Cerebral disorders not involving Heschl's gyrus are referred to as non-auditory reception (NAR) lesions.

The present paper will focus on two aspects of the SSW Test in patients with documented brain lesions: 1) The relationship of damage to the auditory reception (AR) center and the C-SSW score; and, 2) which area of the brain when disrupted causes the type of response bias which is called "reversals."

Anatomical and Physiological Considerations

Anatomically, the cerebrum is made up of four lobes; however, there is a disadvantage relying on these landmarks when we are concerned with physiology and pathological symptoms. For example, it is recognized that Heschl's gyrus is the primary auditory reception center (Brodmann's area 41). Figure 2 shows Brodmann's area 41 (Elliott, 1963).

Luria (1970) describes various auditory functions in the temporal lobe. Other areas of the brain are involved in auditory integration association, and memory (Schiller and Haymaker, 1969, Schiller, 1969). It is reasonable that auditory tests can gather clues about functions in different parts of the temporal lobe and in centers outside of the temporal lobe.

The SSW Test appears to challenge various processing skills and thereby may be of help in identifying lesions in a variety of auditory or auditory-related centers. It is on the one hand sufficiently complex to test many functions but easy enough in other ways to be applicable to diverse populations. The simplicity is the two spondaic words which are presented slowly, loudly and clearly: while the complexity is the four monosyllables, the two ears and the staggered delivery. By the use of the SSW test or other procedures, it is hoped that patterns of disturbance can be related to specific dysfunction in the nervous system. This would enable the audiologist to contribute further to the differential diagnosis of the brain and brainstem pathology.

FIGURE 2 ▬▬▬▬▬▬▬▬▬▬▬▬▬▬▬▬▬▬▬▬▬▬▬▬▬▬▬▬▬▬
The location of Brodmann's area 41 "according to Brodmann's original plan..." (After Eliott, 1963, Figure 22-5, p. 357).

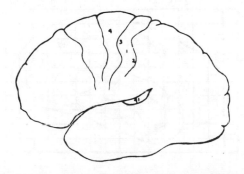

Recording the Presence of Brain Lesions

In previous SSW research, cerebral lesions were marked by a neurologist or neurosurgeon on a generalized brain diagram. Eventually, left and right hemispheres were represented laterally and an anterior-posterior view was available to record the depth of the lesion.

For the present project, we attempted to study fewer cases with more refined localization of lesions in a three-dimensional field. An average sized human brain was obtained and cut saggitally in one centimeter sections. There were 12 sections across the brain from left to right. The photograph of the extreme left section was labled plate 31 and the extreme right section plate #XII. All sections were viewed from left to right. Figure 3 shows the left lateral plate superimposed on a diagram of the brain for purposes of orientation. The abscissa was subdivided into 1 cm units labeled 1 through 16. The ordinate was also subdivided into centimeter units and labeled A through J.

Figure 4 is plate #111, the third one from the left. By placing a template over any of the marked plates, the damaged cube of brain tissue could be located from the neurologist's drawing. This method permitted a brain pathology analysis into approximately 1000 1 cm cubes.

We considered the possibility that 1) the analysis method was more specific than the brain itself; that 2) there was too much variation in structure from one person to the next, or that 3) the neurologist might be unable to represent the involved area with sufficient accuracy from

---

FIGURE 3 ▬▬▬▬▬▬▬
Plate number 1 showing a photograph of the extreme left lateral section of a brain superimposed on a diagram of a brain for purposes of orientation.

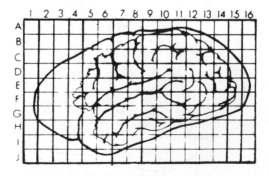

FIGURE 4

A photograph of plate number III which is the third section in the
left hemisphere and represents the first plate of the medial section.

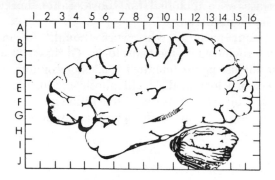

the available data to suit this method. We assumed that the data would
tell us if we have overstepped one or more of these limits in that there
would be lack of correspondence between the SSW test and the
anatomical drawings. This method would be feasible only if there was
consistency of performance. If we see some uniformity of response in
patients with similar lesions, then the technique could be a useful
method for identifying even fine differences for purposes of differential
diagnosis.

Procedures

Over the past 13 years, we have utilized the SSW test with various
populations, both clinically and under experimental conditions. We obtained information about auditory reception lesions and have had a
high degree of accuracy in identifying them clinically (Katz, 1968). An
interesting response on the test was the reversal which seemed to carry
diagnostic information. In the present study, we tried to determine if
our previous hunches were correct and to see if they could be narrowed
down further, anatomically. By having one neurologist who was well
oriented to the project and the SSW test, we assumed that we could
maintain a higher level of standardization.

The routine hearing test battery was administered prior to the
SSW test and word discrimination scores (WDS) were obtained on the
same day. The subjects were given at least 40 SSW items on the EC list.
Some of the cases who were given list 1B (52 items) were completely
rescored using only the 40 EC items.

The study was double blind, in that the audiologist was unaware of the specific neurologic diagnosis and the neurologist was unaware of the audiological findings. No cases of brainstem or brainstem plus cerebral disease were included for consideration nor were strictly cerebellar cases considered.

Seventy-four patients who were thought to have cerebral disorders were reviewed by the neurologist. Of these, 44 were rejected primarily for not having sufficiently focal lesions or not sufficient information to be clearly localized. The diagnosis and localization of the lesion was based on one or more of the following: autopsy, surgery, radiologic studies, EEG, or neurologic examination, as well as case history.

Subjects

The 30 patients who were chosen for this study had a mean age of 48 years. Two subjects exceeded the 11 to 60 year age limits for normal adult performance (Katz, 1968). One was 65 and the other 76 years of age. Sixteen of the subjects were males and 14 females.

Since the SSW test is relatively free from effects of hearing loss, no individuals were excluded because of hearing loss. The test is a binaural procedure so we would have eliminated a patient with no hearing in one ear or close to 0% discrimination, but there were none with such extreme conditions in the sample. The mean speech reception threshold was 3 dB in each ear ranging from 10 to 48 dB HL. Word discrimination was 92% in the right ear and 91% in the left. The scores ranged from 68% to 100%.

The final diagnoses revealed that 16 of the 30 cases had tumors; 9 had vascular disease; 3 had damage due to trauma; and 2 primarily as a result of surgery. The main type of confirmation of the locus of the lesion was specified by the neurologist. Specification of the lesion was made primarily on the basis of autopsy in two cases; on surgery in 18 patients; on various radiological procedures in 9 subjects; and on neurological examination in one case. Thirteen of the subjects were diagnosed as having lesions in the right hemisphere and 17 in the left hemisphere.

Auditory Receptions (AR) vs. Non-Auditory Reception (NAR) Lesions

The first phase of this study was to evaluate the effects of auditory reception (AR) lesions as compared with those lesions sparing the reception (NAR) centers on each side. The effect was studied in the contralateral ear for the corrected SSW score. Our previous research suggested that AR lesions would result in moderate to severe scores (a score of 21 or more in the contralateral ear).

Figure 3 shows the brain diagram with a grid super-imposed on it. The square labeled E9, which corresponds roughly to Brodmann's area 41, was felt to represent the most sensitive area of the brain (in either hemisphere) for producing errors on the SSW test. Two neurologists concurred that this represented the auditory reception area, Heschl's gyrus. Therefore, damage to E9 was considered evidence of an AR lesion and lesions sparing this area were considered NAR pathology. In a previous study, SSW scores agreed closely with the site of lesion as drawn by a neurologist (Dr. Arthur W. Epstein) (Katz, 1968, Figure 3, p. 144).

Since Heschl's gyrus is a cortical area, only the two lateral plates were considered for each side in the present study. Plates I and II represented the left hemisphere, and plates XI and XII, the right hemisphere. Taken together, these plates represent 2cm on each side and are referred to as the lateral sections.

Thirteen of our cases had lesions involving E9 laterally and were thus classified as AR subjects (three had right hemisphere lesions and 10 left). The remaining 17 did not involve E9 laterally and were labeled NAR cases. The mean C-SSW score in the ear contralateral to the damage was 53 (severely depressed) for the auditory reception cases as compared with a score of 5 (upper limit of normal) for the non-auditory reception subjects. The difference between the groups was statistically significant (t = 9.45) at <.01 level of confidence.

All of the AR cases had the expected moderate or severe C-SSW scores in the contralateral ear. They ranged from 34 (moderately depressed) to 77 (severely depressed). Figure 5A shows the means and standard deviations for the 13 AR cases and Figure 5B the means and standard deviations for the 17 NAR cases for the four C-SSW conditions. The conditions were arranged for the contralateral and ipsilateral ear. The group varied in their contralateral C-SSW ear score from −4 (normal) to 18 (mildly depressed).

We have contended for a number of years that the peak errors in NAR cases is a weak indicator of the damaged hemisphere (Katz, 1968). Only in auditory reception cases can we have reasonable assurance of the damaged hemisphere. The present sample provided an opportunity to test this observation. Figure 5B shows that there is little difference between the contralateral and ipsilateral ears for the NAR cases. Table 1 shows whether the peak was in the RC or LC condition in relation to the damaged hemisphere. Twelve of the 17 cases were correctly

**Graphic representation of the four SSW conditions organized
according to the ear ipsilateral and contralateral to the damaged
hemisphere for the thirteen AR subjects. Means and standard
deviations are shown.**

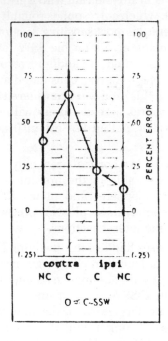

identified, three were incorrectly identified and two were equivocal.
Seventy-one percent of the cases in this sample were correctly identified, 18% were incorrectly located and 12% were without indications
of a hemisphere. In previous samples, we had as few as 50% correct (no
better than chance). At this time, we do not feel that we could say with
confidence which hemisphere is involved in non-auditory reception
cases although we might gather qualitative information to show where
the dysfunction occurs within one of the hemispheres.

In order to see if our hit-miss performances could be equalled
using any other cube besides E9 in the lateral plates, we checked the
surrounding coordinates and those in the medial and central plates and
found none of them to be as critical in separating the AR from the NAR
cases.

FIGURE 5B.

Graphic representation of the four SSW conditions organized according to the ear ipsilateral and contralateral to the damaged hemisphere for the seventeen NAR subjects. Means and standard deviations are shown.

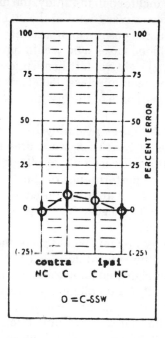

TABLE 1.

Distribution of 17 subjects relative to the damaged hemisphere and the ear with the poorer competing condition.

	Non-Auditory Reception Cases			
Damaged Hemisphere	C-SSW Competing Condition R>	L>	R = L	Total
Left	5	2	1	8
Right	1	7	1	9
Total	6	9	2	17

Cases Eliminated from Study

Had all 74 cases been included in the study, the hit-miss ratio would not have been as favorable as was found in the 30 clearly localized cases. The neurologist eliminated cases which were not accurately localizable or not focal. This included cases who would have been correctly identified 1) AR vs.NAR, 2) right vs. left hemisphere, but there were also cases that would have been misclassified. Thus by sorting out the less clear neurological cases, some of the less clear audiological cases were also eliminated.

Twenty-five of the cases probably had left hemisphere lesions (mostly aphasics due to CVA's); 6 were probably right hemisphere cases, and 13 were either diseased bilaterally or the side was not clear.

Table 2 shows the performance of the 44 patients who were excluded from the study. They are distributed according to the damaged hemisphere, their C-SSW category for the poorer competing condition and in which ear it was.

A perfect diagnosis record would have shown all moderate and severe SSW scores in the contralateral ear ("R>" for left hemisphere cases and "L>" for the right hemisphere). There should be no particular pattern for the bilateral or non-diagnosed cases.

Since we do not obtain important information about the side of lesion for normal or mild scores, we would anticipate a random distribution of scores in the "R>" and "L>" categories.

From Table 2, we see that all of the right hemisphere cases with moderate or severe scores were correctly identified and 11 of the 16 moderate or severe left hemisphere cases were similarly identified. Thus, 76% of these difficult cases were correctly categorized as to hemisphere if they had moderate or severe scores. When we add the 13 AR cases from the main part of this study, the correct identification goes up to 85%. As expected, the NAR's are about equally divided between correct and incorrect identifications.

Sparks and Geschwind (1968) have demonstrated that the performance in the left ear on a dichotic competing or dichotic integrating task is severely depressed when the corpus callosum is sectioned. Dr. Lynn has already described the performance of his patients who have lesions in the corpus callosum.

Interestingly, none of the clearly localized cases had moderate or severe peaks in the left ear without a corresponding lesion to the opposite reception center. However, four of the rejected left hemisphere cases had C-SSW peaks in the left ear. Some of these cases could have had callosal lesions but the lack of certainty in diagnosis precluded this conclusion.

TABLE 2. ▬▬▬▬

Distribution of 44 patients eliminated from the study because of
insufficient information to locate the lesion accurately or the
medical criteria showed widespread damage. Patients are classified
by the apparent side of lesion, the C-SSW category for the poorer
competing condition and whether it is in the right ear, left ear or if
they are equal.

	Cases Excluded from Primary Study			
Apparent Lesion	Category	R>	C-SSW Competing Condition L>	R = L
Left	N, Mi	3	5	1
Hemisphere	Mo, S	11	4	1
Right	N, Mi	0	1	0
Hemisphere	Mo, S	0	5	0
Both				
Hemispheres	N, Mi	2	4	1
or Unknown	Mo, S	4	2	0

We are experimenting with a competing environmental sounds
test in an effort to differentiate AR cases from those with corpus
callosum lesions.

Another unexplained finding was the case with a severe C-SSW
score in each ear for the competing condition. Several hypotheses can
be put forth but because of the poor localization of lesion, they must remain unexplained at this time. 1) The effect of aphasia might have in-
terfered with all speaking activities. We could expect this to be about
equal in each ear if the auditory reception centers were intact and the
problem was primarily in the processing or output stage. 2) The
auditory reception center on the left might have been damaged producing a depressed score in the right ear and the corpus callosum was also
disrupted on the left causing a poor score in the left ear. 3) The bilateral
depression could be caused by a generalized, bilateral disorder. We
have seen this in some very old patients (Balas, 1962) and possibly some
chronic alcoholics. This particular patient was only 33 years of age, but
he has been considered a chronic alcoholic (who later suffered a
stroke). We have no evidence that there is generalized brain dysfunction in this patient.

Although we know of no studies with chronic alcoholic patients,
Young (1971) tested the acute effects of alcohol on the SSW test. The effects were bilateral and more depressed in the competing conditions.
As the patients took more and more alcohol, their scores were more
and more depressed, bilaterally and eventually even affecting the noncompeting conditions. The early effects of alcohol seem to resemble an

"inattention pattern" and then an "immature pattern" as seen in children (Katz and Illmer, 1972). Eventually, when all four conditions are depressed, the problem is obviously a generalized one and not specifically related to dichotic competition.

McClellan, Wertz and Collins (1973), showed that their left hemisphere cases (all aphasics) had peak C-SSW scores in the left ear or bilaterally. Their results with a Veterans Administration Hospital population are similar but more exaggerated than the population of 25 left hemisphere cases (who were excluded from this study) from private hospitals. The problem did not influence the 15 right hemisphere (non-aphasic) cases who were correctly identified regardless of the category. Our findings tend to support their observation. The three right hemisphere AR cases in the main study all had peaks in the left ear, as well as 7 of the 9 NAR cases. The two cases that did not conform had normal C-SSW conditions in both ears. One was "T>," the other "R = L." To the right hemisphere cases we could add the six poorly localized cases who all peaked in the left competing condition. Thus, 16 out of 18 right hemisphere cases did have peaks in the left ear.

While the problem with left hemisphere aphasic patients does tend to reduce the capacity of the SSW test and the other similar tests, there are other sources of information which might help out until a test is devised to identify lesions in the corpus callosum.

The Use of Word Discrimination Scores (WDS) and Other Tests

In the 30 subjects included in the main aspect of this study, there was a strong relationship between the C-SSW score and the status of Heschl's gyrus on the opposite side. In the 44 subjects with more widespread damage or difficulty in specifically locating the site of lesion, there were some cases having bilateral peaks (difficulty) or peaks in the ear ipsilateral to the damaged hemisphere. It has been established that this could be due to a lesion in the corpus callosum (depressed performance in the left ear regardless of where the corpus callosum is damaged).

A brief tone, monaural test such as proposed by Baru and Karaseva (1972) could be a valuable procedure in eliminating the likelihood of a right auditory reception lesion. However, other procedures could be more definitive in demonstrating the presence of a lesion in the corpus callosum.

Music centers and the identification of environmental sounds are primarily functions of the right hemisphere (Curry, 1972, Shankweiler, 1966, Kimura, 1964). While competing speech tests will be depressed in the left ear when the corpus callosum is sectioned, the right (non-dominant) ear will be depressed for competing music or other sounds.

By comparing the performance of a speech test with a music or environmental sound test, we can see that the opposite ears are depressed when there is a callosal lesion—the non-dominant ear in each case. Thus, we can see that both reception centers are intact but the connection between hemispheres is damaged.

Until these tests are worked out for clinical use, the audiologist is at a loss to say if a lesion is in the right AR center or somewhere in the corpus callosum. Indeed, there could also be some confusion with damage to the left brainstem. The SSW test is not always sufficient to unravel this dilemma. Fortunately, the audiologist has other information available to him.

In order to differentiate an AR lesion on the right and a brainstem lesion on the left, tests of tonal decay can be of greatest help (Katz, 1970). We have suspected that WDS can help to identify which cases are true AR and which are NAR, but peak in the non-dominant ear because of damage to the communication between the right and left hemispheres. The present study provided an opportunity to investigate this.

Our purpose was to determine if WDS was poorer in AR cases and whether the contralateral ear was more depressed than the ipsilateral.

A t-test was computed between the mean bilateral discrimination score $\frac{(R + L)}{(2)}$ for AR and NAR subjects. The mean WDS for the respec- group was 87% vs. 96%. The mean difference of 10.4% was statistically significant ($t = 4.96$) at the .01 level of confidence. Thus, the AR cases appeared to be more depressed than NAR cases. There seemed to be no difference between right and left hemisphere damage in the AR cases or NAR cases. A matched t-test was computed to compare the contralateral and ipsilateral ears for the AR group. The WDS in the contralateral ear was 85% and on the ipsilateral side, 89%. The mean difference of 4.7% was significant ($t = 2.59$) at the .05 level. There was no difference between ears for the NAR group when they were calculated for contralateral and ipsilateral ears.

Although the mean difference was small, we can expect WDS to be depressed and a bit poorer in the ear contralateral to the damaged hemisphere in AR cases. If a patient with a severe peak in the left ear on the SSW test has good WDS bilaterally, we have some evidence that this may be a corpus callosum lesion rather than an AR lesion.

It may be appropriate to mention here that the SSW test cannot be separated out of the audiological battery because it must be interpreted in light of the other findings. For example, a brainstem lesion on the left is most easily distinguished from an AR lesion in the right hemisphere by the presence of tone decay in the left ear rather than any other single factor.

Localizing Cerebral Lesions Using Reversals

For the past 12 years, reversals have been recorded in patients responding on SSW items. By a reversal, we mean a response in which the monosyllables are repeated in a re-arranged order. Even when the words are reported correctly, the listener might say them in a different sequence. For example, in the item "upstairs, downtown," the response could be "downtown, upstairs," "downstairs, uptown," or any other permutation.

At first, only items with four correct monosyllables and a reversal of order were counted. These are called "true reversals." Over the years, we have continued to relax our criteria for reversals because some of the same subjects tended to make sequencing errors, as well as performing incorrectly on one of the monosyllables. A reversal with one word in error (a substitution or distortion) is called a probable reversal. If the one error is an omission with the remaining words misordered as well, this is called a questionable reversal. We are presently studying to see if questionable reversals add diagnostic sensitivity to the SSW test (for example for AR cases) or if it introduces contamination. Because there is reasonable expectation that the three types of reversals can be combined, the reversal information in this study (unless otherwise specified) will refer to the total of any or all of these types. This is referred to as *maximum reversals*.

Reversals on the SSW test are not limited to patients with brain lesions. We have noted them in conductive hearing loss cases, cochlear hearing loss cases (more so in unilaterals) and in more than one-half of the non-organics. If there is no hearing loss in the speech frequencies, nor a lack of motivation to respond accurately, reversals could be considered evidence of cerebral dysfunction. Eighth nerve and brainstem cases typically do not have reversals.

The literature contains information which could be related to reversals. Efron (1963) studied temporal order for paired 10 msec. signals of 250 and 2500 Hz. They were presented monaurally with varying time delays between them. The patient indicated whether the high or low frequency signal came first.

The right hemisphere stroke patients were probably less efficient than normals at this task but they were superior to the left hemisphere, aphasic patients. One patient with left hemisphere damage but no aphasia behaved much like the right hemisphere cases on this task. The left hemisphere group was divided into two sub-groups. Those who were more "expressive aphasic" had greater difficulty on the auditory sequencing task. These patients tended to have lesions in the fronto-temporo-parietal region.

Luria (1970) also noted sequential difficulty in aphasic patients. He did not find these peculiarities in non-aphasic patients. He stated, "...most clear-cut impairment of sequential integration occurs with lesions in *the anterior parts of the temporal area*" (p. 268). By impairment of sequential integration, he means "the...patient is unable to retain a series of auditory signals in their original order" (p. 178).

The same author noted a similar phenomenon occurring with lesions in the "marginal" parts of the premotor area. Luria (1970) explained, "the patient no longer utters a whole meaningful complex ...Instead, the unit becomes the individual *word* or *syllable*" (p. 176). There is "...a loss of sentences in which the order of words does not correspond to the order of thoughts" (p. 177).

The auditory sequencing area of Efron (1963) as represented by Masland (1969, p. 108) and the regions described by Luria (1970) have been adapted to the brain diagram used in this study. Figure 6 shows Luria's premotor area (a), his sequencing integration area (b), and Efron's auditory sequencing area (c).

Prior to this study, we considered columns #6 and #7 (especially from row C to I), plus row #5 in the temporal lobe (rows, G, H and I) as the tentative "reversal strip." It is interesting to note that this conforms closely to the composite of Efron's and Luria's sequencing areas.

A fascinating study by Andrews, Pinheiro and Moore (in press) may shed light on the physiology of reversals. Auditory evoked responses (AER) were recorded in normal right-handed subjects. They were presented three signals (e.g., soft-loud-soft) in any one of six combinations. If the subject indicated a "mirror image," loud-soft-loud, this was called a reversal.

FIGURE 6. ══════════════════════════════════
Approximate regions of the brain associated with phenomena similar to reversing on the SSW test as described by Luria (1970), areas a and b, and Efron (1963), area c.

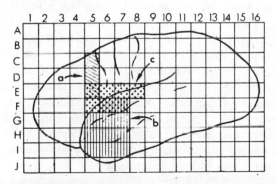

There were differences in the averaged AER's for correct responses as compared with the averaged AER's when the subjects had reversals. Of great interest was the observation that the differences in pattern were present *before the first signal was completed.* The patient could not have known at that time whether it was going to be the loud signal or the soft tone. This suggests that electrophysiological activity during or before the onset of the signal determines the perceived order. This fascinating approach by Andrews, Pinheiro and Moore appears to have considerable promise for studying reversals in normal and pathologic cases.

In the present study, we analyzed the performance of the 17 NAR cases on the SSW test. The AR cases were excluded from this analysis because the amount of errors could adversely influence the number of reversals. Nine of the 17 NAR subjects had reversals. They ranged from one maximum to 28 with a mean of 11.

It was our purpose to relate the site of lesion to the tentative reversal strip and the adjacent area: 1) to determine the hit-miss ratio based on the presence of reversals or no reversals; 2) to determine the region in which lesions are associated with the most reversals whether there is a gradient in the mean number of reversals.

In our previous work, we found no difference in the incidence of right or left hemisphere cases who had reversals. Neither was there any obvious difference in the number of reversals. For this reason, we felt justified in combining the information for patients with lesions in either hemisphere. To be sure that the entire reversal strip was analyzed, data were tabulated for columns #5 through #8 (see Figure 3) for the lateral and medial plates separately, as well as combined. Later, the analysis was extended to Column #4.

Table 3 shows the hit-miss ratio for each column (from row B to I). The data for the lateral plates (1 to 2cm deep), medial plates (3 to 4cm deep) and the combined lateral and medial sections are presented for the 17 NAR cases.

The table shows that column #6 has the best hit-miss ratio for the lateral plates. There were nine correct positives (correct hits). This shows that each subject in the sample who had a reversal was shown to have a lesion in at least one of the eight, 1cm boxes in column #6, laterally. There were four correct negatives. Thus, four subjects were correctly identified as not having a lesion in column #6 since they had no reversals. Another four cases were false negatives. This means that the test did not detect or signal the fact that column #6 was damaged, laterally. Finally, there were no false positive cases. A false positive error would be the worst type since it would identify a lesion as being in one place when it was indeed in another.

By combining the correct positive and correct negative cases, we find that 13 of the patients would have been properly classified (9 with damage to column #6 and 4 as sparing column #6). The total false cases (misdiagnosed) is four. Since the four were false negatives, we can assume that the presence of reversals is an excellent indicator of a lesion in the reversal strip but the absence of reversals cannot be taken as strong evidence that there is no dysfunction in the precentral gyrus.

Column #7 was almost as successful for purposes of diagnosis as #6 except for one false positive case. Since the most sensitive areas for reversals in the lateral plates are right next to each other (the pre- and post-central gyri), it is difficult to say if both are sensitive, if just one is sensitive, or whether the difference of 1 cm is too refined for this phase of the study.

The analysis of the medial plates shows that the diagnosis which was based on reversals would be less successful than the analysis of the lateral plates. Like E9, (the auditory reception center), the cortical region seems more sensitive than the deeper structures.

TABLE 3. ═══

The number of NAR subjects with correct positive (reversal strip column is damaged and the patient has reversals); correct negative (no damage in the particular reversal strip column and no reversals); false negative (damage to the reversal strip column but no reversals); and false positive responses (no damage in the particular reversal strip column but there are reversals). The hit-miss information is listed for the lateral and medial plates separately and combined.

Hit-Miss Ratio for Reversals with Lesions
in the Fronto-Temporo-Parietal Area

Plates	Column	Correct Positive	Correct Negative	False Negative	False Positive
Lateral	4		(Did Not Tabulate)		
	5	7	6	2	2
	6^	9	4	4	0
	7	8	4	4	1
	8	6	2	6	3
Medial	4		(Did Not Tabulate)		
	5	5	6	2	4
	6*	7	5	3	2
	7*	7	5	3	2
	8	4	4	4	5
Lateral	4	4	6	2	5
and	5	8	6	2	1
Medial	6*	9	4	4	0
	7	8	5	3	1
	8	6	4	4	3

*Column with best hit-miss ratio for diagnosing the lesions base on the presence of reversals.

The bottom portion of Table 3 shows the hit-miss relationship for the lateral and medial plates combined. Mean reversals for column #4 are shown here. It is clear that reversals provide very little diagnostic information about this area of the frontal lobe. There is some overall improvement in column #5, #7 and #8, but there is no change in the success for column #6. Since columns #6 and #7 are the best ones, we tried to obtain better predictability by combining them but there was no combination better than column #6, laterally.

The present results tend to support our previous finding with reversals and lesions in the area of the Fissure of Rolando. The motor and sensory strips, as well as the anterior temporal lobe appear to make up the reversal strip. There is some suggestion that the motor strip is more critical than the post central gyrus, however, this will require additional cases for confirmation. For the time being, we can consider the strip to be columns #6 and #7.

The presence of reversals is closely related to damage to the reversal strip. Our previous data suggested further specification of the level in the reversal strip based on the number of reversals. The region corresponding approximately to C6 and C7 was thought to be the most sensitive region. The cases with the greatest number of reversals had lesions in that area of the brain (and perhaps slightly below). The total reversals (questionable reversals were not counted) associated with that area was 12 or more. Below this zone but above the lateral fissure was the 6 to 12 zone and below this in the anterior temporal area we expected six or fewer reversals.

The mean number of maximum reversals for the 17 NAR subjects were calculated for a lesion involving each square. Figure 7 shows that the greatest number of reversals were found in cases who had lesions in row C.
The four subjects with the most reversals (10 to 28) had lesions in C6 or C7. Above and below row C, there were fewer mean reversals.

Figure 8 shows the same diagram with means based on only those subjects who had one or more reversals.
We can see a general trend for the scores to decrease from row C (or row B) down to row I. If the present means tend to hold up with additional cases, then there will be a slight change in the number of maximum reversals associated with the reversal strip.

The literature suggests that there are aphasia-related phenomena which are similar to the reversals seen on the SSW test. Efron (1963) and Luria (1970) indicate that these are found when there is damage to the left hemisphere. We therefore divided up the 17 NAR cases to see if more of the patients with left hemisphere lesions had reversals. On the contrary, six of the cases had damage to the right hemisphere and three

FIGURE 7 ▄▄▄▄▄▄▄▄▄▄▄▄▄▄▄▄▄▄▄▄▄▄

Means of maximum reversals on the SSW test for the 17 NAR cases. The reversals, if any, were averaged for each subject whose lesion involved each of the squares. The smallest dots show boxes with mean reversals of three to five; the middle size dots represent six to seven reversals; and the largest dots stand for eight to nine reversals.

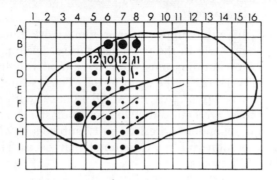

FIGURE 8 ▄▄▄▄▄▄▄▄▄▄▄▄▄▄▄▄▄▄▄▄▄▄▄▄▄▄▄▄▄▄▄▄

Mean performance for the nine NAR subjects average for each square. The dots represent boxes with two or fewer entries.

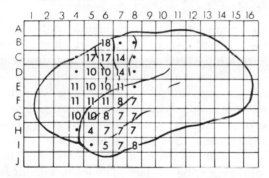

to the left. Four right and four left hemisphere cases were free of reversals. When the AR subjects were added, there was an equal number of reversal cases in both hemisphere groups (7). Six right hemisphere cases and 10 left had no reversals.

Many brain lesion patients have reversals. Our data suggest that the audiologist can have reasonable confidence that such cases have involvement in columns #6 and/or #7, laterally in either hemisphere. The number of reversals can give some further clues in localizing the lesion.

Summary and Conclusion

This study investigated a sample of 30 patients with well-localized lesions in the cerebrum. The lesion was drawn in a three-dimensional field by a neurologist based primarily on surgical and autopsy information. The SSW test of central auditory function was administered and the results were compared.

In general, this study supports our previous work, but also permits refinements not possible in the previous studies. Lesions to Heschl's gyrus (labeled E9 on our diagrams) produced a moderate to severe corrected SSW (C-SSW) score in the opposite ear. These subjects are referred to as auditory reception (AR) cases. All 13 cases with moderate or severe C-SSW scores were judged by the neurologist as having damage to E9 based on independent criteria. The 17 subjects in which E9 was spared were called non-auditory reception (NAR) cases. They had normal or mild C-SSW scores.

The literature suggests that corpus callosum lesions will produce a decreased score in the non-dominant ear for language. Such cases and those having bilaterally depressed performance were not included in the main part of the study because they were questionable neurological cases. It is thought that word discrimination scores and other standard hearing tests can help to differentiate corpus callosal lesions (NAR problem) from true AR disorders.

Reversals are an intriguing phenomenon noted on the SSW test. They (and other forms of response bias, not included in this paper) seem to contain information which can help to localize brain lesions outside of the AR centers. There is a "reversal strip" which grossly speaking involves the pre- and post-central gyri, as well as the anterior temporal lobe. The number of reversals can aid in narrowing down the diagnosis. The presence of reversals can be considered good evidence that the brain lesion affects this area but the absence of reversals does not necessarily mean that the reversals strip is spared. The tendency to reverse does not seem to be influenced by lesions in one hemisphere or the other.

Additional subjects are needed before final criteria can be established for reversals. The "tentative" norms for the C-SSW scores (Katz, 1968) seem to have held up well for several years of clinical practice. The present data show that they are appropriate for identifying AR lesions. We can safely delete the word "tentative."

The use of the brain diagram divided into 1cm cubes seems to be a useful approach for studying pathological effects on the auditory system. There is little doubt that the SSW test can be a differential diagnostic aid in the evaluation of patients with cerebral disorders.

Acknowledgements

The authors would like to acknowledge the guidance of Arthur Epstein for setting up the study criteria, and Deanie Kushner, Max McClellan, and Iris Shur for contributing cases used in this investigation.

References

1. Andrews, L. T., Pinheiro, M. L. and Moore, A. R.: Auditory evoked potentials in accurate and reversed pattern perception. In press.

2. Balas, R. F.: Results of the staggered spondaic test with an old age population. Unpublished Masters Thesis, Northern Illinois University, 1962.

3. Baru, A. V. and Karaseva, T. A.: The brain and hearing: Hearing disturbances associated with local brain lesions. New York Consultants Bureau, 1972.

4. Bocca, E. Calearo, C. and Cassinari, V.: A new method for testing hearing in temporal lobe tumors; preliminary report. *Acta Otolaryngol.*, 44:210, 1954.

5. Brunt, M. A.: The staggered spondaic word test. In Katz, J. (Ed.) *Handbook of Clinical Audiology.* Baltimore, Maryland, Williams and Wilkins Co., 1972, p. 334–356.

6. Brunt, M. A. and Goetzinger, C. P.: A study of three tests of central function with normal subjects. *Cortex,* 4:288, 1968.

7. Curry, F. K. W.: A comparison of left-handed and right-handed subjects on verbal and non-verbal dichotic listening tasks. *Cortex,* 3:343, 1972.

8. Efron, R.: Temporal perception, aphasia and deja vu. *Brain,* 86:402, 1963.

9. Elliott, H. C.: *Textbook of Neuroanatomy,* second edition. Philadelphia, Pennsylvania, J. B. Lippincott Company, 1963, p. 357.

10. Goetzinger, C. P.: The Rush Hughes test in auditory diagnosis. In Katz, J. (Ed.), *Handbook of Clinical Audiology.* Baltimore, Maryland, Williams and Wilkins Co., 1972, p. 325–333.

11. Goldman, S. O. and Katz, J.: A comparison of normal hearing subjects on the SSW test given under four conditions—dichotic, diotic, monaural (dominant ear) and monaural (non-dominant ear). Paper presented at American Speech and Hearing Association Convention, Chicago, Illinois, 1966.

12. Katz, J.: The use of staggered spondaic words for assessing the integrity of the central auditory nervous system. *J. Aud. Res.,* 2:327, 1962.

13. Katz, J.: The SSW test: An interim report. *J. Speech Hear. Disord.,* 33:132, 1968.

14. Katz, J: Audiologic diagnosis: cochlea to cortex. *Menorah Med. J.,* 1:25, 1970.

15. Katz, J., Basil, R. and Smith, J.: A staggered spondaic word test for detecting central auditory lesions. *Ann. Oto. Rhino. Laryngol.,* 72:908, 1963.

16. Katz, J. and Illmer, R.: Auditory perception in children with learning disabilities. In Katz, J. (Ed.), *Handbook of Clinical Audiology.* Baltimore, Maryland, Williams and Wilkins Company, 1972, pp. 552–554.

17. Kimura, D.: Cerebral dominance and the perception of verbal stimuli. *Can. J. Psychol.,* 15:166, 1961.

18. Kimura, D.: Left-right differences in the perception of melodies. *Q. J. Exp. Psychol.,* 16:335, 1964.

19. Luria, A. R.: Traumatic Aphasia. *The Hague & Paris:* Mouton Co., 104–141, 267–268 (1970).

20. Masland, R. L.: Paper presented to Orton Society. "Brain Mechanisms Underlying the Language Function." Reprinted in *Human Communication and Its Disorders—An Overall View.* National Advisory Neurological Diseases and Stroke Council, 85–109, 1969.

21. Matzker, J.: Two new methods for the assessment of central auditory functions in cases of brain disease. *Ann. Otol. Rhinol. Laryngol.*, 68:1185, 1959.

22. McClellan, M. Wertz, R. T. and Collins, M. J.: The effects of interhemispheric lesions on central auditory behavior. Presented at the American Speech and Hearing Association Convention, Detroit, Michigan, 1973.

23. deQuiros, J. B.: Accellerated Speech Audiometry. An examination of Test Results. In Translations of the Beltone Institute for Hearing Research, 17. 1964. Based on Interpretation de los resultados obtenidos con logoaudiometrica accolerada. Revista Fonoaudiologica, 7, 128–164, 1961.

24. Schiller, F.: Dysarthria, aphasia and apraxia. *In* Haymaker, W. (Ed.), *Bing's Local Diagnosis in Neurological Diagnosis* (15th edition). St. Louis, Missouri, C. V. Mosby Co., 1969, pp. 397–403.

25. Schiller, F. and Haymaker, W.: Disturbances of behavior, memory, awareness, smell, taste and hearing. *In* Haymaker, W. (Ed.), *Bing's Local Diagnosis in Neurological Diagnosis* (15th edition). St. Louis, Missouri, C. V. Mosby Co., 1969, pp. 379–396.

26. Shankweiler, D.: Effects of temporal-lobe damage on perception of dichotically presented melodies. *J. Comp. Physiol. Psychol.*, 62:115, 1966.

27. Sparks, R. and Geschwind, M.: Dichotic listening in man after section of neocortical commissures. *Cortex*, 4:3, 1968.

28. Walsh, T. and Goodman, A.: Speech discrimination in central auditory lesions. *Laryngoscope*, 65:1, 1955.

29. Young, E.: Personal Communication, 1971.

The Use of Competing Speech (SSW) and Environmental Sound (CES) Tests for Localizing Brain Lesions

Jack Katz, Deanie Kushner and Gary Pack

SSW Test

To evaluate central auditory function. Different spondees go to each ear, partially overlapped in time. Listener repeats all words heard.

SSW Test: identifies lesions in various parts of the brain and brainstem. It indicates intrahemispheric dysfunction but frequently gives no indication of

Poster Session, ASHA Convention, Washington, D.C., 1975

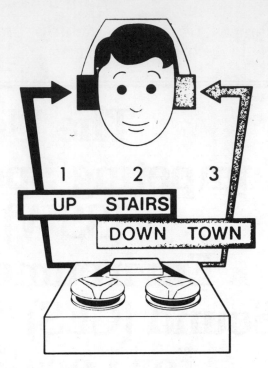

the damaged hemisphere. In some cases (presumably due to corpus callosum lesions) performance is depressed in the nondominant ear regardless of which hemisphere is involved.

Competing
Environmental Sound (CES) Test

Supplements the SSW Test as a measure of central auditory function. Different familiar sounds are presented to each ear at the same time.

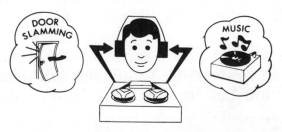

Advanced Use of the Staggered Spondaic Word Test

Two choices from four pictures facilitate the response to each of the 20 items.

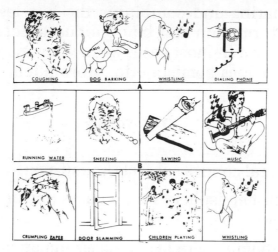

Music and environmental sounds are thought to be dominant in the right hemisphere (better in the left ear). This could aid in identifying lesions to interhemispheric pathways because CES Test errors would peak in one ear and SSW Test errors would peak in the other ear.

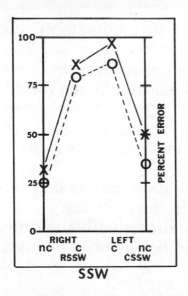

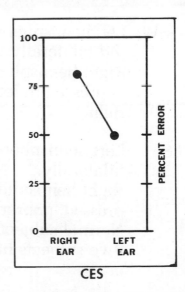

Relationship Between SSW & CES

By comparing and combining the two tests, additional information can be obtained to identify the side of lesion in most cases even when neither test, alone, provides hemispheric information.

Subjects

27 Normal control subjects (mean age—32 years)

10 Right hemisphere lesion cases (mean age—52 years)

10 Left hemisphere lesion cases (mean age—48 years)
(pathological cases had strokes, tumors and traumatic lesions).

Results (median values)

R-SSW: Left hemisphere cases moderately depressed bilaterally.
Right hemisphere cases severely depressed in left ear, mildly depressed in right.

CES: Left hemisphere cases mildly depressed bilaterally.
Right hemisphere cases moderately depressed, poorer in the right ear.
Normal subjects almost without error (two subjects had one error in the right ear).

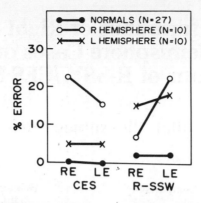

MEDIAN SCORES FOR NORMALS AND RIGHT AND LEFT HEMISPHERE
LESION CASES. THE R-SSW RESULTS FOR NORMALS ARE FROM
10 SUBJECTS RANDOMLY SELECTED FROM ANOTHER STUDY (M.
BRUNT). THE MEAN AGE FOR THE LATTER GROUP WAS 50 YEARS.

There was considerable overlap between pathological groups. However, certain relationships among the CES/R-SSW scores were noted which distinguished the right from the left hemisphere cases.

SSW & CES Scores

The percent of error for R-SSW and CES are compared separately for each ear.

TEST	RE	LE
R–SSW	A	B
CES	-C	-D
DIFFERENCE	Δ_R	Δ_L

Eight comparisons helped to differentiate the two pathological groups. Odd numbered comparisons resemble right hemisphere lesion cases and even numbered resemble left hemisphere cases.

Performance of Right and Left Hemisphere Cases on Eight Comparisons of R-SSW/CES Scores

A "+" shows that the subject met the stated criterion.

Side of Lesion Typified	Comparison	Hemisphere of Lesion Right					Left				
		1	2	3	4	5	1	2	3	4	5
	S's	6	7	8	9	10	6	7	8	9	10
1. R	$B+C \geqslant (A+D) + 10$	+	+	+	−	+	−	−	−	−	−
		+	+	−	+	−	−	−	−	−	−
2. L	$A+D \geqslant (B+C) + 10$	−	−	−	−	−	−	−	+	−	−
		−	−	−	−	−	−	−	−	+	−
3. R	$\Delta_R - \Delta_L \leqslant -10$ (ie, −10, −11...)	+	+	+	−	+	−	−	−	−	−
		+	+	−	+	+	−	−	−	−	−
4. L	$\Delta_R - \Delta_L \geqslant -0$ (ie, 0, 1...)	−	−	−	−	−	+	+	+	−	−
		−	−	+	−	−	+	+	−	+	+
5. R	$\Delta_R + \Delta_L \leqslant -10$ (ie, −10, −11...)	+	+	+	−	+	−	−	−	−	−
		+	+	−	+	−	−	−	−	+	−
6. L	$\Delta_R - \Delta_L \geqslant -25$ (ie, 25, 26...)	−	−	−	−	−	+	−	+	+	−
		−	−	−	−	−	−	−	+	−	−
7. R	$(A+B) - (C+D) \leqslant -25$ (ie, 25, 26...)	−	+	−	−	−	−	−	−	−	−
		−	−	−	+	−	−	−	−	−	−
8.* L	$(A+B) - (C+D) \geqslant 25$ (ie, 25, 26...)	−	−	−	−	−	−	+	+	−	+
		+	−	−	−	−	−	−	+	−	−

* #8 can be positive because of poor discrimination (regardless of involved hemisphere) as was noted in one right hemisphere case. If #8 is positive but the other signs are for the right hemisphere and the patient has poor discrimination, the left hemisphere sign can be disregarded.

Hit/Miss Ratio Using SSW/CES Comparisons

Each subject is listed separately. The hit number listed for each S represents the number of "+s" correctly indicating the damaged hemisphere (a possible total of four). Miss number indicates the total "+s" that indicated a dysfunction in the wrong (opposite) hemisphere (a possible total of four).

The hemisphere receiving the greater number of "+s" was considered the resulting diagnosis.

10 right hemisphere cases: eight correctly identified, one incorrect, and one case was so normal on SSW and CES that no indicators were significant.

10 left hemisphere cases: all 10 were correctly identified.

Right Hemisphere	Cases										Resulting
Indicators	# 1	2	3	4	5	6	7	8	9	10	Diagnosis
Hits (Indicating R-Hemis.)	3	4	3	0	3	3	3	0	4	1	8
Misses (Indicating L-Hemis.)	0	0	0	0	0	1	0	1	0	0	1

Left Hemisphere	Cases										Resulting
Indicators	# 1	2	3	4	5	6	7	8	9	10	Diagnosis
Hits (Indicating L-Hemis.)	2	2	4	1	1	1	1	2	2	1	10
Misses (Indicating R-Hemis.)	0	0	0	0	0	0	0	0	1	0	0

The damaged hemisphere was correctly identified in 90% of the cases using the SSW/CES comparisons. 10% were not identified at all or the wrong hemisphere was identified. It is interesting that the patient who was mislabeled was left handed. The patient for whom there were no hemispheric indications had no difficulty on either SSW or CES.

Case Study

A 37-year-old male had experienced increasing seizures with temporal lobe automatisms. ⓛ arteriovenous malformation was the diagnosis.

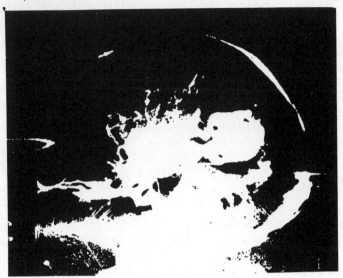

SSW results: severely depressed bilaterally. CES results: one error in each ear.

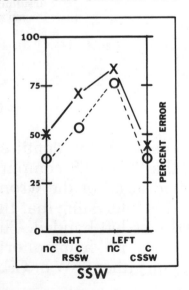

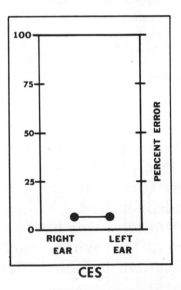

Advanced Use of the Staggered Spondaic Word Test

Since the central speech test was depressed bilaterally and the central environmental sound test was almost normal bilaterally, we can presume that left hemisphere function was impaired (speech) and that the right hemisphere was essentially intact (environmental sounds). In order to check this, eight comparisons were made of the R-SSW/CES tests.

	RE		LE
	59		66
	− 5		− 5
	54		61

1	R	71	⩾ 74	−
2	L	64	⩾ 81	−
3	R	−7	⩽ −10	−
4	L	−7	⩾ 0	−
5	R	115	⩽ −10	−
6	L	115	⩾ 25	+
7	R	115	⩽ −25	−
8	L	115	⩾ 25	+

There were two indicators of left hemisphere disorder and none supporting right hemisphere involvement.

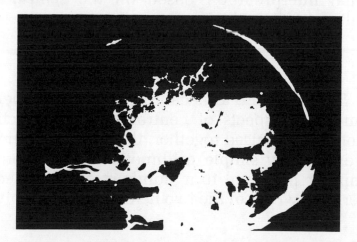

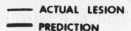

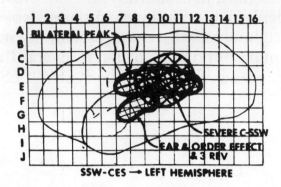

SSW-CES → LEFT HEMISPHERE

The SSW scores and response bias suggested a dysfunction in the area shown below. This agrees with the drawing made of the area of dysfunction by the audiologist.

The blue area (circular area in columns 8–12 and rows C–F) is the neurosurgeon's (S. Rengachary, M.D.) drawing of the lesion and the red area (the two eliptical areas defined in columns 7–12, rows C–E and columns 7–8 rows F–G) represents the audiological interpretation based on the central test results.

Summary

The SSW and CES tests can be used independently to measure aspects of central auditory function. When they are used together, there is an additional advantage. By simple arithmetic computation (or computer program) four numbers can be used to determine which of the two hemisphere is involved.

AUDIOLOGIC DIAGNOSIS: COCHLEA TO CORTEX [*]

Jack Katz, Ph.D.

For a number of years Jerger (1960) and others have recommended the test battery approach to audiologic diagnosis. This concept is based on the knowledge that no one test can be relied upon to signify the underlying pathology without error. The reasons for this limitation include: a) the inaccuracies of the tests themselves; b) the error introduced by the patient's inattention and response set; c) contamination of the results by more than one locus of lesion; and d) the lack of positive findings due to a mild loss of hearing function.

In recent years the demand for comprehensive audiologic evaluation has grown. As new anatomical, physiological and pathological information about the auditory system is revealed the investigators attempt to gather evidence to locate or rule out these conditions. New tests and combinations of test results have been used to make these finer discriminations. Presently, the studies of the auditory system are geared toward problems from the outer ear up to and including the primary reception centers of the brain. The present paper will discuss hearing test procedures and their use in analyzing the system from the

---

[*] Based on a paper presented at the American Speech and Hearing Association Convention, November 13, 1969, Chicago, Illinois.

Menorah Medical Journal, 1, 25–38, 1970.

cochlea to the temporal lobe into five categories. The procedures will include classical techniques like Fowler's (1936) test of recruitment as well as newer tests such as the continuous tone masking test, developed at Menorah Medical Center (Katz, 1969).

In the past 25 years there has been considerable refinement in auditory analysis. After World War II the audiologist had only to contend with conductive and "nerve" (now called sensory-neural) problems. Since 1948 (Dix, Hallpike and Hood), nerve losses have been subdivided functionally (and anatomically) into sensory (cochlear) and neural (retrocochlear) dysfunction. Dix, Hallpike and Hood (1948) showed that individuals with cochlear problems like Meniere's disease demonstrate recruitment while patients with retrocochlear disorders like VIII nerve tumors do not. In 1954, Bocca, Calearo and Cassinari reported that temporal lobe tumors could be localized by auditory tests although there was no hearing loss for pure tones. Performance was depressed on "difficult-speech" tests of hearing, primarily in the ear contralateral to the damaged hemisphere. Further study revealed that the reception center (Heschl's gyrus) rather than the entire temporal lobe was the area most easily isolated by the auditory tests (Katz, 1968).

Based on recent findings retrocochlear disease can be divided into three parts (Cozad and Katz, 1968). Thus we presently have a five-category analysis of the sensory-neural system. This does not include the conductive system, peripheral to the cochlea, nor the cortical system beyond the reception centers.

The Test Battery

Before any special tests are given pure tone air and bone conduction tests are administered. These two techniques have been the mainstay of audiology for many years and remain valuable measures for diagnosis and description. With the addition of word discrimination testing (WDS) we have a good indication whether further diagnostic study is necessary. Subtle problems may not be revealed by the basic test battery. Therefore, the case history, information from medical tests or the physician's suspicions are critical for selecting the proper tests.

Two common special tests for cochlear disease are the loudness balance and short increment sensitivity index (SISI) tests. When the binaural loudness balance (ABLB) test (Fowler, 1936) cannot be given, the monaural (MLB) test (Reger and Kos, 1952) may be used. The SISI test (Jerger, Shedd, and Harford, 1959) can be used with patients having unilateral or bilateral hearing loss of at least 40 to 45 dB ISO (Owens, 1965).

Bekesy audiometry (Bekesy, 1947) can designate either cochlear or retrocochlear disorders (Jerger, 1960). Bekesy audiometry also provides another dimension. Unlike most of the other tests the intensity of the signal is automatically changed by the patient's response. While the earlier tone decay tests (Carhart, 1957) were used to identify retrocochlear problems, the Owens (1964) procedure may be used to evaluate both cochlear and retrocochlear disease.

Because of the insensitivity of auditory tests to mild losses the continuous tone masking (CTM) test was developed (Katz, 1969). This procedure is based on Bekesy audiometry except that a continuous tone and a pulsed tone of the same frequency are presented to the same ear. The patient tracks his sensitivity to the pulsed tone by use of the Bekesy response switch. The patterns may reveal cochlear and/or retrocochlear signs even with very mild lesions. Hopefully, this will enable early identification of these disorders.

Cerebral function may be analyzed by use of the Rush Hughes difference test (Goetzinger and Angell, 1965) which is a difficult-speech test. Another approach is the SSW test (Katz, 1962, 1968) a competing message procedure for measuring central auditory function. It was designed to study cerebral reception but also provides information about other areas of the auditory system.

Five Auditory Subdivisions

The area from the cochlea to the temporal lobe can be divided by auditory test patterns into five categories (with the aid of the caloric test). Figure 1 shows the five subdivisions.

The Cochlea.

The cochlear subdivision, which includes the sensory apparatus within the boney shell, is the first step in the sensory-neural process. At this point mechanical energy is translated into bioelectrical signals.

The VIII Nerve.

The VIII nerve portion is shown to include the ipsilateral cochlear nuclei of the brain stem as well as the VIII nerve proper. This has been done because of our inability to differentiate these two areas at the present time.

The Lower Brain Stem.

The nerve fibers in the lowest portion of the auditory brain stem beyond the cochlear nuclei are known to split into two bundles. It is thought that the majority of the fibers cross over and ascend the contralateral brain stem. It is not clear how high this subsection goes giving a consistent audiologic picture. It is fair to say that it reaches at least to the superior olivary area.

FIGURE 1.
Five functional subdivisions from the cochlea to the cortex.

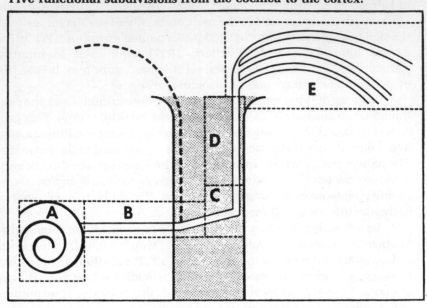

	Diseased Area and Ear under Test	Tests Giving Positive Results
A	Cochlear Ipsilateral Ear	Alternate Binaural Loudness Balance (ABLB). A monaural (MLB) procedure is used when ABLB is not appropriate. Short Increment Sensitivity Index (SISI) Bekesy Audiometry (Bekesy). Cochlear pattern (Type II). Tone Decay (TD)—Cochlear Pattern on Owens test. Continuous Tone Masking Test (CTM)—Cochlear Pattern.
B	VIII Nerve Ipsilateral Ear	Bekesy Audiometry—Retrocochlear pattern (Type III). Tone Decay—Retrocochlear pattern on Owens test. Continuous Tone Masking. Retrocochlear pattern. Word Discrimination Score (WDS) (Using recorded W-22 lists) Score severely depressed relative to pure tone thresholds. Vestibular Tests (V)—Such as

		caloric (given by physician) or electronystagmography.
C	**Lower Brain Stem Ipsilateral Ear**	Bekesy Audiometry—Retrocochlear pattern (Type III).
		Tone Decay—Retrocochlear pattern on Owens test.
		Continuous Tone Masking—Retrocochlear pattern.
		Word Discrimination Score—severely depressed relative to pure tone thresholds.
D	**Upper Brain Stem Primarily Ipsilateral Ear when bilaterally affected**	Beksey Audiometry—Retrocochlear pattern (Type III).
		Tone Decay—Retrocochlear pattern on Owens Test.
		Continuous Tone Masking—Retrocochlear pattern.
		Word Discrimination Score—Moderately depressed relative to pure tone thresholds.
		Staggered Spondaic Word Test (SSW). Corrected (C-SSW) depressed in ipsilateral ear.
E	**Cerebral Reception Contralateral Ear**	Staggered Spondaic Word Test. Corrected (C-SSW) depressed in contralateral ear.
		Rush Hughes Test (RH). Score depressed relative to WDS also filtered speech and other tests.

The Upper Brain Stem.

The upper functional limit of the upper portion of the auditory brain stem is no doubt the medial geniculate body. This segment of the brain stem when damaged shows a different audiologic picture from the lower portion.

The Primary Auditory Reception Center.

The auditory radiations and the primary auditory reception centers are often considered the highest area in the auditory hierarchy. Functionally this subsection starts in the area of the basal ganglion and ends in the middle and posterior portion of the superior temporal gyrus.

For the purpose of this paper we shall limit our discussion to these five units although we feel that auditory damage can be recognized in other parts of the CNS. Research into other auditory centers is in progress.

Auditory Tests Useful in Identifying Each of Five Subdivisions

Figure 1 and the associated chart show the audiologic procedures which may be used to identify lesions in the five auditory areas. These tests characteristically show positive results with lesions in the specific area. In addition, we expect negative findings on all other tests. Of course, where multiple auditory lesions exist the results of a lesion not under investigation may cause confusion. By judicious use of various tests at various frequencies the portions of the loss corresponding to each locus usually can be isolated.

Cochlear Dysfunction   Hearing loss (reduced sensitivity for sound such as on a pure tone test) is most easily produced by damage to the cochlea. The loss of clarity for speech (word discrimination problem) is related to the extent of the hearing loss and to the specific tones involved. Before positive results are expected on the SISI and Bekesy tests there needs to be a moderate loss of hearing sensitivity. The ABLB test and especially CTM are valuable because they show positive results even with mild conditions. Cochlear problems of 30 dB ISO or even less can be detected by means of the CTM test.

VIII Nerve Dysfunction   Hearing sensitivity for pure tones is less vulnerable with VIII nerve lesions. Sometimes a large tumor produces only a mild or moderate loss of hearing for pure tones but WDS and tone decay may be greatly affected. The breakdown on these two tests are out of proportion to the amount of hearing loss. However, VIII nerve disease can affect WDS and tone decay even when pure tone thresholds are relatively normal.

Lower Brain Stem Dysfunction   For lower brain stem lesions as in the previous subdivisions, hearing loss is shown in the ipsilateral ear. As with VIII nerve lesion the discrimination problem is great compared to the pure tone loss. Tone decay is also highly significant in that the tone continues to fade away or becomes a noise. A lesion to one side usually spares hearing on the other side (Horrax, 1927), especially when the lesion is small. Low brain stem lesions are often difficult to differentiate from VIII nerve lesions on the same side. The caloric test can be used to differentiate the VIII nerve from lower brain stem lesions because vestibular function is more often intact in brain stem cases.

High Brain Stem Dysfunction   High brain stem lesions on one side typically affect the ipsilateral ear more than the other. This is the highest level to affect the ipsilateral ear. As the lesion increases in size, the contralateral system may become involved too. For high brain stem disease, significant tone decay is present but WDS is not as severely affected as for VIII nerve and low stem lesions. When simple discrimination ability remains fairly good in high brain stem cases, Rush Hughes-difference and other difficult-speech tests are effective in breaking down performance, ipsilaterally. We have found the SSW test a good indicator of high stem lesions. The SSW test score remains depressed ispilaterally even after correction for the WDS (C-SSW score). In high brain stem lesions we see that both the cerebral and the retrocochlear tests are positive in the same ear. The diagnosis would be much different if the cochlear (or retrocochlear) tests were positive for one ear and the cerebral tests positive in the other ear. This suggests a vascular lesion on the side of the peripheral problem which also affects the brain on that side:

Primary Auditory Reception   The fifth level, that of cerebral auditory reception, does not involve hearing loss per se (except perhaps in the rare instance of a bilateral lesion). The patient has normal results for pure tones and even for WDS. However, he has difficulty on the SSW test, the Rush Hughes-difference test, filtered speech tests and others. Our findings and those at other centers (Berlin, Chase, Dill and Hageponos, 1965; Lynn and Gonzalez, 1969) show that the SSW test is extremely sensitive to superior temporal gyrus lesions and is rarely positive in the contralateral ear unless this area is functioning improperly, regardless of dominance for language. This contralateral effect is demonstrated on all cerebral reception tests except on ones in which langauge dominance tends to overshadow the presence of a lesion (Kimura, 1961).

Case Studies

Case A.   Cochlear-Meniere's Disease

Meniere's disease is often considered the prototype for cochlear impairment. The results of the special tests in this case are similar to those obtained with other cochlear problems like noise-induced hearing loss, certain ototoxic lesions and vascular disease. Figure 2 shows the audiometric results for a 42-year-old woman who was diagnosed as having right, Meniere's disease. Hearing loss, WDS, SISI, tone decay (cochlear type) were all positive in the right ear and indicated the cochlear disease. An equivocal finding was partial recruitment.

FIGURE 2.

Case A, age 42, female, diagnosis: Right Ear, Meniere's Disease (Cochlear Pathology).

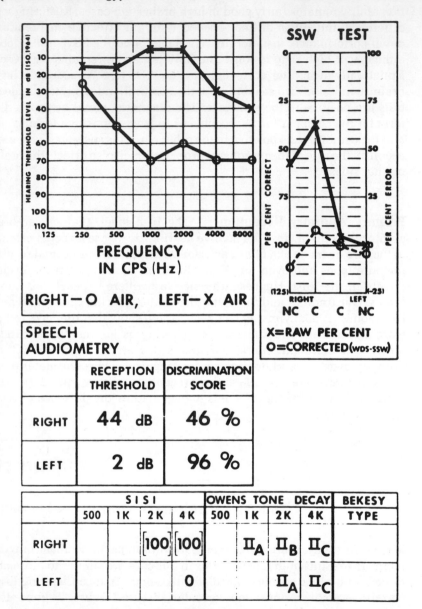

RIGHT—O AIR, LEFT—X AIR

SPEECH AUDIOMETRY

	RECEPTION THRESHOLD	DISCRIMINATION SCORE
RIGHT	44 dB	46 %
LEFT	2 dB	96 %

	SISI				OWENS TONE DECAY				BEKESY
	500	1K	2K	4K	500	1K	2K	4K	TYPE
RIGHT			[100]	[100]			II$_A$	II$_B$	II$_C$	
LEFT				0			II$_A$	II$_C$	

A.B.L.B.=PARTIAL RECUITMENT

Case B.   VIII Nerve-Tumor.

Tumors in the cerebellopontine region are used to typify VIII nerve disease. The results are consistent with those of vascular lesions and ototoxic disorders of the auditory nerve. Figure 3 demonstrates the results of a 32-year-old woman whose left VIII nerve tumor was confirmed at surgery. Hearing level for pure tones, WDS, tone decay, CTM and Bekesy audiometry were all positive in the left ear and demonstrate the retrocochlear condition. Contaminating results were on the SISI and ABLB tests which suggest a cochlear overlay for the high frequencies.

Case C.   Low Brain Stem-Tumor.

The audiologic and otologic literature are very sparse on the topic of brain stem pathology. This is surprising since brain stem problems often mimic VIII nerve lesions. Aside from vascualr pathology, multiple sclerosis affects this region not infrequently. Figure 4 presents the audiometric results for a 43-year-old man who had low brain stem tumor on the left side which was visualized during exploratory surgery. Hearing loss, WDS, tone decay and Bekesy audiometry identified the retrocochlear lesion. The caloric test was negative. There were no equivocal or conflicting results.

Case D.   Upper Brain Stem-Tumor.

Because the brain stem is so compact it is difficult to determine which lesion or lesions produced specific effects on diagnostic tests. We have both vascular and tumor cases to support our diagnostic conclusions. Figure 5 shows audiometric findings for a 15-year-old girl with a left tumor involving the fourth ventricle confirmed at autopsy. Hearing loss, WDS, apparent tone decay (noted on standard pure tone test) ;and SSW were positive in the left ear.

Case E.   Cortical Auditory Reception-Tumor.

Since the middle 1950's audiologists have concerned themselves with disorders of auditory reception but only recently has there been wide interest in this problem. Auditory tests are sensitive to space-occupying lesions as well as vascular insufficiency to Heschl's gyrus. Subcortical disorder as low as the basal ganglion can be noted on these tests in the ear contralateral to the disease. Figure 6 illustrates the results for a 47-year-old man with a lesion in the left tempro-parietal-occiptal region which was confirmed at surgery. The SSW result was highly positive in the right ear indicating the left reception lesion. As in some of these severe cases WDS was also affected to some extent.

FIGURE 3.
Case B, age 32, female, diagnosis: Left Ear, VIII Nerve Tumor.

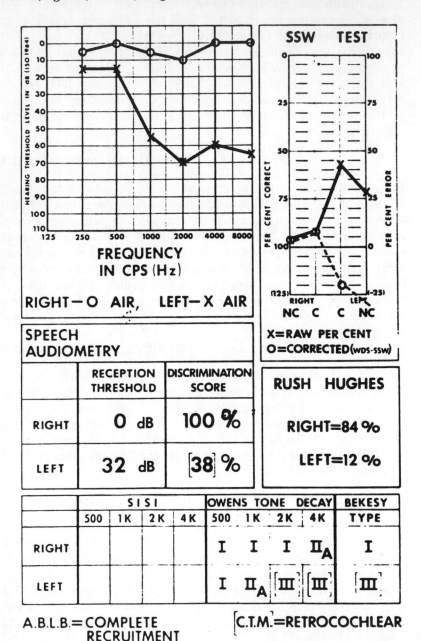

Advanced Use of the Staggered Spondaic Word Test

FIGURE 4. ═══════════════════════

Case C, age 43, male, diagnosis: Left Sided, Low Brain Stem Tumor.

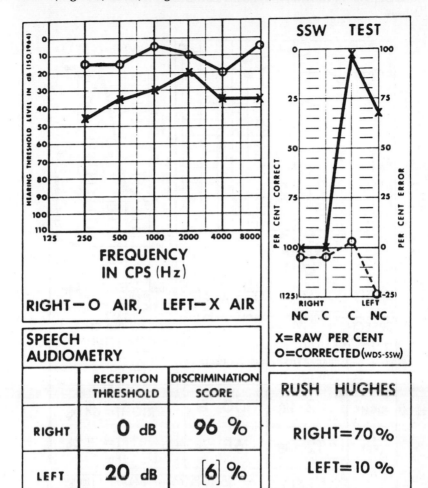

RIGHT—O AIR, LEFT—X AIR

SSW TEST

X=RAW PER CENT
O=CORRECTED(WDS-SSW)

SPEECH AUDIOMETRY	RECEPTION THRESHOLD	DISCRIMINATION SCORE
RIGHT	0 dB	96 %
LEFT	20 dB	[6] %

RUSH HUGHES

RIGHT=70 %

LEFT=10 %

	SISI				OWENS TONE DECAY				BEKESY
	500	1K	2K	4K	500	1K	2K	4K	TYPE
RIGHT		0		0					I
LEFT	0	0	15	5	[III]	[III]	[III]	[III]	[III]

A.B.L.B.=NEGATIVE

FIGURE 5.

Case D, age 15, female, diagnosis: Left Sided, High Brain Stem Tumor.

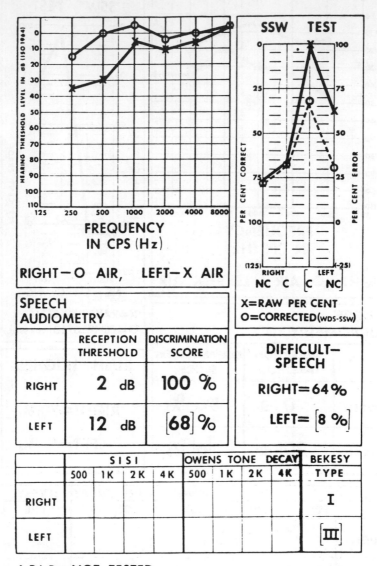

RIGHT—O AIR, LEFT—X AIR

SSW TEST

X=RAW PER CENT
O=CORRECTED(WDS-SSW)

SPEECH AUDIOMETRY	RECEPTION THRESHOLD	DISCRIMINATION SCORE
RIGHT	2 dB	100 %
LEFT	12 dB	[68] %

DIFFICULT— SPEECH

RIGHT=64%

LEFT= [8 %]

	SISI				OWENS TONE DECAY				BEKESY
	500	1K	2K	4K	500	1K	2K	4K	TYPE
RIGHT									I
LEFT									[III]

A.B.L.B.=NOT TESTED

FIGURE 6.

Case E, age 47, male, diagnosis: Left Tempro-Parietal-Occiptal Tumor, Involving the Auditory Reception Center

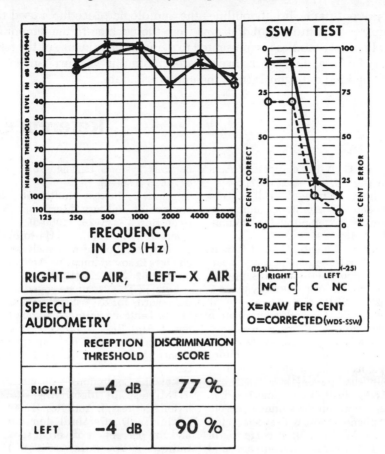

RIGHT—O AIR, LEFT—X AIR

SSW TEST

X=RAW PER CENT
O=CORRECTED (WDS-SSW)

SPEECH AUDIOMETRY

	RECEPTION THRESHOLD	DISCRIMINATION SCORE
RIGHT	−4 dB	77 %
LEFT	−4 dB	90 %

	SISI				OWENS TONE DECAY				BEKESY
	500	1K	2K	4K	500	1K	2K	4K	TYPE
RIGHT									
LEFT									

A.B.L.B.=NOT TESTED

Summary

The present paper briefly outlines the audiologic procedures used to identify lesions in five subdivisions from the cochlea to the temporal lobe. Five case studies are presented to demonstrate the use of the test battery for localizing lesions in each area. A simplified chart is given to aid in making a diagnosis from the audiologic data.

References

Bekesy, G., A new audiometer. Acta Otolaryng. 35, 411–422 (1947).

Berlin, C., Chase, R., Dill A., and Hagepanos, T., Auditory findings in patients with temporal lobectomies. ASHA 7, 386 (1965).

Bocca, E., Calearo, C., and Cassinari, V., A new method for testing hearing in temporal lobe tumours; preliminary report. Acta Otolaryng., 44, 219–221 (1954).

Carhart, R., Clinical determination of abnormal auditory adaptations. Arch. Otolaryng., 65, 32–39 (1957).

Cozad, R., and Katz, J., Auditory symptoms of brain stem pathology. Unpublished paper (1968).

Dix, M., Hallpike, C., and Hood, J., Observations on the loudness recruitment phenomenon, with special reference to the differential diagnosis of disorders of the internal ear and eighth nerve. Proc. Roy. Soc. Med., 41, 516–526 (1948).

Fowler, E., A method for the early detection of otosclerosis: A study of sounds well above threshold. Arch. Otolaryng., 24, 39–49 (1965).

Goetzinger, C., and Angell, S., Audiological assessment in acoustic tumors and cortical lesions. EENT Monthly, 44, 39–49 (1965).

Horrax, G., Differential diagnosis of tumors primarily pineal and primarily pontile. Arch. Neurol. Psych. 17, 179–192 (1927).

Jerger, J., Audiological manifestations of lesions in the auditory nervous system. Laryngoscope, 70, 417–425 (1960-a).

Jerger, J., Bekesy audiometry in analysis of auditory disorders. J. Sp. Hear. Res. 3, 275–287 (1960-b).

Jerger, J., Shedd, J., and Harford, E., On the detection of extremely small changes in sound intensity. Arch. Otolaryng., 69, 200–211 (1959).

Katz, J., The use of staggered spondaic words for assessing the integrity of the central auditory nervous system. J. Aud. Res., 2, 327–337 (1962).

Katz, J., The SSW test: An interim report., J. Sp. Hear. Dis., 33, 132–146 (1968).

Katz, J., Continuous tone masking (CTM) test for identifying site of lesion. In press, J. Aud. Res. (1960).

Kimura, D., Cerebral dominance and the perception of verbal stimuli. Canad. J. Psychol., 15, 166–171 (1961).

Lynn, G., and Gonzales, S., Auditory test findings in documented cases of CNS disorder. Unpublished paper presented at ASHA convention in November 1969, Chicago, Illinois.

Owens, E., Tone decay in VIIIth nerve and cochlear lesions. J. Sp. Hear. Dis., 29, 14–22 (1964).

Owens, E., The SISI test and VIIIth nerve versus cochlear involvement. J. Sp. Hear. Dis., 30, 252–262 (1965).

Reger, S., and Kos, C., Clinical measurements and implications of recruitment. Ann. Otol. Rhin. and Laryng., 61, 810–823 (1952).

Author's Note:

Audiologic Diagnosis: Cochlea to Cortex shows some advanced concepts for 1970, but does not reflect the advances that we have seen in the past decade. Without benefit of ABR or acoustic reflex testing, we were well aware of the ipsilateral brainstem effect from our work with the SSW. There is mounting electrophysiological evidence to support my behavioral observations over a period of years.

Although the pathophysiology did not follow the accepted anatomical arrangement, I did show a standard drawing of the ipsilateral and contralateral pathways. It would have been more consistent to show the system that was revealed by neurological, radiographic, and autopsy information in patients who had tumors and strokes involving the brainstem. The figure below shows the cochlea on the left side giving rise to the VIIIth nerve on the left, which then leads to the brainstem on the left side. The decussation to the right side is not shown because the brainstem lesion effect is felt to be primarily ipsilateral and not contralateral. We have found this to be true for almost all of our brainstem cases, whether the lesion was within the brainstem or involved the brainstem from without. Although the lower portion of the brainstem showed more specifically ipsilateral involvement, the cases with upper brainstem lesions showed more dysfunction contralaterally than ipsilaterally.

The ipsilateral brainstem effect and the distinction between the upper and lower brainstem responses are still largely unrecognized by audiologists. This will certainly change in the coming years because of ABR and acoustic reflex testing, along with greater interest in brainstem disorders than in the past.

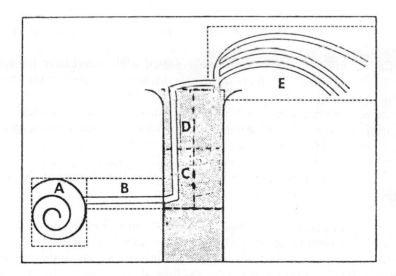

Reversible Neuroaudiologic Findings in a Case of Right Frontal Lobe Abscess With Recovery

Frank E. Musiek, PhD and Ernest Sachs, Jr., MD

A patient with a large right frontal lobe abscess was administered a battery of audiologic and neuroaudiologic tests. Results indicated a definite central auditory processing deficit with essentially normal peripheral hearing. The same test battery was given three months later, after the abscess had completely resolved. The neuroaudiologic results on retest were essentially normal for the entire test battery. The specific central auditory processing deficit noted in this case is discussed, along with details of the neuroaudiologic assessment.

Lesions confined to the frontal lobe often do not show any major effect on the central processing of auditory information.[1]

We have recently evaluated a case, summarized below, in a patient with a right frontal lobe brain abscess in which neuroaudiologic testing indicated an interference with interhemispheric auditory processing. With aspiration of the frontal lobe abscess and the instillation of antibiotics, the lesion completed disappeared, and the neuroaudiologic test results showed a return to normal.

Archives of Otolaryngology, May 1980, Volume 106

We believe this is an instance in which a frontal lobe lesion resulted in compression of the right side of the interhemispheric auditory pathway. This was reflected by depressed left-ear scores on various central auditory tests. The background of this case, auditory findings, and underlying neuroauditory mechanisms are reported.

Report of a Case

A 59-year-old, highly intelligent, right-handed woman suffered a spontaneous subarachnoid hemorrhage 36 hours prior to admission. The patient's neurologic history was negative, but she had suffered a chronic medical illness with long-standing psoriasis, secondary psoriatic arthritis, and depressed immune responses. The day prior to admission to the Mary Hitchcock Memorial Hospital, she had the abrupt onset of headache followed by loss of consciousness. Except for the decreased level of consciousness, there were no lateralizing neurologic signs. A lumbar puncture revealed 400,000 RBCs per cubic millimeter in her spinal fluid. She remained without neurological signs, and her state of consciousness gradually improved after initial mild confusion. She was treated with aminocaproic acid to prevent further hemorrhage, and reserpine and oral kanamycin sulfate[2] to prevent intracranial vasospasm. On her 11th posthemorrhage day, when she was alert and oriented, a right frontal craniotomy was carried out, occluding her proximal right anterior cerebral artery for an arteriographically proven anterior communicating artery aneurysm. Her postoperative course was complicated by a subgaleal staphylococcus wound infection, requiring removal of her bone flap on the fifth postoperative day. Subsequently, a right frontal lobe brain abscess developed, which was treated with antibiotics and repeated aspiration and instillation of bacitracin. Serial computerized axial tomographic scans revealed progressive diminution and finally disappearance of the brain abscess over a three-month postoperative course. During the presence of and recovery from her brain abscess, neuroaudiologic tests were conducted, with follow-up testing three months later.

Test Description and Results

Test Administration

All tests were conducted with the patient seated in a sound-treated room. Neuroaudiologic test items were taken from a dual-channel tape recorder, fed through the speech circuit of an audiometer, and presented to the subject through earphones. Appropriate calibration of all test material was carried out prior to testing.

Basic Audiologic Tests

The patient's pretreatment pure-tone thresholds indicated borderline normal hearing for the left ear and a flat, very mild sensorineural hearing loss for the right ear. Speech discrimination ability was excellent bilaterally (i.e., greater than 90%, using the Northwestern University phonetically balanced word list [NU No. 6 PB]).

Posttreatment, there was essentially no change in pure-tone sensitivity or speech-discrimination ability for either ear.

Neuroaudiologic Tests

Northwestern University No. 20 Competing Message Tapes (NU No. 20) Competing Message Tapes

The NU No. 20 tapes[3] are composed of phonetically balanced monosyllabic words from the NU No. 6 list in competition with intelligibility sentences (Bell Laboratories): For example, the word "read" is presented to the right ear, and the phrase "why do boys like to go barefooted?" is presented to the left.

Fifty monosyllabic words are presented at a 30-dB sensation level (i.e., 30 dB above the threshold for speech) to one ear while the sentences are presented simultaneously at a 45-dB sensation level to the opposite ear.[4] The patient's task is to repeat the monosyllabic words and ignore the competing sentences. Referring to the example, the patient is required to repeat only the word "read."

Pretreatment results for the NU No. 20 showed a 0% score for the left ear and essentially normal findings for the right ear (84%). Posttreatment results show approximately normal scores for the two ears (Figure 1).

Dichotic Digits

In this text,[5,6] 40 sets of two digits are presented simultaneously to each ear at a 40-dB sensation level. The patient is required to repeat all four digits presented. Pretreatment results again indicated a severe deficit for the left ear, whereas posttreatment scores were excellent bilaterally (Figure 2). These findings are similar to those obtained from "split-brain" subjects.[7-9]

Staggered Spondaic Words (SSW)

The SSW test, introduced and developed by Katz,[10,11] provides test items made up of two spondaic words that are presented in partially overlapping fashion. For example, the word "daylight" is presented to the right ear, and "lunchtime" is presented to the left.

FIGURE 1. ══════════════════════════
Results on Northwestern University phonetically balanced word list
dichotic competing message test. Circles and solid lines are pretreatment; squares and broken lines are posttreatment.

FIGURE 2.
Results of dichotically presented digits test. Circles and solid lines
are pretreatment; squares and broken lines are posttreatment.

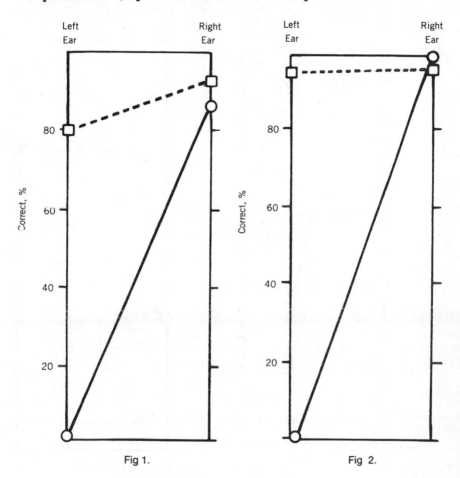

Fig 1.

Fig 2.

The words "light" and "lunch" are in dichotic competition, while
the words "day" and "time" are presented in a noncompeting condition. The 40-item test is presented at a 50-dB sensation level. Results are
expressed in Figure 3 as the percentage of errors for the right and left
ears in both the competing and noncompeting conditions.

FIGURE 3.
Results on staggered spondaic words test (raw score). Circles and solid lines are pretreatment; squares and broken lines are post-treatment.

FIGURE 4.
Results on low-pass filtered speech test. Circles and solid lines are pretreatment; squares and broken lines are posttreatment.

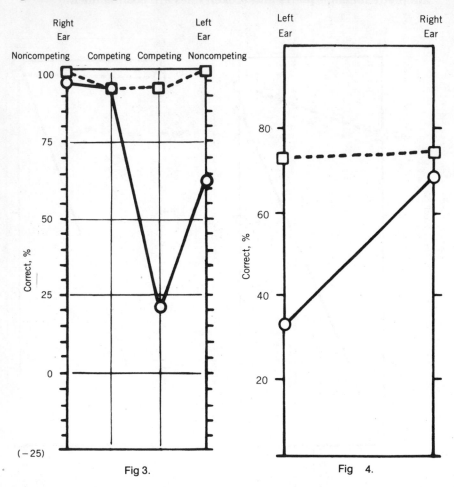

Fig 3.   Fig 4.

There was a high percentage of errors, especially for the competing condition for the left ear on the pretreatment SSW test. A portion of these errors occurred when the first spondee was presented to the left ear. When the first spondee was presented to the right ear and the second spondee to the left ear, the difference between the two ears was not as great. Posttreatment results were within normal limits for all conditions bilaterally.

256   Advanced Use of the Staggered Spondaic Word Test

FIGURE 5
**Results on frequency pattern recognition test. Circles and solid lines
are pretreatment; squares and broken lines are posttreatment.**

FIGURE 6.
**Auditory pathways to cortex, with dashes indicating weaker,
ipsilateral route and single arrow and double arrows showing
stronger, contralateral route for right and left ear, respectively.**

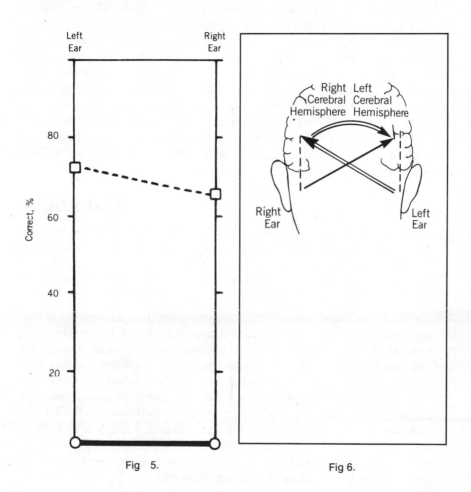

Fig 5.   Fig 6.

Low-Pass Filtered Speech (LPFS)

Low-pass filtered speech has been a popular test for some time in the
assessment of central auditory dysfunction.[12,15]

In this study, 50 phonetically balanced monosyllabic words were
presented monaurally to each ear at a 50-dB sensation level. NU No. 6

words were passed through a filter with a cutoff frequency at 500 Hz and a 24-dB per octave roll-off. Pretreatment scores again showed a left-ear deficit, while after treatment, the results were normal and bilaterally symmetric (Figure 4).

Frequency Patterns

Thirty auditory pitch patterns were presented monaurally at a 40-dB sensation level.[16] Patterns were composed of three successive tone bursts that were either 880 Hz (low) or 1,222 Hz (high). The tones were pseudorandomized to allow six types of patterns (i.e., HHL, HLL, HLH, LHL, LLH, and LHH, with H meaning high and L meaning low). The duration of each of the tones was 150 ms, and the interval between tones was 200 ms. The subject was required to verbally reproduce the pattern presented. Prior to treatment, the subject was completely unable to perform this task for either ear. After treatment, the subject could perform the task relatively well, although scores were slightly below normal (Figure 5).

Comment

The major finding in this case was the severe deficit for the left ear shown on various dichotic auditory tests. The improved scores after treatment for the left ear would indicate the returned function of a specific auditory process. We feel there is strong evidence that this returned function is that of interhemispheric transfer of acoustic information.

Various investigators[7,8,17,18] have observed that in a dichotic listening situation the weaker, ipsilateral neural pathway is suppressed in favor of the stronger contralateral pathway to the cortex. Hence, in a dichotic listening task, the preponderance of auditory information presented to the left ear goes to the right cerebral hemisphere and vice versa (Figure 6). Stimuli reaching the right cerebral hemisphere are transferred to the left cerebral hemisphere by fibers of the corpus callosum for linguistic processing and speech responses if needed. Stimuli introduced to the right ear in a dichotic condition go primarily to the left cerebral hemisphere, hence eliminating the need for hemisphere transfer for linguistic labeling (Figure 6).

In the case presented, the right frontal lobe abscess may have resulted in the compression of the neurons that course from the right temporal lobe to the corpus callosum. Therefore, dichotic speech stimuli presented to the left ear/right cerebral hemisphere could not be adequately transferred to the left cerebral hemisphere. Therefore, no linguistic processing or speech response could be mediated. Stimuli to the right ear, however, would be unaffected by this lesion, as the right ear

Advanced Use of the Staggered Spondaic Word Test

route to the left cerebral hemisphere does not involve the corpus callosum and adjacent connecting fibers.

After treatment of the right cerebral hemisphere abscess, apparent decompression of the neurons connecting the right temporal lobe to the callosal pathway took place. This restored interhemispheric transfer of acoustic information and neuroaudiologic test scores improved dramatically.

In the test battery, only two tests were not dichotic in nature (the LPFS and frequency pattern tests). The decreased score pretreatment for the LPFS test may be indicating some right temporal lobe disruption from either the abscess or previous vascular problem.

Classically, tests like the LPFS test show reduced function for the ear contralateral to the hemisphere affected,[13,15] which was what was demonstrated in this case. Another possible explanation for depressed LPFS test scores in the left ear is degradation of the stimulus that reaches the left cerebral hemisphere by the ipsilateral route. The contralateral routing of the left ear signals (e.g., left ear to right cerebral hemisphere to corpus callosum to left cerebral hemisphere) may provide more accurate processing of the signal than the ipsilateral route (e.g., left ear to left cerebral hemisphere). It seems that this concept is a feasible one, based on certain physiologic and psychophysical studies.[19,20]

Frequency Patterns

A unique finding was the 0% scores for pattern recognition for both ears' pretreatment. It has been postulated by Pinheiro[21] that the recognition and verbal response to auditory patterns require interhemispheric interaction.

More specifically, the right cerebral hemisphere identifies the contour of the pattern while the left cerebral hemisphere seems responsible for sequencing and initiating the verbal response. Supportive data for this concept have been obtained from subjects with complete commissurotomy.[22] These "split-brain" subjects could not verbally report various auditory patterns presented to either ear. In the case reported, the same phenomenon is seen before treatment (0% scores), with marked improvement posttreatment. This again implicates breakdown of interhemispheric transfer of acoustic information.

Conclusion

Neuroaudiologic test data from this case indicate the possible occurrence of a frontal lobe lesion affecting interhemispheric auditory processing. Information from this case study also shows the sensitivity of selected auditory tests to detect such problems.

The type of auditory deficit portrayed by this patient coincides well with findings on split-brain patients on similar tasks.[7,9] This lends considerable support to the notion that neurons carrying acoustic information to the corpus callosum from the auditory reception area in the right hemisphere may have been compressed pretreatment. This resulted in auditory response behavior similar to that seen in patients with commisurotomy. Proper treatment resulted in the decompression of these neurons and essentially normal performance on selected central auditory tests.

Acknowledgement

Research for this article was supported in part by grant 65 from the Hitchcock Foundation, Hanover, NH.

References

1. Lynn G, Gilroy J: Effects of brain lesions on the perception of monotic and dichotic speech stimuli, in Sullivan M (ed): *Proceedings of a Symposium on Central Auditory Processing Disorders.* Omaha, University of Nebraska Medical Center, 1975, pp 47–81.

2. Zervas, N, Heros R C, Lavyne M H: Frequency and reduction of infarction in stable aneurysm patients awaiting operation. Presented at the 45th annual meeting of the American Association of Neurological Surgeons, Toronto, April 27, 1977.

3. Tillman T, Carhart R: Effect of competing speech on aided discrimination of monosyllabic words, abstracted. *J Acoust Soc AM* 35:1900, 1963.

4. Burke M, Noffsinger D: Dichotic performance by cortical lesion subjects utilizing meaningful and meaningless competition. Presented at the American Speech and Hearing Association Convention, Houston, Nov 21, 1976.

5. Kimura D: Cerebral dominance and the perception of verbal stimuli. *Can J Psychol* 15:166–171, 1961.

6. Sparks R, Goodglass H, Nickel B: Ipsilateral versus contralateral extinction in dichotic listening resulting from hemisphere lesions. *Cortex* 6:249–260, 1970.

7. Sparks R, Geschwind N: Dichotic listening in man after section of the neocortical commissures. *Cortex* 4:2–16, 1968.

8. Milner B, Taylor L, Sperry R: Lateralized suppression of dichotically presented digits after commissural section in man. *Science* 161:184–186, 1968.

9. Musiek F, Wilson D, Pinheiro M: Audiological manifestations in split brain patients. *J Am Aud Soc* 5:25–29, 1979.

10. Katz J: The use of staggered spondaic words for assessing the integrity of the central auditory nervous system. *J Aud Res* 2:327, 1962.

11. Katz J: Audiological diagnosis: Cochlea to cortex. *Menorah Med J* 1:25, 1970.

12. Bocca E: Clinical aspects of cortical deafness. *Laryngoscope* 68:301–309, 1958.

13. Bocca E, Calearo C: Central hearing processes, in Jerger J (ed): *Modern Developments in Audiology.* New York, Academic Press Inc, 1963.

14. Jerger J F: Observations on auditory behavior in lesions of the central auditory pathways. *Arch Otolaryngol* 71:797–806, 1960.

15. Hodgson W: Filtered speech tests, in Katz J (ed): *Handbook of Clinical Audiology*. Baltimore, Williams & Wilkins Co, 1972.

16. Pinheiro M: Auditory pattern perception in patients with right and left hemisphere lesions. *Ohio J Speech Hear* 12:9–20, 1976.

17. Speaks C: Dichotic listening: A clinical or research tool? in Sullivan M (ed): *Proceedings of a Symposium on Central Auditory Processing Disorders*. Omaha, University of Nebraska Medical Center, 1975, pp 1–24.

18. Rozenzweig M: Representation of the two ears at the auditory cortex. *Am J Physiol* 167:147–158, 1951.

19. Brugge J, Merzenich M: Patterns of activity of single neurons of the auditory cortex in monkey, in Moller A (ed): *Basic Mechanisms in Hearing*. New York: Academic Press Inc, 1973, pp 745–763.

20. Berlin C, Lowe-Bell S, Cullen J, et al: Dichotic speech perception: An interpretation of right-ear advantage and temporal offset effects. *J Acoust Soc Am* 53:699–709, 1973.

21. Pinheiro M: Tests of central auditory function in children with learning disabilities, in Keith R (ed): *Central Auditory Dysfunction*. New York, Grune & Stratton Inc, 1977.

22. Musiek F, Pinheiro M, Wilson D: Processing of temporal patterns by split brain patients. Presented at the 95th meeting of the Acoustical Society, Providence, RI, May 17, 1978.

SSW and Dichotic Digit Results Pre- and Post-commissurotomy: A Case Report

Frank E. Musiek and Donald H. Wilson

A 19-year-old right-handed male with normal peripheral hearing bilaterally, was tested on the SSW and dichotic digits before and after commissurotomy. SSW results showed a definite deficit for words presented to the left ear in both the competing and noncompeting conditions. Dichotic digit results showed complete inability on the part of the subject to report the digits presented to the left ear. These findings are similar to other dichotic test results previously reported on split-brain patients.

The Staggered Spondaic Words (SSW) test developed by Katz (1962, 1968) has been shown to be a valid test for detecting central auditory dysfunction (Katz, Basil, and Smith, 1963; Katz, 1970; Brunt, 1972; Katz and Pack, 1975). This test requires the dichotic presentation of two spondees overlapping in time as shown in the example.

RE:	race horse
LE:	street car

TIME———>

Journal of Speech and Hearing Disorders November 1979, Vol. 44, No. 4

In the example, *race* is presented to the right ear in a noncompeting condition, while *horse* and *street* are presented simultaneously to the right and left ears respectively in a competing or dichotic condition. *Car* is then presented to the left ear in a noncompeting condition. The test is designed so that the lead word is introduced alternately to the right or left ear. Test items are presented at a sensation level (SL) of 50 dB and the listener is asked to repeat all the words heard.

Though there has been wide use of this test for various central auditory pathologies, there is a paucity of data for patients with lesions of the corpus callosum (Katz, 1977). To alleviate this specific lack of data, we administered the SSW to a patient who had undergone surgical section of the corpus callosum (Wilson, Reeves, Gazzaniga, and Culver, 1977).

We also elected to administer a dichotic digit test of our own composition but based on the work of Kimura (1961). This test involves the presentation of paired single digits to each ear simultaneously as shown in the example.

RE: 2,6
LE: 5,1

The listener's task is to repeat all four digits verbally. In this case the digits were presented at a 50 dB HL. There were a total of 40 digits (20 pairs) presented to each ear from which a percentage correct was derived.

Previous Auditory Data Involving Dichotic Listening

Milner, Sperry, and Taylor (1968) and Sparks and Geschwind (1968) were the first to report auditory data for split-brain subjects. Both of these investigations used words or numbers presented dichotically to test their patients. Generally, there was a definite left ear deficit for these types of stimuli. Springer and Gazzaniga (1975) presented consonant-vowel pairs dichotically to patients with differing portions of the cerebral commissures sectioned. Again, a general deficit was noted in the ability to respond to stimuli presented to the left ear.

Surgical Aspects

The corpus callosum, from rostrum to splenium, and the hippocampal commissure, which attaches to its undersurface, were the only commissures divided in this patient, by a refined, extraventricular method that used the operating microscope and two small craniotomies

(Wilson, Reeves, Gazzaniga, and Culver, 1977). Anterior commissure and fornix were left intact. The patient recovered promptly from surgery; his convalescence was uncomplicated. The precision afforded by microsurgery and the restriction of division to the corpus callosum reduced the variables in postoperative testing; that is, the variables of peripheral trauma to the brain and division of multiple commissures (Wilson, Reeves, and Gazzaniga, 1978).

Method
Subject

The subject was a 19-year-old, right-handed male who demonstrated normal hearing on pure-tone thresholds (250–8000 Hz), speech reception thresholds (20 dB HL or better) and speech discrimination tests (90% or better on Northwestern University Auditory Test No. 6) bilaterally. He was tested just before surgery, and one and one-half weeks postsurgery. At the time of testing, he was alert, oriented, and cooperative during assessment procedures.

Test Administration

The SSW was administered in the traditional manner (Brunt, 1972). For the dichotic digits, individuals are asked to repeat all four digits, and if they are unsure they are encouraged to guess. The subject was tested in a sound-treated room with the stimuli being presented through TDH-49 earphones with appropriate calibrations being carried out before testing.

Analysis of Data

The results obtained (from the commissurotomized patient) were analyzed along several parameters. Primarily the so-called corrected scores (C-SSW), reversals, ear effect, order effect, and total ear and condition (TEC) were analyzed. Details for the scoring procedures can be found elsewhere (Katz, 1977, 1976, 1973; Katz and Pack, 1975).

As mentioned earlier, for dichotic digits, the number of correct responses for each ear were used to derive a percentage score. Reversals of digit order were not computed.

Results

Before surgery, SSW scores for all conditions bilaterally for this subject were well within normal limits. Postoperatively, the corrected SSW score showed a marked decrease in performance for the left ear (see Figure 1). Specifically, the majority of errors occurred in the left competing condition (LC). However, a considerable number of errors were also noted in the left noncompeting condition (LNC). Right ear results were within normal limits for competing and noncompeting conditions postoperatively. Postoperatively as well as preoperatively no response bias was noted (that is reversals, ear or order effects).

The TEC scores for this patient were in the severe range. The use of mild, moderate, and severe classification denotes the degree of deficit for total score, poorest ear, and poorest condition score (Katz, 1976).

Dichotic Digits

Dichotic digit scores before surgery were well within normal limits bilaterally (that is, better than 90%). However, after surgery, the subject was totally unable to repeat digits presented to the left ear (see Figure 2). Postoperatively, right ear scores were within normal limits.

Discussion

Comparison with Other Dichotic Tests on Split-Brain Patients

In comparing the SSW and dichotic digits results with other dichotic listening tasks for split-brain patients, a common trend is noted (Sparks and Geschwind, 1968; Milner, Sperry, and Taylor, 1968; and Musiek,

FIGURE 1.
SSW scores pre- and postcommissurotomy

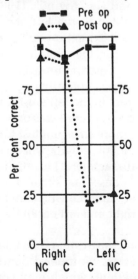

FIGURE 2. ════════════════════════════════
Dichotic digit results pre- and postcommissurotomy

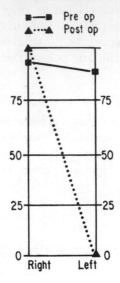

Pinheiro, and Wilson, in press). Specifically, there is a consistent and marked left ear deficit. The degree of deficit, however, varies depending upon the type of test.

Historically, probably the most common test used with these patients has been dichotic digits (Kimura, 1961) or words (Sparks and Geschwind, 1968). Sparks and Geschwind's (1968) patient could not repeat digits or words presented to the left ear. Milner, Sperry, and Taylor (1968) showed complete extinction of left ear responses for two of their seven subjects. However, the overall mean correct for left ear responses in their study was approximately 20%.

In this investigation the postoperative SSW scores for this split-brain patient were 20% correct in the left ear for the competing condition while for dichotic digits a 0% score was observed. Hence, it seems that dichotic digits may be a more stringent test for this clinical population. The lower scores for dichotic digits when compared to the SSW may be attributed to two main factors: (1) the dichotic digits are in more direct opposition in regard to onset and offset of the acoustical stimuli; and (2) the SSW may provide some acoustical and contextual cues from the words presented to the right and left ear in the noncompeting situation.

Undoubtedly, there are also other considerations such as the nature and extent of the lesion, peripheral hearing loss, and overall neurological status of the patient, which may contribute to the slight differences and results among various investigators. However, we think, at least with our patient, that these aspects are not significant factors in comparing the SSW to other dichotic tasks.

Neurological Aspects

It has been shown that acoustical stimuli presented to the left ear are received primarily at the right hemisphere (Rosenzweig and Rosenblith, 1953; Kimura, 1967; Speaks, 1975). Under at least certain ditions, the auditory information must be transferred across the corpus callosum to the left hemisphere to allow linguistic processing (Sparks and Geschwind, 1968). If the corpus callosum is sectioned, this process either cannot be accomplished, or it is severely degraded. This deficit takes place only for the left ear because stimuli presented to the right ear reaches the left hemisphere without crossing the corpus callosum. The left ear deficit is best demonstrated when dichotic acoustic stimuli are used, as this type of presentation seems to result in suppression of information by way of the ipsilateral route (Berlin, Cullen, Lowe-Bell, and Thompson, 1972).

Conclusion

It seems that the SSW and the dichotic digit tests show similar effects for this particular split-brain subject. However, the left ear deficit noted on the SSW is not quite as dramatic as has been seen on the dichotic digit tests. This observations is also supported by other auditory studies on split-brain patients (Sparks and Geschwind, 1968; Milner, Sperry, and Taylor, 1968; Musiek, Wilson, and Pinheiro, in press).

Implications from our clinical research can be viewed in the following ways: (1) that the SSW and dichotic digit results support the concept that in general, these types of tests are valuable in demonstrating interhemispheric transfer of acoustic information; and (2) that severe left ear deficits on dichotic listening tasks requiring verbal report may be an indication of involvement of the neural system responsible for transferring acoustic information from one hemisphere to the other.

Acknowledgement

Requests for reprints should be directed to Frank E. Musiek, Hitchcock Clinic, Dartmouth Medical School, Dartmouth-Hitchcock Medical Center, 2 Maynard St., Hanover, New Hampshire 03755.

References

Berlin, C., Cullen, J., Lowe-Bell, S., and Thompson, C., Dichotic speech perception: An interpretation of right ear advantage and temporal offset effects. *J. Acoust. Soc.*, 53, 699–709 (1972).

Brunt, M., The staggered spondaic word test. In J. Katz (Ed.), *Handbook of Clinical Audiology*. Baltimore: Williams and Wilkins Co. (1972).

Katz, J., The use of staggered spondaic words for assessing the integrity of the central auditory nervous system. *J. Aud. Res.*, 2, 327–337 (1962).

Katz, J., The SSW test—An interim report. *J. Speech Hearing Dis.*, 33, 132–146 (1968).

Katz, J., Audiologic diagnosis: Cochlea to cortex. *Menorah Medical Journal*, 1, 25–28 (1970).

Katz, J., SSW Workshop. Greenfield, New Hampshire (1976).

Katz, J., The staggered spondaic word test. In R. Keith (Ed.), *Central Auditory Dysfunction*. New York: Grune and Stratton (1977).

Katz, J., Basil, R., and Smith, J., A staggered spondaic word test for detecting central auditory lesions. *Annals of Otology*, 72, 908–918 (1963).

Katz, J., and Pack, G., New developments in differential diagnosis using the SSW test. In H. Sullivan (Ed.), *Proceedings of a Symposium on Central Auditory Processing Disorders*. University of Nebraska Medical Center (1975).

Kimura, D., Cerebral dominance and perception of verbal stimuli. *Can. J. Psychol.*, 15, 166–171 (1961).

Kimura, D., Functional asymmetry of the brain in dichotic listening. *Cortex*, 3, 163–178 (1967).

Milner, B., Sperry, R., and Taylor, L., Lateralized suppression of dichotically presented digits after commissural section in man. *Science*, 161, 184–186 (1968).

Musiek, F., Wilson, D., and Pinheiro, M., Audiological manifestations in split-brain patients. *J. Amer. Aud. Soc. (in press)*.

Rosenzweig, M., and Rosenblith, W., Responses to auditory stimuli at the cochlea and at the auditory cortex. *Psychology Monographs*, 67, 1–26 (1953).

Sparks, R., and Geschwind, N., Dichotic listening in man after section of neocortical commissures. *Cortex*, 4, 3–16 (1968).

Speaks, C., Dichotic Listening: A clinical or research tool? In M. Sullivan (Ed.), *Proceedings of a Symposium on Central Auditory Processing Disorders*. University of Nebraska Medical Center (1975).

Springer, S., and Gazzaniga, M., Dichotic testing of partial and complete split brain subject. *Neuropsychologica*, 13, 341–346 (1975).

Wilson, D., Culiver, C., Waddington, M., and Gazzaniga, M., Disconnection of the cerebral hemispheres: An alternative of hemispherectomy for the control of intractable seizures. *Neurology*, 25, 1149–1153 (1975).

Wilson, D., Reeves, A., Gazzaniga, M., and Culver, C., Cerebral commissurotomy for control of intractable seizures. *Neurology*, 27, 708–715 (1977).

Wilson, D., Reeves, A., and Gazzaniga, M., Division of the corpus callosum for incontrollable epilepsy. *Neurology*, 28, 649–653 (1978).

Audiological Tests for Evaluation of Central Auditory Disorders

Richard G. Winkelaar, M.A., and Terry K. Lewis, M.A.

Three audiological tests (Competing Sentences, Rapidly Alternating Speech, Staggered Spondaic Words) currently being used to evaluate central auditory dysfunction are discussed. Audiological and neurological findings on three patients with central auditory lesions are presented, with special reference to their performance on these central auditory tests. Results suggest the tests are of value in identifying and/or corroborating central lesions, and in providing a more complete explanation of patient communicative difficulties.

Audiological tests which assess central auditory integrity can provide valuable information in diagnosis and/or corroboration of lesions affecting the central auditory pathways. Conventional speech audiometric tests are not sensitive enough to identify these lesions as they do not sufficiently tax the capabilities of the auditory system. In fact, patients with central auditory pathology will often demonstrate normal performance on conventional word discrimination tasks.

Decreasing speech signal redundancy makes the listening task more difficult. This can cause a breakdown in performance if the central auditory pathways are affected. Bocca[1,2] and his associates in Italy first reported using word discrimination tests in which signal redundancy was reduced through high frequency filtering. They found that patients with temporal lobe lesions obtained lower word discrimination scores in the ear contralateral to the lesion than in the ipsilateral ear when these modified tests were used.

Subsequently, Jerger[3,4], Antonelli[5], Willeford[6], and Lynn[7] used a variety of monotic low redundancy word discrimination tests to evaluate patients with temporal lobe lesions. Their findings were similar to Bocca's, indicating reduced ability to correctly identify words in the ear contralateral to the lesion.

The use of dichotic speech tasks, in which different signals are simultaneously presented to each ear (Matzker[8], Kimura[9], Jerger[10-12], Willeford[13], Lynn[14,15], Ivey[16], Smith and Resnick[17]) has also supplied additional information in the assessment of brainstem and central auditory function.

The purpose of this paper is to describe some of the central auditory tests currently used in the Audiology Clinics at the University Hospital and the University of Western Ontario in London, Ontario. In addition, the diagnostic utility of these tests will be discussed through the presentation of audiological-neurological findings on three patients with lesions in the central auditory pathways. The tests being used are briefly described below.

The Staggered
Spondaic Word Test (SSW)

This is a dichotic task which utilizes two-syllable words like "day-light" and "lunch-time" (Katz[18,19], Brunt[20]). The second half of the first spondee is overlapped with the first half of the second spondee and the words are presented at a 50 dB sensation level to each ear (Figure 1). Patients with intact auditory reception areas have no difficulty repeating the competing items (e.g., "light" and "lunch") and have error scores of less than 10 per cent. Patients with lesions affecting auditory reception have difficulty repeating the competing syllables in the ear contralateral to the affected hemisphere. They obtain error scores in excess of 15 percent. In addition to this quantitative scoring method, Katz[21] also suggests qualitative scoring procedures (ear effects, order effects). An ear effect occurs when the error score for one ear is +5 or greater than the other ear for both competing and non-competing items, indicating the possibility of diffuse lesions involving the

TIME SEQUENCE

	1 ⟶	2 ⟶	3
RE	DAY	LIGHT	
LE		LUNCH	TIME

LE	FOR	GIVE	
RE		MILK	MAN

anterior areas of the temporal and parietal lobes. An order effect occurs when the first spondee is correctly identified less often than the second or *vice versa*. A significant order effect is +5 or greater errors and indicates the possibility of diffuse lesions involving the frontal lobes. The SSW can be used for patients 12–65 years of age, the results are not contaminated by the effects of peripheral hearing loss, and it is essentially free of contamination due to language dominance (Brunt and Goetzinger[22]).

The Competing Sentence Test

This test was developed by Willeford[23] and consists of a series of sentences presented dichotically (Figure 2). Patients are required to repeat the quieter primary message and ignore the louder secondary one. Ten pairs of sentences are presented, the RE receiving the primary

FIGURE 2. ▬▬▬▬▬▬▬▬▬▬▬▬▬▬▬▬▬▬▬▬▬▬▬▬▬▬▬▬▬▬▬▬▬▬▬▬
Sample items for Competing Sentence Test.

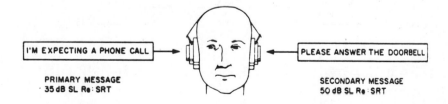

I'M EXPECTING A PHONE CALL	PLEASE ANSWER THE DOORBELL
PRIMARY MESSAGE 35 dB SL Re: SRT	**SECONDARY MESSAGE** 50 dB SL Re: SRT

message at 35 dB SL and the LE receiving the secondary message at 50 dB SL. This procedure is then reversed. Patients with intact temporal lobes repeat the primary message with no difficulty (70–100 per cent correct) while patients with damaged temporal lobes have difficulty repeating the primary message when it is presented to the ear contralateral to the affected hemisphere. A RE-LE difference of greater than 10 per cent is considered significant especially when both scores are 70 per cent or less. Age range for the test is approximately 10–60 years.

Rapidly Alternating
Speech Perception Test (RASP)

This is a test of binaural "resynthesis" (Lynn and Gilroy[24]), being based on an earlier technique of Bocca and Calearo[25]. A sentence "Do you want to go on the picnic" alternates between the ears every 300 msec. (Figure 3). Integration of these 300 msec. segments occurs in the brainstem where the central auditory pathways first come together (Matzker[26], Hall[27]). The segments from one ear are minimally intelligible to normals but the segments from both ears fuse together into an easily intelligible message, scores being 95–100 per cent for a series of 10 sentences. Lowered scores suggest a breakdown in brainstem processing of auditory stimuli. Age range for the test is approximately 10–75 years.

FIGURE 3. ━━━━━━━━━━━━━━━━━━━━━━━━━━━━━━━━
Sample items from the Rapidly Alternating Speech Perception Test (RASP).

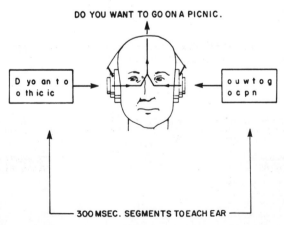

Advanced Use of the Staggered Spondaic Word Test

Case Report

The following three patients illustrate the usefulness of central auditory tests in providing information on site of lesion and in helping to explain patient complaints which were not determined with conventional audiological tests.

Patient 1: Age 62, had a history of three strokes within a period of 18 months prior to the examination. Complained of difficulty understanding speech in noise or in the presence of competing speech. No tinnitus

---

FIGURE 4.
Audiological and Neurological Findings on Patient No. 1 A: Audiogram, speech audiometry, B: SSW test, C: Neurologist's drawing of lesion site from EEG indicating involvement of the left temporo-parietal area.

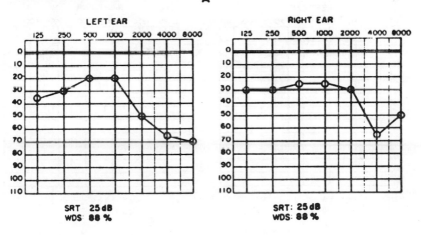

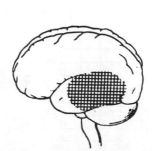

or dizziness were noted. Conventional audiological tests (Figure 4-A) revealed moderate bilateral steeply sloping high frequency sensorineural hearing losses for pure tones with excellent word discrimination ability bilaterally. The peripheral hearing loss was not of sufficient degree to explain the patient's complaints. The SSW test (Figure 4-B) revealed central auditory dysfunction involving the left temporal lobe. The moderate degree of error in the Right Ear—Competing Items with normal performance on the other items suggested involvement of the primary auditory reception area. The greater number of right-ear-first item errors also suggested that this lesion was diffuse, involving the anterior areas of the temporal lobe as well (Katz[28]).

FIGURE 5.
Audiological and Neurological Findings on Patient No. 2 A: Audiogram, speech audiometry, B: SSW test, C: Neurologist's drawing of lesion area from EEG indicating involvement of the left temporal lobe.

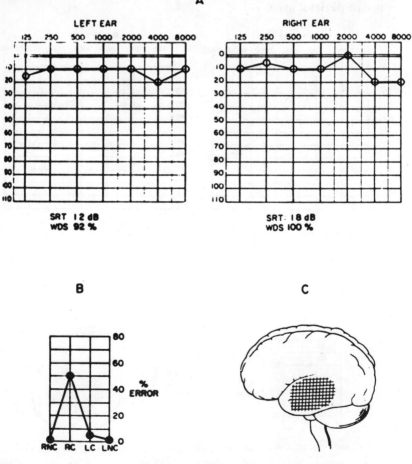

Advanced Use of the Staggered Spondaic Word Test

Subsequent neurological examination (Figure 4-C) identified the area of the Heschl's gyrus and the anterior and inferior areas of the temporal lobe of the left hemisphere as the areas of dysfunction. The patient returned for re-assessment six months after the first visit. Results indicated no change in peripheral sensitivity and SSW scores were identical to the first evaluation. The patient continues to have great difficulty in noise or in the presence of competing speech.

Patient 2:   Age 45, had a history of aneurysmal rupture and hemorrhage with subsequent aphasic-like symptoms. No tinnitus or dizziness were reported and the patient complained of difficulty understanding speech in noisy environments. Conventional audiological tests (Figure 5-A) revealed normal peripheral hearing bilaterally with word discrimination being excellent. The SSW test (Figure 5-B) revealed central auditory dysfunction involving the left temporal lobe. The moderate degree of error suggested involvement of the primary auditory reception area (Heschl's gyrus). The greater number of right-ear-first item errors also suggested the lesion was diffuse, involving anterior areas of the temporal lobe. Subsequent neurological examination (Figure 5-C) identified the lesion site in the temporal lobe of the left hemisphere, with diffuse involvement consistent with that predicted by the SSW results.

Patient 3:   Thirty-eight years of age and mildly retarded. Originally seen at age 16 when a right hemiparesis, visual difficulty, and bilateral papilledema were noted. An arteriorgram and pneumonencephalogram done at that time suggested a tumor deep in the left thalamic region. A surgical shunting procedure was performed and the papilledema and visual difficulties disappeared. The patient was seen 16 years later after seeking assistance at a centre for social difficulties. At that time skull x-rays revealed a large densely calcified mass in the region of the left thalamus. EEG's were asymmetrical with left temporal lobe activity being abnormal and period eliptiform activity noted in the anterior temporal region (Figure 6-C).

Audiological findings indicated a mild bilateral loss sloping from 25 dB at 250 Hz to 80 dB at 4,000 Hz. Word discrimination was borderline in the right ear and severely impaired in the left (Figure 6-A). SSW test results indicated mildly reduced scores in the right ear for competing items, suggesting the lesion was not in the area of Heschl's gyrus. The Competing Sentence Test gave scores of 70 percent in the RE and 60 per cent in the LE, these scores being below normal for both ears. The RASP (Rapidly Alternating Speech Perception) gave an overall score of 50 per cent (Figure 6-B). While the effects of the peripheral lesion on the CST and RASP must be considered, the diagnosed lesion in the thalamic region still appeared to have a diffuse effect on auditory abilities, causing difficulty with competing messages (Competing Sentence Tests, SSW and the ability to synthesize incoming auditory signals (RASP). In this case, the audiological results did not identify the site of lesion but are especially interesting as they rather effectively demonstrate the broad effects this specific lesion had on auditory performance. The results also help to explain the difficulties the patient was encountering in everyday listening situations.

FIGURE 1. ━━━━━━━━━━━━━━━━━━━━━━━━━━━━
Audiological and Neurological Findings on Patient No. 3 A: Audiogram speech audiometry, B: Central auditory tests, C: Neurological report.

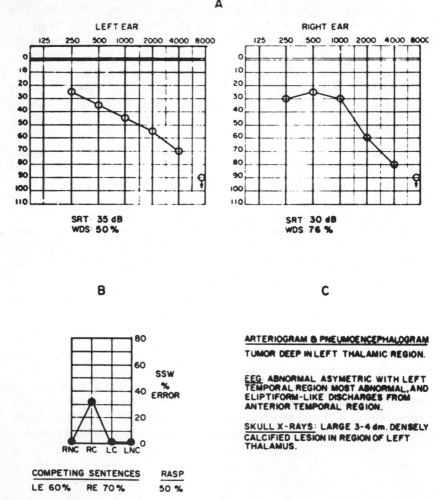

A

SRT 35 dB
WDS 50 %

SRT 30 dB
WDS 76 %

B

SSW % ERROR

COMPETING SENTENCES
LE 60%   RE 70%

RASP
50 %

C

ARTERIOGRAM & PNEUMOENCEPHALOGRAM
TUMOR DEEP IN LEFT THALAMIC REGION.

EEG: ABNORMAL ASYMETRIC WITH LEFT TEMPORAL REGION MOST ABNORMAL, AND ELIPTIFORM-LIKE DISCHARGES FROM ANTERIOR TEMPORAL REGION.

SKULL X-RAYS: LARGE 3-4 dm. DENSELY CALCIFIED LESION IN REGION OF LEFT THALAMUS.

The clinical findings previously presented demonstrate the effectiveness of central auditory tests in identifying and/or corroborating lesions in the central auditory nervous system. Patients 1 and 2 provide examples of the specific effects of temporal lobe lesions while patient 3 provides an interesting example of the diffuse auditory symptomatology caused by a thalamic lesion.

As pointed out by Lynn and Gilroy[29] the effects of peripheral lesions on central auditory test performance are not completely understood. As these effects cannot be subtracted out from the scores of the central tests in all cases, some caution in central test interpretation is indicated. Nevertheless, the tests appear to be a valuable addition to the standard audiological test battery. They can often more fully explain patient complaints not identified with conventional speech audiometric tasks, and, when used in conjunction with neuro-otological information, help insure accurate diagnosis of lesions in the central auditory pathways. Further research with these and other tests designed to evaluate central auditory function is now in progress.

Acknowledgement

The authors wish to express appreciation to C. Amaral and V. Peruchko for their assistance in data collection and compilation. This study was supported in part by a grant from the University of Western Ontario Foundation (New York), London, Ontario, and by the Oxford Regional Center, Woodstock, Ontario.

References

1. Bocca E, Calearo C, Cassinari V: A new method for testing hearing in temporal lobe tumors. *Acta Otolaryngol (Stockh)* 44: 219–221, 1954.

2. Bocca E, Calearo C, Cassinari V, et al: Testing "cortical" hearing in temporal lobe tumors. *Acta Otolaryngol (Stockh)* 45: 289–304, 1955.

3. Jerger J: Observations on auditory behavior in lesions of the central auditory pathways. *Arch Otolaryngol* 71: 797–806, 1960.

4. Jerger J: Auditory tests for disorders of the central auditory mechanism. In Field WS, Alford BR (eds.), *Neurological Aspects of Auditory and Vestibular Disorders,* New York: C. Thomas, pp 105–119, 1964.

5. Antonelli A, Calearo C: Further investigations on cortical deafness. *Acta Otolaryngol (Stockh)* 66:97–100, 1968.

6. Willeford J: Competing messages for diagnostic purposes. *Unpublished material.* Colorado State University, Fort Collins, Colorado, 1968.

7. Lynn GE, Gilroy J: Neuro-audiological abnormalities in patients with temporal lobe tumors. *J Neuro Sci* 17: 167–184, 1972.

8. Matzker J: Two methods for the assessment of central auditory functions in cases of brain disease. *Ann Otol (St. Louis),* 68: 1185–1197, 1959.

9. Kimura D: Some effects of temporal lobe damage on auditory perception. *Can J Psych* 15: 166–171, 1961.

10. Jerger J: op. cit. 1964.

11. Jerger J, Speaks C, Trammell J: A new approach to speech audiometry. J. Speech Hear Dis 33: 318–328, 1968.

12. Jerger J, Jerger S: Clinical validity of central auditory tests. Scan Aud 4: 147–163, 1975.

13. Willeford J: op. cit., 1968.

14. Lynn GD, Gilroy J: op. cit., 1972.

15. Lynn GE, Benitez JT, Eisenbrey AB, et al: Neuro-audiological correlates in cerebral hemisphere lesions, temporal and parietal lobe tumors. Audiology 11: 115–134, 1972.

16. Ivey RG: Tests of CNS auditory function. Unpublished Master's Thesis, Colorado State University, Fort Collins, Colorado, 1969.

17. Smith BB, Resnick DM: An auitory test for assessing brain stem integrity: Preliminary report. Laryngoscope 82: 414–424, 1972.

18. Katz J.: The use of staggered spondaic words for assessing the integrity of the central auditory nervous system. J Aud Res 2: 327–337, 1962.

19. Katz J: The SSW—an interim report. J Speech Hear Dis 33: 132–146, 1968.

20. Brunt M: The Staggered Spondaic Word Test. In Katz J (ed), Handbook of Clinical Audiology, Baltimore: Williams and Wilkins, Chp't. 18, 1972.

21. Katz J: Staggered Spondaic Word Test: Workshop. Menorah Medical Center, Kansas City, Mo., 1974.

22. Brunt M, Goetzinger CP: A study of three tests of central function with normal hearing subjects. Cortex 4: 288–297, 1968.

23. Willeford J: op. cit., 1968.

24. Lynn CE, Gilroy J: Effects of brain lesions on the perception of monotic and dichotic speech stimuli. In MS Sullivan (ed.), Central Auditory Processing Disorders: Proceedings of the Conference. Nebraska Medical Center, Omaha, Nebraska, pp 47–84, January, 1975.

25. Bocca E, Calearo C: Central hearing processes. In J Jerger (ed.), Modern Developments in Audiology, New York: Academic Press, p 337, 1963.

26. Matzker J: op. cit., 1959.

27. Hall JL: Binaural interaction in the accessory superior olivary nucleus of the cat. J Acoust Soc Amer 37: 814–823, 1965.

28. Katz J: op. cit., 1974.

29. Lynn GE, Gilroy J: op. cit., January, 1975.

Related Readings

J. Katz Clinical use of central auditory tests. Handbook of Clinical Audiology, 2nd edition, Baltimore: Williams & Wilkins (1978), 233–243.

J. Katz The Staggered Spondaic Word Test. Central Auditory Dysfunction, R. Keith (ed.), New York: Grune & Stratton (1977), 103–128.

G. E. Lynn, J. T. Benitez, A. B. Eisenbrey, J. Gilroy, and H. I. Wilner Neuroaudiological correlates in cerebral hemisphere lesions. Audiology, 11 (1972), 115–134.

G. E. Lynn and J. Gilroy Evaluation of central auditory dysfunction in patients with neurological disorders.

Central Auditory Dysfunction, R. Keith (ed.), New York: Grune & Stratton (1977), 177–222.

G. E. Lynn and J. Gilroy Neuro-audiological abnormalities in patients with temporal lobe tumors. *Journal of* the Neurological Sciences, 17 (1972), 167–184.

L. Weisenberg and J. Katz Neurological considerations in audiology. *Handbook of Clinical Audiology,* 2nd edition, Baltimore: Williams & Wilkins (1978), 23–38.

One of the unique characteristics of the SSW Test is that it has a correction procedure which accounts for peripheral distortion. The first two studies in this section consider the effectiveness of this procedure when evaluating patients with cochlear hearing loss. The importance of using the C-SSW score is emphasized along with the need to evaluate the test in conjunction with other audiologic tests.

Another unusual facet of the SSW Test is that it has been prepared in a number of different languages. Foreign language versions include: English (American, Indian, English), Turkish, Japanese, Portuguese, Danish, Spanish, French, and Hebrew. The last three papers of this section deal with two of those versions–Hebrew and Japanese–and the necessity to consider the patient native language before interpreting test results. Rawiszer's paper suggests that even after practice with the test items, non-native English speakers do not perform at expected norms.

5

Effects of Hearing Loss and Dialect on the Staggered Spondaic Word Test

SSW Test Results by Patients With Meniere's Disease

Denise L. Cafarelli, M.S., Richard H. Nodar, Ph.D.,
Mary Collard, M.A., and Deborah A. Larkins, M.A.

One of the largest obstacles in the assessment of central auditory function is the interference of peripheral pathology.

In 1960, Katz developed the Staggered Spondaic Word Test (SSW). The purpose of the test is the delineation of disorders along the auditory pathway. In 1968, he revised the test with the corrected (C-SSW) score to compensate for reduced word discrimination scores (WDS) in peripheral sensory neural hearing losses. Katz reported that patients with Meniere's Disease would obtain mild, normal, or over-corrected scores on the SSW, since Meniere's is localized to the cochlea, i.e., it is peripheral.

The present study was developed following the observation that a patient with a medical diagnosis of Meniere's Disease presented a moderate score on the SSW, suggesting a central lesion. The purpose of the study was to answer the following questions:

1. Does this Meniere's patient have a concomitant central disorder?
2. Are the SSW Test results confounded by the asymmetry and/or severely reduced speech discrimination scores associated with Meniere's?
3. Are these SSW Test result patterns common among patients with Meniere's?

ASHA Convention, Chicago, Illinois, 1977

Method

Twelve subjects ranged in age from 23 to 57 years. Each presented a case history of fluctuating hearing loss, tinnitus, and rotary vertigo, with no significant history of noise exposure, viral infection, or foreign language background. All were medically diagnosed as having Meniere's Disease.

The data collected represents 16 discrete test batteries, since two subjects were tested in active and remissive stages of the disease and two were tested twice during the active stage of the illness.

A control group consisted of ten individuals, 25–56 years old, with a medical diagnosis of unilateral cochlear pathology (not Meniere's).

Each group received an audiologic evaluation that included tympanometry, pure tone thresholds, speech reception thresholds, speech discrimination tests, threshold tone decay, electronystagmography (ENG), otolaryngologic examination, and the SSW. Patients with normal tympanometric or tone decay test results were excluded.

Results

Inter- and intragroup SSW Test results, particularly the total ear condition (TEC) score, were compared on the basis of speech discrimination scores (WDS) and stage of the illness, as well as degree and configuration of the pure tone loss.

Overall, the results were negative. For the Meniere's gorup, no relationship was found between the combined TEC score and the pure tone average (PTA), the audiometric configuration, or between the stage of the disease.

Despite the wide dispersion of speech discrimination scores, there was little variation in TEC scores in either group. This supports the use of the corrected TEC score in diminishing artifacts due to peripheral hearing loss which is one of the most important outcomes of this study.

In the majority of subjects, the total-ear-conditon score lies within the *Over-corrected* category. None of the subjects demonstrated severely depressed TEC scores. Reversals in word sequence were made by 31.3% of the Meniere's group, while the control group had none. Response bias was observed in 50% of the Meniere's subjects, while 30% of the control subjects demonstrated order effects and/or ear effects.

In general, SSW test results by the Meniere's subjects revealed a greater variability of scores. In fact, one subject achieved an over-corrected TEC score and ear effect within the active stage; SSW results made by this same patient fell within the *Mild* category when tested during remission.

Of particular interest was the result that two Meniere's subjects (S_5, S_6) presented moderately depressed TEC scores, suggesting central auditory pathology at the level of the brainstem (Figure 2).

Both subjects were tested in the remissive stage and had good to excellent speech discrimination scores, which were noncontributory to the severity of the SSW results. Both subjects demonstrated response bias, although one had an order effect (S_5) and the other had both ear and order (S_6) effects. Subject 6 had unilateral symptoms, with a depressed TEC score in the same ear. Subject 5 had asymmetrical bilateral findings and also demonstrated "deviant ENG findings suggestive of retrolabyrinthine findings." Polytomography and EMI studies had been administered and interpreted as normal. Neurologic evaluations were recommended and scheduled; since both patients lived a considerable distanced from the clinic, they were unfortunately lost for follow-up.

Discussion and Conclusion

The question of concomitant central disorders in the two Meniere's subjects remains unanswered at this time. However, since only these two subjects (16%) had moderate SSW TEC scores, this work supports the use of the C-SSW score in diminishing contamination of the SSW test results by a peripheral impairment. However, greater inter- and intrasubject variability of the SSW test results was demonstrated within the Meniere's group; ;therefore, no pattern of SSW test results was considered characteristic of this disease. In addition, conservative interpretation of the SSW test results is still advocated when testing patients with Meniere's Disease.

Acknowledgement

The authors wish to express their appreciation to Willard Parker, M.D., Sam E. Kinney, M.D., John Conomy, M.D., and the staffs of the Otolaryngology and Neurology Departments of the Cleveland Clinic Foundation for their cooperative efforts in the otoneurologic evaluation and diagnosis of the subjects presented.

FIGURE 1.
Comparison of SSW Results by Meniere's subjects and control group

	TEC Category						Response Bias			
	O-S	OC	WNL	Mi	Mo	Sev	OE	EE	Type A	Rev
Meniere's S's (N = 10)		50% (8)	25% (4)	12.5% (2)	12.5% (2)	0%	37.5% (6)	18.8% (3)	12.5% (2)	31.3% (5)
Controls (N = 10)	10% (1)	70% (7)	10% (1)	10% (1)	0%	0%	10% (1)	30% (3)	0%	0%

FIGURE 2.
Comparison of two Meniere's subjects with moderate TEC scores.

	Affected Ear	Duration of Illness	Stage of Illness	PTA (dB) R/L	Audio Config	WDS (%) R/L	OE	EE	Type A Pattern	Rev
S₁	Left	10 yrs	Remission	0/35	Flat	96/86	Low/High	—	Yes	—
S₂	Bilateral (Asymm)	31 yrs	Remission	65/20	Flat	76/96	Low/High	High/Low	—	2

SSW Test Results With Peripheral Hearing Loss

Dennis James Arnst, Ph.D.

The Staggered Spondaic Word (SSW) Test was introduced by Katz in the early 1960s as a means of assessing central auditory function. The test paradyme consists of dichotically presented spondee words, which are overlapped partially. The result is a series of competing and noncompeting monosyllables in each word sequence.

The dichotically-paired spondee words are presented alternately to the right and left ears—20 items to the right (REF); 20 items to the left (LEF). Errors on the SSW are evaluated both quantitatively and qualitatively. First, two types of quantitative scores are determined. The *raw score* (R-SSW) represents the total percent error. The *corrected score* (C-SSW) reflects the percent error after accounting for any peripheral component. This is accomplished by subtracting the WDS error from the R-SSW. Any remaining error reflects problems related primarily to central dysfunction. Consequently, the SSW Test attempts to account for the influence of cochlear hearing loss and thereby isolate results due to central problems. This procedure is unique to the SSW.

Second, a qualitative analysis of performance is made and is represented collectively by response bias. It includes ear effects, order effects, and reversals. An *ear effect* represents the total number of errors scored when the word sequence was started REF compared with LEF. *Order effect* represents total errors scored on the first spondee versus the second spondee. *Reversals* indicate the number of times the word

Presented at the American Speech-Language-Hearing Association Convention November 21–24, 1980 Detroit, Michigan sequence was altered. Since its introduction, the SSW Test has been shown to be helpful in identifying areas of dysfunction from the cochlea to the cortex due to various types of etiology.

The purpose of the present study was to evaluate the effect of cochlear hearing loss on SSW Test performance in light of the correction step incorporated into the scoring procedures.

Fifty male subjects (mean age: 45 years; see Figure 1) were selected for this study. The mean pure tone audiogram for both ears is shown in Figure 2. All subjects had bilaterally symmetrical sensory-neural hearing loss. The difference between the right and left three-frequency pure tone average (PTA) was required to be no greater than 10 dB. The mean PTA for the right ear was 33.8 dB and 34.2 dB for the left ear. The mean WDS was 83.6% for the right ear and 84.0% for the left ear.

The SSW Test was administered according to standard procedures using a dual channel clinical audiometer. The scores shown in Figure 3 are the mean raw and corrected scores for the competing and noncompeting conditions for the right and left ears. These results are drawn on an SSW-gram (Figure 4). Note the difference between the raw and corrected scores across the listening conditions. This type of separation between results is typical when a cochlear problem exists. The mean ear scores for the C-SSW were within the normal range defined by Katz. Therefore, results were consistent with a lack of central dysfunction in this group.

The ear and order effects obtained with this group are shown in Figure 5. Note the fact that over 50% of the subjects showed no significant ear or order effects. However, when ear effect was significant, most of the subjects showed a tendency to make more errors when word sequence was started LEF (i.e., Ear Low/High). Also, significant order effects tended to show more errors were made on the first spondee than on the second spondee (i.e., Order High/Low).

FIGURE 1. ━━━━━━━━━━━━━━━━━━━━━━━━━━
Distribution of Subjects by Age

	20–29	–	4		
	30–39	–	11	Mean Age	= 45.8 years
N = 50	40–49	–	16	SD	= 10.4
	50–59	–	15	Range	= 22–60
	60	–	4		

FIGURE 2. ▬▬▬▬▬▬▬▬▬▬▬▬▬▬▬▬▬▬▬▬▬▬▬▬▬▬▬
Mean, Pure Tone Audiogram

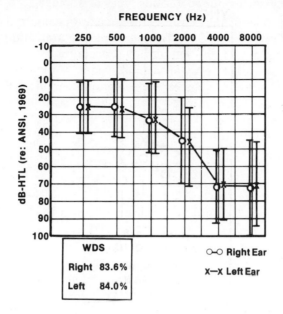

	Condition			
	RNC	RC	LC	LNC
R-SSW	18.6 (22.9)	26.6 (24.2)	33.0 (27.5)	19.9 (21.8)
C-SSW	0.8 (13.0)	8.8 (13.9)	15.8 (18.2)	4.4 (14.2)

In terms of reversals (see Figure 6), 45 subjects (or 90% of the group) changed the sequence on less than four of the dichotic word pairs. Consequently, this group tended to show no significant central problems on the C-SSW and no outstanding response bias pattern. These findings are consistent with the results reported by Katz and the norms established for the test.

We now need to consider the WDS-correction factor and the effect of varying amounts of hearing loss on test results. Katz (1973) reported that the WDS and the R-SSW were highly correlated. The Pearson product–moment correlation for his data was r = 0.86.

FIGURE 4.
SSW-gram

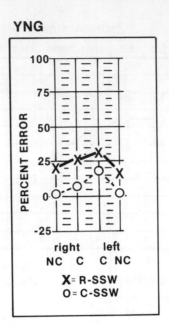

YNG

X= R-SSW
O= C-SSW

FIGURE 5.
Response Bias (N = 50)

Category	Ear Effect	Order Effect
NS	29 (58%)	31 (62%)
Low/High	19 (38%)	6 (12%)
High/Low	2 (4%)	13 (26%)

A similar comparison was made using the results obtained with the present group. The correlation coefficient was calculated to be $r = 0.82$. Consequently, these data support the Katz contention that the WDS and R-SSW are highly related. The next question is, what happens to that relationship when WDS decreases?

As shown in Figure 7, WDS and R-SSW have a fairly linear relationship—poor WDS parallels poor R-SSW. A one-way ANOVA with a Duncan Multiple Range post-hoc test supported this observation at the 0.01 level of significance. As a result, these two scores are highly

FIGURE 6. ━━━━━━━━━━━━━━━━━━━━━━━━━━━━━
Response Bias: reversals ($N = 50$)

Mean Number of Reversals = 1.8		
0	– 32	(64%)
1	– 5	(10%)
2–6	– 8	(16%)
7–12	– 2	(4%)
≥13	– 3	(6%)

FIGURE 7. ━━━━━━━━━━━━━━━━━━━━━━━━━━━━━

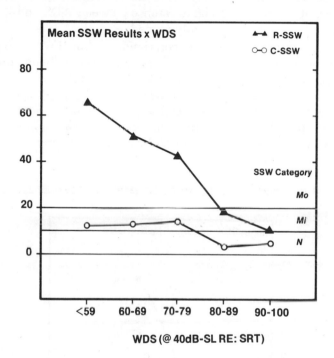

WDS (@ 40dB-SL RE: SRT)

related, regardless of the WDS level. Therefore, if WDS error is sub-tracted from the R-SSW, the correction effect should be consistent across all levels of WDS.

In Figure 7, the C-SSW was added and plotted as a function of WDS. A one-way ANOVA showed no significant differences to exist. Moreover, the Pearson Product Moment Correlation between the WDS and C-SSW was found to be $r = 0.15$. Therefore, the SSW correction procedure appears to equalize results across all levels of WDS.

We now need to consider the effect of amount of hearing loss (HL) on the SSW Test results. First, let's consider the R-SSW as HL increases. Note the data represented with triangles in Figure 8. A one-way ANOVA indicated that as the three-frequency PTA increased, so did the R-SSW. A Duncan post-hoc test, however, revealed that a grouping of the data occurred. Hearing loss had no significant effect until the PTA reached 40 dB. Furthermore, once HL reached 50 dB, differences in R-SSW were also not significant.

A similar break in the data occurred when the difference between R-SSW and WDS as a function of PTA was analyzed (i.e., the difference between the triangles and the filled circles). Apparently, HL has an effect on the relationship between WDS and R-SSW. With HL less than 40 dB, these two scores are highly related, in fact, almost identical. However, above this level the difference between WDS and R-SSW is greater and may not be as highly related.

If we assume the $r = 0.82$ correlation obtained with the present data to be average for this group, the correlation is better than 0.82 below 40 dB HL and poorer than 0.82 above 40 dB HL.

Finally, we need to consider the effect of hearing loss on the corrected SSW score. As can be seen in Figure 8, an inflection in the data occurs at 40 dB HL. This increase in C-SSW is significant, based on a one-way ANOVA and a Duncan post-hoc probe. Therefore, it is con-

FIGURE 8.

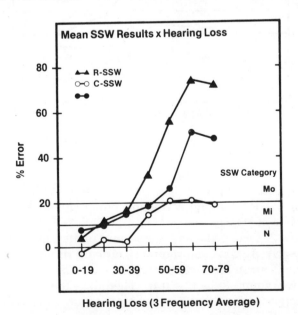

Hearing Loss (3 Frequency Average)

Effects of Hearing Loss and Dialect on the SSW Test

FIGURE 9.

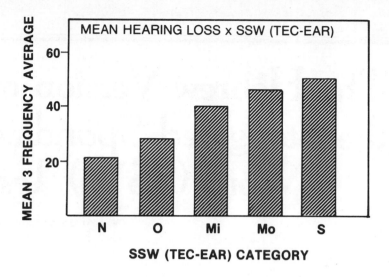

cluded that the WDS-correction procedure is necessary for a reasonable interpretation of the SSW Test. However, above 40 dB HL, caution must be used, since a higher C-SSW may result due to the amount of HL.

As can be seen in Figure 9, as the SSW category became poorer—decreased from *Normal* to *Severe*—the PTA increased. Therefore, in cases of bilateral cochlear hearing loss in excess of 40 dB *Moderate* and *Severe* SSW categories are possible. In the present study, only 12 (24%) of the 50 subjects obtained these two categories. The remaining 38 (76%) scored either *normal*, *Over-corrected*, or *Mild*—the expected result as reported by Katz.

Consequently, it is imperative that for a true picture of the ear's function, C-SSW results should be interpreted in the context of other audiometric findings to avoid false-positive conclusions indicating central dysfunction. The influence of HL above 40 dB does not invalidate the C-SSW score, since central dysfunction patterns have been found to emerge clearly despite cochlear dysfunction. Rather, the user must beware of this influence to avoid erroneous judgments.

The Hebrew Version of the Staggered Spondaic Word (SSW) Test

Bilha Keydar and Jack Katz

Introduction

The Staggered Spondaic Word (SSW) Test has been used in the United States for the past 15 years as a measure of central auditory function (Katz, 1962; Brunt, 1972). This test is used to locate disorders of the brain and brain stem. One important feature of the SSW Test is that it is not limited to the study of lesions involving Heschl's gyrus. Rather it can be used to differentially indicate lesions in various parts of the brain (Katz and Pack, 1975). The test has been shown to have a high degree of reliability (Katz and Arndt, 1974), and is widely applicable in age (Balas, 1962; Myrick, 1965), intelligence (Hadaway, 1969) and for various hearing and central pathology groups (Katz et al, 1966; Katz, 1968; Brunt, 1972; Katz and Illmer, 1972).

Bocca et al (1954) indicated that audiometric measurement could identify brain lesions. Distorted speech can be used to challenge the brain's capacity to integrate information (Bocca et al, 1955; Calearo and Lazzaroni, 1957). Dichotic speech tests have been used to evaluate the brain's ability to handle competing messages (Feldmann, 1962, 1967; Katz, 1962; Sparks et al, 1970). Patients with lesions in Heschl's gyrus of the temporal lobe exhibit particular difficulty in processing information from one ear when both ears are stimulated (Katz, 1968). The dysfunction is primarily demonstrated in the ear contralateral to the le-

The Journal of Auditory Research, 1976, 16, 135–142

Effects of Hearing Loss and Dialect on the SSW Test

sion regardless of the cerebral test being used (Kimura, 1961; Hodgson, 1967; Jerger, 1970; Lynn and Gilroy, 1975).

A wide variety of techniques has been found to be useful in testing central auditory function. Among them are filtered speech (Bocca et al, 1955; Matzker, 1959), compressed speech (Calearo and Lazzaroni, 1957; Quiros, 1961), synthetic sentences (Jerger, 1970), brief tones (Baru and Karaseva, 1972) and others (Walsh and Goodman, 1955; Broadbent, 1956; Goetzinger and Rousey, 1959; Carhart, 1969).

The SSW Test appears to be particularly challenging to patients with brain lesions because it combines both a dichotic test with a complex presentation method. Nevertheless, it is quite an easy task for individuals who have normal brain and brain stem function.

Each of the 40 SSW items is composed of two spondaic words. English spondaic words are compound, two, one-syllable words like *baseball*, and *airplane*, which are spoken with equal stress. The words are presented in a partially overlapping manner (see Figure 1). The odd-numbered items start in the R ear and the even-numbered ones in the L (or vice versa).

Many languages do not have spondaic words per se; however, familiar 2-word combinations can be used for the SSW Test. Each of these "compound words" preferably will be made up of two monosyllabic words. In some languages this may not be practical because of the language makeup. In such cases it would be best to have monosyllabic words for the competing portions. In some languages even the competing words might need to be of 2 syllables.

Each item will have a Right noncompeting (RNC) word, (e.g., "up" in Figure 1); a Right competing word (RC) word (e.g., "stairs"); Left competing (e.g., "down") and Left noncompeting (e.g., "town"). The patient is instructed to repeat all of the words that he hears except for the "Are you ready?" which precedes each item. The words are presented at 50 dB SL.

The number of errors on the 4 conditions (RNC, RC, LC and LNC) are summed separately and the raw percent of error (R-SSW) is ob-

FIGURE 1. ▰▰▰▰▰▰▰▰▰▰▰▰▰▰▰▰▰▰▰▰▰▰▰▰▰▰
A sample SSW item. Each item is made up of two spondaic words. One is presented to each ear but in a staggered manner so that only two of the four monosyllabic words compete in time.

| | Time Sequence | | |
	1	2	3
Right ear	up	stairs	
Left ear		down	town

tained. Since the correlation between the R-SSW score and word discrimination score (such as on the CID W-22 lists) is .92 or .93 in cases with peripheral hearing loss, a correction factor should be used (Katz et al, 1963; Katz, 1968). These corrected SSW (C-SSW) scores therefore compensate for peripheral distortions which the patient may have.

Patients with lesions to Heschl's gyrus tend to have numerous errors in the ear contralateral to the disorder. Individuals with dysfunction in other parts of the brain may have fewer errors but often demonstrate some form of response bias. Response biases may be an alteration in the order of the words or various other peculiarities (Katz and Pack, 1975; Brunt, 1977).

Because of the C-SSW scores, the presence of a hearing loss will not invalidate the test although it might limit the interpretation in some cases. In other situations the hearing loss information can provide valuable data for interpreting problems in the brain stem (Katz, 1970, 1977; Weisberg and Katz, 1977).

Variations of the SSW test have been adapted in other languages and dialects. The present project was undertaken to adapt the staggered dichotic technique to the Hebrew language. It was the hope that the Hebrew version would be roughly comparable to the American test (List EC), despite the lack of spondees in Hebrew. The equivalency of the two tests were evaluated by use of bilingual Ss, both Americans and Israelis.

Construction of the Hebrew SSW Test

The Hebrew SSW Test was designed to parallel the EC list. It was made up of 40 items with two compound words in each. The odd-numbered items begin in the R ear and terminate in the L. The even items are routed the opposite way. Figure 2 shows the phonetic transcriptions of one Hebrew item.

FIGURE 2. ━━━━━━━━━━━━━━━━━━━━━━━━━━━━━━
An example of a Hebrew SSW item, transcribed in phonetics and translated into English.

| | **Time Sequence** | | |
	1	2	3
Right ear	bet	/ imu /		(bathroom)
Left ear		sɛfɛl	kafɛ	(cup of coffee)

As in the American version, the items were designed so that the two noncompeting words also formed a familiar combination. In this example the words {bet kaf } (coffee house) was formed.

In order to arrive at a group of 40 familiar items, a list of 45 potential items was devised. The list was shown to 10 Israelis who were living in the United States. These individuals were mothers or other individuals who were familiar with the vocabulary of Israeli children. The raters were asked to assign a number to each of the 90 compound words based on their familiarity to 8- and 9-yr-old children. A rating of 1 was "extremely familiar"; 2 was "familiar"; 3, "fairly familiar"; 4, "slightly familiar"; and 5 was for "unfamiliar" words. Items containing mean ratings of over 3 for either compound word were excluded. The mean ratings for the remaining 80 words was 1.8, and thus were quite familiar to 8- and 9-yr-olds.

Eighty compound test words (160 individual words and some practice words) were recorded on tape. Half of each item was recorded on one of two monophonic tape recorders by a native female Israeli speaker (BK). To construct each item equal-sized tape loops were made for corresponding words and were run continuously. In order to get the competing conditions to overlap in time, one of the loops was slowed in relation to the other until simultaneity appeared to be achieved (Berlin and Lowe, 1972). The outputs from the tape recorders were then routed to a stereophonic tape recorder on which the carrier phrase had been prerecorded. If the competing words sounded overlapped when played to both ears, to one ear, passed very slowly across the playback head and visually on the VU meters, the item was used. If not, the previous steps were repeated until a useable item was obtained. On rerecording the test, the peak energy for the competing words were matched for each item.

Method

Subjects

Two groups of bilingual Ss were selected, all with HLs≤20dB at 0.5–2 kc/s, bilaterally. No S had significant otological or neurological histories.

The native American speaking group and the native Hebrew speaking group each contained 5 men and 5 women. Mean age for the Americans was 22 yrs, for the Israelis 29 yrs. Above-normal ability was expected of each S in his native language and fluent communication in the foreign language.

Design

A calibrated Maico 24 audiometer was used for the pure-tone testing. A Sony stereophonic tape recorder was routed through the audiometer for all speech testing. Speech tests were given in a counterbalanced order. A word discrimination test was given in one language followed by the SSW test in the same language. Then the discrimination and SSW tests were given in the other language. Half of each SSW test was given at 50 dB SL (the standard clinical level) and 15 dB above the pure-tone speech average. The 15 dB SL was used to obtain more errors in evaluating the relative difficulties of the two tests since few errors are made by normals at 50 dB SL.

The English language tests were the recorded CID W-22 List 3C using 25 words for each ear. The SSW test was List EC. The Hebrew language discrimination test was developed for this study and recorded by the same speaker as the Hebrew SSW test; 25 words were delivered to each ear. Both discrimination tests were presented at 40 dB above the pure-tone speech average.

Results

The mean performance of the American and Israeli Ss on the discrimination test, the SSW at 50 dB SL and the SSW at 15 dB SL for both languages are shown in Table 1. The results for the R and L ears were combined in each case.

The performance on the English discrimination task was quite similar for both American and Israelis. The same was true for both groups on the Hebrew discrimination test.

A 4-way ANOVA was computed to determine whether there were any statistically significant differences among the means for the two groups for the R-SSW results in the two languages, at the two presentation levels for the individual ears.

TABLE 1.
Results for Americans and Israelis on 3 Conditions in Each Language Results for the 2 Ears were Combined for the Discrimination Task and the 15 dB SL and 50 dB SL Conditions for Each Language. Discrimination Task is in Per Cent Correct, the SSW Test in Per Cent Error

	Discrim-ination	R-SSW /15	R-SSW /50	Discrim-ination	R-SSW /15	R-SSW /50
Americans	97.6	5.1	2.3	99.0	6.3	1.3
Israelis	96.4	13.8	8.3	98.8	1.7	0

Importantly, the difference between the performance of the Americans on the English test and the Israelis on the Hebrew test was not significant ($F = 3.35$). There was a difference in the performance of the Israelis on the English vs the Hebrew SSW test ($F = 43.64$, $p < .01$) but this was not true for the American Ss. The major difference for the Israelis was their difficulty with the American version of the SSW test at 15 dB SL. At the 50 dB (standard clinical) level there was no difference between the groups.

Table 2 shows the performance of the Americans and Israelis on both SSW tests at both presentation levels separately for each ear. It can be seen that for each language each group performed similarly in the two ears when the test was given at the 50 dB (standard) level. However, at the 15-dB level there is a statistically significant difference ($F = 10.11$, $P < .01$).

Discussion

The SSW test is an excellent procedure for evaluating central auditory function. It was the purpose of this work to develop a similar complex dichotic test in Hebrew in the hope that the method is generally applicable and not specific to English. To be maximally useful the two tests should be equated in difficulty and in diagnostic indicators. In this way the growing literature can be applied to people in various countries. Developing a comparable SSW test in Hebrew was not without its problems in devising appropriate items.

The first and most important concern was whether Israelis would perform comparably on the Hebrew SSW as Americans perform on the English EC list when the materials are presented at the standard 50 dB SL. While there was a tendency for the Israeli version to be slightly easier at both the 15 and 50 dB levels, the differences were not significant. The patterns of responses were also similar for the 4 conditions (RNC, RC, LC, LNC). Therefore, for normal Ss we can assume that the two tests are equivalent for native speakers.

TABLE 2.

Results for Americans and Israelis on the English and Hebrew SSW Tests at 15 and 50 dB SL for Each Ear Separately. Data are in Per Cent Error

	R-SSW English Language				R-SSW Hebrew Language			
	15 dB SL		50 dB SL		15 dB SL		50 dB SL	
	RE	LE	RE	LE	RE	LE	RE	LE
Americans	2.0	8.2	2.5	2.2	3.8	9.0	1.5	1.0
Israelis	9.0	18.5	7.5	9.0	.5	3.0	0	0

By correcting for discrimination we see that the SSW tests are compatible with various studies on the English SSW test (Brunt, 1972). For the Americans the EC list yielded a C-SSW total score of −.1 and for Israelis the Hebrew version yielded a score of −1.2. Brunt shows that studies with comparable aged Ss varied in the C-SSW scores from −1.3 to +1.4 (Brunt, 1972).

An interesting sidelight to this study is the cross-language use of the SSW test. That is, on occasion a foreign-born speaker was tested on the SSW test for clinical or research purposes. We would hope that the evaluation in the second language would not be greatly altered if the individual was fluent in the second language. This was not supported in the present study in which the mean total C-SSW was within the mild range for the Israelis on the English test; 4 Israelis had total C-SSW scores of 5 or greater (showing mild abnormality). These are presumably false positive responses. None of the Americans had a total C-SSW score of 5 or more on the Hebrew version. While the Hebrew version appears appropriate for fluent non-native speakers, further evaluation of the American version is needed to see if it is too difficult for the non-native.

One explanation of the inability of the Israelis on the English version is that by use of only monosyllabic words the task is more difficult. The Americans frequently had 2-syllable competing words. This gave them more phonetic and linguistic cues, a longer signal and there was more information that was not overlapped by information coming from the other side. While these cues may be useful to the normal listener it might not benefit the patient with a brain lesion. This is yet to be studied.

An important clinical feature of the SSW test is that it is comparatively free from laterality effects (Brunt, 1972). While the R ear is often the better one on the SSW test, the difference in most normal groups is not statistically significant. Even when statistical significance has been shown (Brunt and Goetzinger, 1968), the difference between ears (<1 %) was not of any clinical significance.

The present study gave us an opportunity to study laterality effects on both SSW tests. At the 50 dB level neither test showed a significant difference. However at 15 dB SL Ss had significantly more difficulty in the L ear on both tests. This suggests that the SSW test not be presented at a faint level for fear of contamination by R ear superiority for most Ss. This supports the concept that a central test should be kept easy for normals in order to avoid errors and laterality effects. It has been shown that when the SSW test is made more difficult by routing the entire item to one ear at a time, the R ear performance is superior to the L ear for Right-handed Ss (Goldman and Katz, 1966).

The two discrimination tests used in this study proved to be roughly comparable. The Hebrew version appears to be useful for correcting the Hebrew R-SSW scores.

Further research is underway to determine the applicability of the Hebrew SSW test in the evaluation of patients with CNS disorders.

Summary

The Staggered Spondaic Word (SSW) Test is an English language procedure for evaluating brain and brain stem function. A Hebrew version of the test was constructed and compared to the English test. Twenty bilingual Ss were evaluated on both tests; 10 native Israelis and 10 native Americans. Tests were presented at the standard (50 dB) and at a faint (15 dB) SL.

There was no significant difference between the two nationality groups when tested at 50 dB SL in their native language. No laterality effect was noted. At the 15-dB level the Israelis had more errors on the English test than the Americans had on the Hebrew version. thus, in some ways the English test might be more difficult when there are diminished clues available to the listener. At this faint level the results were significantly poorer for the L ear than for the R.

References

1. Balas, R. Results of the Staggered Spondaic Word Test with an Old Age Population. Unpubl. Master's Thesis, Northern Illinois University, 1962.

2. Baru, A. V. and Karaseva, The Brain and Hearing. N.Y.: Consultants Bureau, 1972.

3. Berlin, C. I. and Lowe, S. S. Temporal and dichotic factors in central auditory testing. In: J. Katz (Ed.) Handbook of Clinical Audiology. Baltimore: Williams & Wilkins, 1972.

4. Bocca, E., Calearo, C. and Cassinari, V. A new method for testing hearing in temporal lobe tumours: Preliminary report. Acta Otolaryngol., 1954, 44, 219–221.

5. Bocca, E., Calearo, C., Cassinari, V. and Migliavaccam, F. Testing "cortical" hearing in temporal lobe tumours. Acta Otolaryngol., 1955, 45, 289–304.

6. Broadbent, D. Successive responses to simultaneous stimuli. Quart. J. Exper. Psychol., 1956, 8, 145–162.

7. Brunt, M. The staggered spondaic word (SSW) test. In: (see Ref. 3).

8. Brunt, M. The SSW test. In: (see Ref. 3, Second Edition, In Press).

9. Brunt, M. and Goetzinger, C. P. A study of three tests of central function with normal hearing subjects. Cortex, 1968, 4, 288–297.

10. Calearo, C. and Lazzaroni, A. Speech intelligibility in relation to the speed of the message. Laryngoscope, 1957, 67, 410–419.

11. Carhart, R. Considerations underlying evaluation of central auditory function. Prog. Amer. Speech Hear. Assoc., Chicago, Ill., November 1969.

12. Feldmann, H. Binaural hearing test. International Audiology, 1962, 1, 222–223.

13. Goetzinger, C. P. and Rousey, C. Hearing problems in later life. Med. Times, 1959, 87, 771–780.

14. Goldman, S. and Katz, J. The SSW Test: Dichotic, diotic and monaural. Progr. Amer. Speech Hear. Assoc., Washington, D.C., 1966.

15. Hadaway, S. An investigation of the relationship between measured intelligence and performance on the Staggered Spondaic Word Test. Unpubl. Master's Thesis, Oklahoma State University, 1969.

16. Hodgson, W. Audiological report of a patient with left hemispherectomy. J. Speech Hear. Dis., 1967, 32, 39–45.

17. Jerger, J. Diagnostic significance of SSI test procedures: Retrocochlear site. In: C. Rojkjaer (Ed.) Speech Audiometry, Denmark, 1970.

18. Katz, J. The use of staggered spondaic words for assessing the integrity of the central auditory nervous system. J. Aud. Res., 1962, 2, 327–337.

19. Katz, J. The SSW Test: an interim report. J. Speech Hear. Dis., 1968, 33, 132–146.

20. Katz, J. Audiologic diagnosis: cochlea to cortex. Menorah Med. J., 1970, 1, 25–36.

21. Katz, J. Clinical use of auditory tests. In (see Ref. 8).

22. Katz, J. and Arndt, W. Split-half reliability of the SSW test. Progr. Amer. Speech Hear. Assoc., Las Vegas, Nevada, 1974.

23. Katz, J., Basil, R. and Smith, J. A staggered spondaic word test for detecting central auditory lesions. Ann. Otol., Rhinol., Laryngol., 1963, 72, 908–917.

24. Katz, J. and Illmer, R. Auditory perception in children with learning disabilities. In (see Ref. 3).

25. Katz, J., Myrick, D. K. and Wynn, B. B. Central auditory dysfunction in cerebral palsy. Progr. Amer. Speech Hear. Assoc., Washington, D.C., 1966.

26. Katz, J. and Pack, G. New developments in differential diagnosis using the SSW Test. In: M. Sullivan (Ed.) Central Auditory Processing Disorders. University of Nebraska Press, 1975.

27. Kimura, D. Some effects of temporal lobe damage on auditory perception. Canad. J. Psychol., 1961, 15, 156–165.

28. Lynn, G. and Gilroy, J. Effects of brain lesions on the perception of monotic and dichotic speech stimuli. In: (see Ref. 26).

29. Matzker, J. Two new methods of assessment of central auditory functions in cases of brain diseases. Ann. Otol., Rhinol., Laryngol., 1959, 69, 1185–1197.

30. Myrick, D. A normative study to assess performance of a group of children ages seven through eleven on the staggered spondaic word test. Unpubl. Master's Thesis, Tulane University, 1965.

31. Quiros, J. B. Interpretation de los Resultados Obtiendos con logoaudiometrica accelerada. Rev. Fonoaudiol., 1961, 7, 128–164.

32. Sparks, R., Goodglass, H. and Nickel, B. Ipsilateral versus contralateral extinction in dichotic listening resulting from hemisphere lesions. Cortex, 1970, 249–260.

33. Walsh, T. and Goodman, A. Speech discrimination in central auditory lesions. Laryngoscope. 1955, 67, 1–8.

34. Weisberg, L. and Katz, J. Neurological considerations of auditory impairment. In: (see Ref. 8).

Abstract

Performance of Non-native English Speakers on the Staggered Spondaic Word Test

Steven J. Rawiszer, M.A.

The purpose of the present study was to evaluate the SSW Test on a population of non-native English speakers. Thirty subjects (20 males; 10 females) from four major geographic areas (Africa, Asia, the Middle East, and South America) were evaluated using the standard SSW Test. All subjects had hearing within normal limits as determined by pure-tone audiometry, impedance audiometry, and speech audiometry. None of the subjects had a history of otologic or neurologic disorders. Scores were also obtained for each subject from the Test of English Language as a Foreign Language (TOEFL), which had been administered as part of their matriculation to an American university (California State University, Fresno). The TOEFL is an entrance measure of English language proficiency for non-native English speakers attending colleges and universities in the United States. All subjects were born and had spent their early childhood outside the United States and had not learned English as their first language.

All subjects were administered the SSW Test with the standard instructions. Then a second test was administered later after a brief instructional period. During that session all subjects were thoroughly familiarized with test items and vocabulary. Both test and retest results were scored according to the standard procedures suggested in the SSW Workshop Manual.

Results indicated that all non-native English speakers performed differently than their English speaking counterparts, as defined by Brunt and others. Significant test–retest differences were found for the entire group as well as males and females. However, males and females did not differ in their retest performance. Despite the improvement following instruction, retest scores remained significantly below data reported in the literature for normal hearing, native English-speaking, young adults. A signficant correlation was found between TOEFL scores and the total R-SSW results.

It appears from the results of this study that non-native English speakers tend to do more poorly with the SSW Test even after thorough exposure to the test vocabulary than native speakers.

Master's thesis, California State University, Fresno, 1979.

Subjects may have considered the two-spondee words in each test item as four unrelated monosyllables. In addition, the dichotic presentation mode may have created an extra distraction for subjects who were already having difficulty with unfamiliar or somewhat familiar words. Consequently, the native language of a patient should be considered prior to administering the SSW Test to point up a potential reason for an inordinately large number of errors not related to central auditory dysfunction.

The Development of a Japanese SSW Test

Floyd W. Rudmin

Introduction

The Staggered Spondaic Word (SSW) Test is a dichotic speech test for evaluating central auditory function (Katz, 1962). The test consists of 40 items each composed of a pair of spondaic words, i.e. "daylight" and "lunchtime." The pairs are matched so that the first part of the first word ("day") can be combined with the last part of the second word ("time") to form a third foil word ("daytime"). Spondaic words encourage correct responses by normals, and foil words encourage errors by abnormals. The two test words are presented dichotically in a partially overlapping manner. For example, as "daylight" is presented to one ear in the first channel, the onset of "lunchtime" to the other ear in the second channel is delayed so that "light" and "lunch" arrive at the same time and compete. The SSW Test is differentially sensitive to disorders in many regions of the cerebrum and brain stem, including cortical reception areas (Katz, 1963; 1968), various cortical non-auditory reception areas (Balas, 1971; Katz and Pack, 1975), cerebral auditory commissural tracts (Katz et al., 1975), auditory regions of the cerebellum (Katz, 1977), and upper vs. lower brain stem (Katz, 1970).

The SSW Test has several clinical strengths because its design includes: (1) common spondaic words, (2) a slow, clear, loud presentation, (3) a time staggered dichotic mode, and (4) a correction factor for

Audiology Japan 22, 36–40, 1979.

word discrimination problems. The SSW is relatively insensitive to peripheral hearing loss and the resulting word discrimination problems. Normal subjects perform essentially without error and show little variability: after corrections for word discrimination, mean SSW scores for normals is about 2 % error, with a standard deviation of about 2 % (Brunt, 1972). Laterality effects due to hemispheric dominance for language is clinically insignificant (Brunt, 1972). The SSW is not sensitive to sex, intelligence, or socio-economic factors (Brunt, 1972). Finally, because the subjects' task is the identification of familiar words, the test is amenable to diverse populations, including children, the aged, the mentally retarded, schizophrenics, and patients hospitalized with CNS disorders (Brunt, 1972).

At present, there is no clinical audiological test in Japanese equivalent to the SSW Test (Tanaka, 1976). The objective of this study was to develop a staggered dichotic speech test in Japanese that will parallel the design of the SSW Test, List EC. The methodology was largely empirical. Two experiments were performed. The purpose of Experiment I was to select a class of Japanese words equivalent to English spondaic words, and to then select words within that class that are both familiar and appropriate for test items. The purpose of Experiment II was to record and dichotically align the test items similarly to the SSW Test, EC, and to then select those items for the final tapes that are most intelligible.

Experiment I

Since Japanese has no class of spondaic words, several feasible classes of words were considered: (1) Numbers with counters, i.e. "ni hiki" (two animals); (2) Two syllable words, with each syllable words a morpheme represented by a single kanji, i.e. "hei wa" (peace); (3) Three syllable words, i.e. "sumi e" (ink painting); and (4) Four syllable words, i.e. "shiro kuma" (white bear). A syllable was defined as a peak of sonorancy, so that double duration vowels, as in "Kyushu," or CVC combinations, as in "konbon," were counted as one syllable each. Most Japanese count syllables on the basis of hiragana orthography and would classify these words as four syllable words, rather than as two syllable words.

With the help of a Japanese language informant, 50 common words were selected for each class and recorded. Each word was preceded by the carrier phrase "tsugi wa" (Next is), and intensities were adjusted to have equal peak intensities, ± 2 dB. The subjects were 8 adult native speakers of Japanese. All had normal hearing. Speech Reception Threshold instructions (in Japanese) and 10 practice items were presented monaurally at 15 dB SL. Subsequent 10 item blocks were presented at successive 5 dB decrements, with the final presentation at −5 dB SL. A questionnaire about the quality of the word lists and of the recording was completed by the subjects after the test.

The resulting intelligibility functions for the four classes of words, as well as for English spondaic words (Hirsh et al, 1952), were graphed. All four intelligibility functions were suitably similar to that of English spondaic words for use with a staggered dichotic speech test. However, four-syllable words were selected as the most appropriate because they had the lowest threshold of intelligibility (−1 dB SL), the greatest mean correct responses for each level (6, 22 out of 10), and the smallest mean standard deviation of errors (1.57). When four syllable words are separated into component segments, i.e. "shiro" and "kuma," each segment is a complete word. The subjects' responses to the post-test questionnaire revealed that the words were common, that the recording quality was good, and that pronunciation speed was average. Five subjects reported the presence of an accent, and four of these felt that the pronunciation seemed unnatural and difficult to understand. Since none of the subjects spoke the same dialect as the speaker, the test results include dialect variables. The high performance of four syllable words, despite dialect effects, indicates that they have some resistance to dialect distortion.

With the help of a Japanese language informant, a list of 90 pairs of matched four-syllable words was compiled. Words were selected to be common and not emotionally loaded (Broadbent et al., 1967). Words were paired so that the non-competing segments could be combined to form a foil word. For example, "yubin kyoku" (post office) paired with "denwa bango" (telephone number) can yield the foil word "yubin bango" (postal code). This list of 90 pairs of four syllable words was sent to 3 survey assistants in Japan. Each assistant interviewed: (1) a child under age 10, (2) a teenager, (3) an adult male, (4) an adult female, and (5) an adult over age 50. These people were asked to select 20 items from the list of 90 that would be familiar and easy for children, and 20 to 30 items that would be unfamiliar or difficult for Japanese in general. Based on their judgments, 30 of the original 90 pairs of four syllable words were eliminated. A recording script was prepared, consisting of the 60 remaining test items, 8 words for practice items, and instructions in Japanese.

Experiment II

An analysis of the SSW Test, List EC, revealed (1) that there is a slight unnatural pause between the two segments of each spondaic word, and (2) that the competing segments are dichotically aligned to have simultaneous centers. For example, the test item "meat sauce"/"base ball" can be perceived as a two-word task (to encourage correct responses by normal subjects) or as a four-word task (to encourage differential errors by abnormal subjects) because there is a slight unnatural pause splitting each spondaic word. Also, the competing segments "sauce" and "base" do not have simultaneous onsets, as is common with dichotic tests, but simultaneous centers, i.e. "base" begins 130 msec after "sauce" but also ends 130 msec before "sauce" ends. The 60 items for the Japanese experimental tape were recorded in standard Japanese by a native speaker. Although pitch contours for four syllable words were maintained, slight pauses were introduced between segments. Thus, by pitch contours, "shiro kuma" can be perceived as one word, yet by the pause it can be perceived as two words. The 60 paired items were aligned dichotically to have simultaneous centers, ± 26 msec. Instructions and practice items were dubbed onto the experimental tape. The carrier phrase "De wa ii desu ka?" (Are you ready?) preceded each test item in the lead channel. Intensity was adjusted so that the competing segments had equal intensity, ± 4 dB.

The subjects were 8 adult native Japanese with normal hearing bilaterally. Instructions in Japanese were presented at 30 dB SL. Practice items and the 60 dichotic test items were presented at 15 dB SL. This low presentation level, rather than the 50 dB SL level used clinically, was necessary to challenge the normal subjects and thereby generate errors. Items were presented alternately left ear first, then right ear first, and so on. Half of the subjects began with the right ear first, half with the left ear first. Errors were noted as omissions or as substitutions, which were transcribed phonetically. With 480 presentations (8 subjects × 60 items) overall mean intelligibility was just over 85%. 27 items were reported correctly by all 8 subjects, and 10 items accounted for over 50% of the errors. These 10 items and an additional 10 items were rejected from consideration for the final tapes. The arrangement of the remaining 40 items for the adult Japanese SSW Test, and the selection and arrangement of the easiest 20 items for the children's version of the test, were decided on the basis of intelligibility and familiarity. Katz (1977) indicates that the difficulty of the SSW Test, List EC, is not uniform, but that the first 10 items and the last 10 items are easier than the middle two blocks of 10 items. The test items for the final versions of the Japanese SSW Test were organized to have a similar difficulty pattern. (Copies of the final scripts and tapes may be obtained from the author, at cost.)

Discussion

Obviously, this study represents a beginning, rather than the completion, of a project to develop a Japanese SSW Test for clinical use. The English and Japanese versions of the test have parallel designs. Errors made by subjects on the 60 dichotic items on the experimental tape were qualitatively similar to those that appear on the SSW Test during clinical use: there were a total of 37 omissions, 60 substitutions (5 involving the use of the foil word), and 3 reversals. Considering the 40 items selected for the adult version of the Japanese test, no laterality effects due to hemispheric dominance for language are apparent: out of 640 presentations per ear, there were 12 errors for each ear.

However, further studies need to be considered before these tapes can be adopted for clinical use. Considering the 40 items selected for the adult version, the leading four-syllable words had more errors (16); than the lagging four-syllable words (2). This type of "lag effect" has been reported by others (Porter et al., 1969; Studdert-Kennedy et al., 1970; Katz, 1977), and may be inherent in dichotic testing. The magnitude of the "lag effect" in this study may be due to low presentation level and/or to the dubbing and alignment techniques. This requires further study. Also, the tapes need to be tested with larger populations of normal subjects to quantify the effects, if any, of age, intelligence, educational background, and dialect. Normal subjects with peripheral hearing loss need to be tested to determine if Japanese SSW dichotic intelligibility correlates with monaural word discrimination scores. Because the SSW scores have a high correlation ($r = .93$) with word dicrimination scores, a correction factor for peripheral disorders is possible (Katz et al. 1963). Finally, it is crucial to establish the ability of the Japanese SSW Test to locate central auditory disorders.

References

Balas, R. F. Staggered spondaic word test: support. Ann. Otol Rhiol. Laryngol. 80: 132–134 (1971).

Broadbent, D. E. and Gregory, M. Perception of emotionally toned words. Nature Lond. 215: 581–584 (1967).

Brunt, M. A. The staggered spondaic word test. In J. Katz (ed.): Handbook of clincial audiology (Williams & Wilkins, Baltimore 1972).

Hirsh, I. J., Davis, H., Silverman, S. R., Reynolds, E. G., Eldert, E. and Benson, R. W. Development of materials for speech audiometry. J. Speech Hearing Dis. 17: 321–337 (1952).

Katz, J. The use of staggered spondaic words for assessing the integrity of the central auditory nervous system. J. Aud. Res. 2: 327–337 (1962).

Katz, J. The SSW test: an interim report. J. Speech Hearing Dis. 33: 132–146 (1968).

Katz, J. Audiologic diagnosis: cochlea to cortex. Menorah Med. J. 1; 26–36 (1970).

Katz, J. Personal communication (1977).

Katz, J., Basil, R. and Smith, J. A staggered spondaic word test for detecting central auditory lesions. Ann. Otol. Rhinol. Laryngol. 72: 908–918 (1963).

Katz, J., Kushner, D. and Pack, G. The use of competing speech (SSW) and environmental sound (CES) tests for localizing brain lesions. Presented at Am. Speech Hearing Assoc. Meeting, Washington, D.C. (1975).

Katz, J. and Pack, G. New developments in differential diagnosis using the SSW test. In M. Sullivan (ed.): Central Auditory processing disorders (U. of Nebraska, Omaha, 1975).

Porter, R., Shankweiler, D. and Liberman, A. Differential effects of binaural time differences on perception of stop consonants and vowels. Proceedings of 77th Annual Meeting of Am. Psychol. Assoc., Washington, D.C. (1969).

Studdert-Kennedy, M., Shankweiler, D. and Schhulman, S. Opposed effects of a delayed channel on perception of dichotically and monotically presented CV syllables. J. Acoust. Soc. Amer. 48: 599–602 (1970).

Tanaka, Y. Personal communication (1976).

No aspect of the SSW test has generated more interest than the application to the study of children. Most of the SSW and CES work thus far has been with adults, relating results to site of dysfunction. By its nature the SSW is well suited to this purpose, because the acoustic task is relatively simple and the competition is not very demanding of a normal adult listener. Thus, it is the person with a central problem who stands out. In its standard form, the SSW would be far too easy to discriminate clearly among normal listeners. The situation is quite different in the case of children.

Because of incomplete language development and limited vocabulary and also because of maturational factors, young normal children make many errors on the SSW Test. How and why they make certain types of errors instead of others provides an opportunity to study the refinement of auditory processing skills. Use of the test for identifying sites of dysfunction must be necessarily more cautious, particularly with young children. Unless there is known brain damage, to which the audiologist is referring, it is inappropriate to refer to "lesions" based on test scores. This is especially true in cases of learning and speech problems.

From the work of White (1977), Kushner, et. al. (1977), Johnson et. al. (1981) and others we see emerging a pattern of normal performance on the SSW. Although it is often the case, we cannot expect a child who is quite young (e.g., 8 years old) to have normal adult performance. It is for this reason that one should not use the adult (i.e., 11–60 years) TEC analyses with children. Should one decide to do this computation, it would not be appropriate to assume that an auditory reception, high brain stem, or corpus collosum problem had been identified. The errors on the SSW could arise from a wide variety of sources, and typically do, in a child who has not yet developed normal adult abilities.

6

Use of the Staggered Spondaic Word Test and Competing Environmental Sounds Test With Children

In the case of children with learning disabilities we must be even more cautious in site of dysfunction statements. While the adult localization information stands as a useful reference and support in the evaluation of normal auditory development, it is further removed from the child with a severe language or learning problem. These children may not be as organized in their cerebral structure and functions as the normal child or adult (Heir, 1980). Indeed, this might be the underlying problem being reflected in poor performance. A child who is developing slowly in one area of function cannot be expected to be developing normally in all other functions. Thus, the typical ages of development might be offset and contribute heavily to the disturbance in SSW and CES performance.

In the area of children we should be especially sensitive to the information that the SSW and CES can provide. On the SSW, the Ear Effect, Order Effect, and other forms of Response Bias are certainly as important as the scores themselves. There is a growing trend to use Response Bias information in making recommendations for therapy and compensations.

One good example of the ways in which the SSW can be applied is shown in the article by Jay Lucker on the Type A pattern. In this work he relates the SSW to spelling and reading. Amy Wetherby and her colleagues show an indepth look at the SSW and CES as they relate to language disorders in autistic children. From the bulk of the work included in this Chapter, there seems to be a great deal of memory (Brunt, 1980) and processing information that one could derive from giving the SSW and CES tests. The information could not only be used in explaining the child's problems to parents and teachers, but also in designing intervention strategies and teaching compensations.

Abstract

A Normative Study to Assess Performance of a Group of Children Aged 7–11 on the Staggered Spondaic Word (SSW) Test

Dean Kent Myrick, M.S.

The present study was designed to assess performance of a group of 50 normal children, aged 7–11 years, on a 20-item Staggered Spondaic Word (SSW) Test adapted for use with children. In addition, a control group of 10 adults was given the 20-item test in order to establish an adult normal baseline for the abbreviated form.

On the basis of the present investigation, the following conclusions are tenable:

1. As chronological age increases, both the number of errors and the size of the standard deviation decreases.

2. The right ear is superior to the left ear in performance on the SSW Test for children, suggesting a significant dominance effect.

3. There is no difference between ears for the adult group indicating that there is no apparent dominance effect operative on this test for adult subjects.

4. The age of 10 appears to be a transitional stage between the performance of children and adults on the SSW Test; however, by the age of 11, performance reaches an adult level.

5. There are no differences between performance of male and female subjects on the SSW Test as young as seven years of age.

6. The use of mental age is not superior to chronological age in predicting SSW score. It is concluded that either or both may be used to specify baseline performance for an individual.

Master's Thesis, Tulane University, New Orleans, Louisiana, 1965.

7. Results of this study replicate previous studies showing
    that normal adults have very few errors and very small
    standard deviations on the SSW Test.

8. The literature indicates normal SSW results as low as eight
    years of age. This level as a general rule is too optimistic.

Abstract

Performance on Three Auditory Tests by Children With Functional Articulation Disorders

Michael Brunt, M.A. (Ph.D.)

Sixty normal hearing children with functional articulation disorders were evaluated on three auditory tests. There were 43 males and 17 females ranging in age from 8–0 to 10–0 years. Each child received the Barker and England Arizona Articulation Proficiency Test (AAPT) and the Ammons Full Range Picture Vocabulary Test. (The AAPT provided a numerical score of articulation proficiency.) These were followed, in randomized order among the subjects, by a Central Institute for the Deaf discrimination list (W-22's) per ear, the Wepman Auditory Discrimination Test (Wepman), and Katz' Staggered Spondaic Word (SSW) Test. All auditory tests were tape recorded.

The data showed no relationship between articulation proficiency and performance on the W-22, Wepman, or SSW tests. The subjects were divided into two groups with respect to mental age and mental age greater than and lesser than chronological age. Analysis of variance of these groups relative to the Wepman, W-22's and AAPT tests suggested that the greater the mental age, the more proficient the

Master's Thesis, University of Pittsburgh, Pittsburgh, Pennsylvania, 1965.

Mean error scores in percent for Raw and Corrected SSW results for 60 subjects.

Raw SSW Scores			
RNC	RC	LC	LNC
14.5	30.3	52.8	23.0
	RE	Total	LE
	22.4	30.2	37.9
Corrected SSW Scores			
RNC	RC	LC	LNC
2.2	17.9	39.1	9.3
	RE	Total	LE
	10.1	17.0	24.1

children were in auditory discrimination and articulatory skills. There was no relationship between mental age and the SSW Test in this study.

There were errors on all conditions on the SSW Test, although the general pattern showed poorer performance for the left ear, especially for the left-competing (LC) items. This pattern was thought to reflect cerebral dominance for language rather than suggestive of cerebral auditory dysfunction. For example, among the 60 subjects, on the corrected competing conditions 54 showed more errors for LC and six for RC. For the corresponding raw competing conditions there were more errors for LC for 50 subjects, more for RC for seven children, and equal errors for three subjects. The table below presents the mean error scores for all seven SSW scores, both raw and corrected.

Central Auditory Dysfunction in Learning Disabled Children

James H. Stubblefield, Ph.D. and C. Ellery Young, Ed.D.

Comparisons of performance on the SSW Test of Central Auditory Function were made between 7- and 11-year-old learning disabled and normally achieving children. Statistically significant performance differences were found between the two groups, with reversal-type errors being a consistent differentiator. The LD group scored well above the top limit of allowable errors (for normal performance) and the control group scored well below the norms standardized for adult performance. It appears reasonable to consider judging the performance of 7-through 11-year-old children by adult performance criteria, and a screening instrument for early detection of central auditory dysfunction appears feasible.

The role of peripheral auditory impairment in learning problems is well known and well documented. Screening procedures are common practice for the early identification of hearing sensitivity problems. Unfortunately, these procedures are not effective for the detection or description of central auditory dysfunction. Central dysacusis is

Journal of Learning Disabilities, 8, 32–37, 1975.

not measured in Hertz or decibels; better dimensions in these areas are to be found in tests which measure speed of perception, synthesis, and understanding of auditory signals. Literally, a child may have perfect peripheral sensitivity but be limited in his "understanding of what he hears"—from only a slight degree to almost total noncomprehension. The necessity for a method of early detection of elements of central auditory dysfunction is urgent since each year lost during the critical early readiness years is irretrievable in terms of learning achievement, language development, and personality adjustment.

Various methods of attempting to identify children with central auditory dysfunction have been used, but with limited success. Since filtered speech procedures have not proven discriminating between children with known specific learning disabilities and control children (Hodgson 1966) and most dichotic tests of undistorted speech have shown a marked laterality effect (Boshes & Mykelbust 1964, Kimura 1961, 1963), it appears that the most promising current evaluative procedure for identifying central auditory dysfunction in children is the Staggered Spondaic Words Test (SSW) developed and standardized by Katz (1962, 1968). Consistent results have been reported in differentiating LD children, and theraputic procedures have been developed and are being used effectively (Katz & Illmer 1972, Katz & Burge 1971). From these tests and from the results of testing performed by Myrick (1965), age adjustment criteria have been developed for children down to age 5, although these criteria represent the extreme upper limits of normal performance and are not intended as means. The right-hand column in Table 1 shows how the error percentage score considered to be normal decreased as the child's age increased.

(Upper score limits for normal performance: Ear = 10; Total = 5)

TABLE 1.
Mean C-SSW ear and total scores from normative study to establish age adjustment criteria (Katz & Myrick 1965).

Age	C-SSW Left Ear (% error)	C-SSW Right Ear (% error)	C-SSW Total (% error)	SD	Upper Limits of Normal ($\bar{x}$.+ one SD)
7 years	12.0	18	11.1	10.4	21.5
8 years	1.5	8	3.6	7.9	11.5
9 years	2.0	8	4.8	6.2	11.0
10 years	0.0	4	1.8	3.2	5.0
11 years	0.0	1	.6	3.7	4.3

Use of the SSW and CES Tests with Children

The purpose of this study was to take the first step toward determining the feasibility of adapting the SSW Test for screening and early identification of children with central auditory dysfunction. Questions asked were: (1) Are there significant and readily identifiable performance differences between LD children and normally achieving children of comparable age, background, and intelligence range? (2) Can performance be evaluated by reference to the standardized normative data presently available for the SSW Test (Katz 1968) for the age range of 11 years to 60 years, or must criteria adjusted for age (Myrick 1965) be used when evaluating children under the age of 11 years?

Method

Subjects.

The study group was composed of 20 children, 10 boys and 10 girls between the ages of 7 and 11 years, who had been referred to a College Educational Evaluation Center for the purpose of psychometric and educational testing. These children were experiencing school difficulties to a degree that had resulted in their being categorized as learning disabled at their schools. Learning disability here refers to deficits in one or more of the specific intellectual processes. Children with learning disabilities demonstrate a discrepancy between expected and actual achievement in spoken, read, or written language, mathematics or other school subjects. The learning breakdown may be in understanding, integrating or using information. It is not primarily the result of sensory, motor, intellectual or emotional handicap, nor lack of opportunity to learn (Kass & Myklebust 1969, Masland 1969).

The comparison group consisted of 20 children from a local elementary school who were judged by their teachers as normally achieving in their studies. All children in both groups were free of physical disabilities, were from equal middle-level socioeconomic backgrounds (rural environments, high school educated parents, no poverty situations), and had IQs in the normal range, 90 to 104 as measured by the WISC. (Normal in this instance was used to mean that intelligence was not a primary factor in the learning disability.)

Subjects for the comparison group were chosen at random from a sample of 50 suitable subjects after the LD children had been tested and age, sex, socioeconomic, and IQ criteria were established for matching.

Procedure.

All testing was performed by an audiologist in a college hearing clinic. Each subject was tested with a standard battery of air conduction pure tone threshold sensitivity tests and speech audiometric procedures (speech reception threshold and discrimination testing in quiet and in noise) to evaluate peripheral hearing sensitivity and to detect any peripheral impairment which could have contaminated the results of central auditory assessment. All procedures were generally accepted clinical methods. All subjects were found to be free of any significant peripheral impairments.

The instrument used to assess central auditory function was the Staggered Spondaic Words Test (SSW) as developed by Katz (1962, 1968) and standardized by Katz et al. (1963), Katz & Fishman (1964), Goldman & Katz (1965); Katz & Myrick (1965), and Brunt (1969). Basically, the SSW is a dichotic listening procedure in that different speech stimuli are presented to each ear simultaneously as competing messages. The subject is expected to repeat both messages in the order presented. The way in which a child is able to handle competing messages will have an important effect on his learning abilities (Katz & Illmer 1972). A person with normal auditory processing and integrating capacities has no difficulty perceiving and repeating the competing messages. A subject with auditory figure-ground differentiation problems will experience difficulty in proportion to his impairment.

Spondaic words (two-syllable words of high familiarity and auditory redundancy) are used to lessen the effects of peripheral hearing impairments and to broaden the range of patient applicability as concerning age, intelligence, education, sophistication, and training. Each test item is composed of two spondees recorded in partially overlapping manner. Different spondees are presented to each ear with the last part of the first-presented spondee being overlapped in time sequence with the first part of the second-presented spondee in the opposite ear. Figure 1 presents an example of two SSW test items illustrating temporal sequence of word presentation and reversal of the leading ear (Brunt 1972). The ear stimulated first changes with each presentation of two spondaic word pairs. To further enhance the difficulty of the task for patients with central auditory problems, the test words are paired so the noncompeting words form yet a third meaningful word. An excellent description of the test and of presentation procedures is found in Brunt (1972). The interested reader is urged to consult this reference for a more complete test explanation.

The SSW Test was administered to standardized instructions (Brunt 1972), and the standard SSW List E on stereophonic tape was utilized. Instructions for the test were the same for all subjects in that the directions were recorded on the SSW tape utilized. Each practice item and each test item ws preceded by the carrier phrase: "Are you ready?" Total test time was approximately 20 minutes with adequate time allowed for subject response. All testing, recording, and scoring were done by the same audiologist. Standard calibration techniques were employed to check the calibration of all audiometric instrumentation to ANSI 1969 standards prior to each day's clinical testing.

Results

Table 2 shows the upper limits of error percentages which can be considered within normal performance. All score interpretation for the study was based on a comparison of obtained-error scores with the standardized norms in Table 2. Table 3 presents the mean corrected SSW scores (whether "competing" or "noncompeting"), ear scores (whether the right or left ear led in presentation), and total scores for both groups of subjects according to age levels. Comparison of the obtained-error percentage scores in Table 4 with the norms in Table 2 shows how each of the LD children consistently made more errors than are considered indicative of normal central auditory processing. Note that *none* of the children in the control group made enough errors to

FIGURE 1. ━━━━━━━━━━━━━━━━━━━━━━━━━━━━━━━━
Example of two SSW Test items illustrating temporal sequence of word presentation and reversal of the leading ear. Each ear receives stimulation in isolation as well as in competition with the other. For example, "up" is heard as a right-noncompeting (R-NC) condition while "stairs" and "down" are heard as right-competing (R-C) and left-competing (L-C) conditions, respectively. Finally, "town" is heard as the left-noncompeting (L-NC) condition. As illustrated, the ear stimulated first changes from item to item (adapted from Katz 1972).

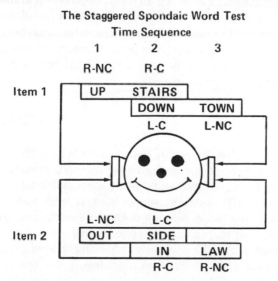

TABLE 2.
Upper limits for corrected SSW scores.*

C-SSW	Normal	Mildly Abnormal	Moderately Abnormal	Severely Abnormal
Total Score	5	15	35	100
Ear Score	10	20	40	100
Condition Score	15	25	45	100

* From Katz (1968).

place him above the "limit-of-error percentage" for normal performance. Standard deviations are shown for group mean scores only. An
analysis of the various scores indicates that there is a substantial difference in the performance levels of the two groups that remains
relatively constant through all age groups. In the summary of means,
standard deviations, and values of t presented in Table 4, note that t
values indicate far greater critical ratios than are necessary to discount
chance occurrence of differences between groups.

Errors made by the LD groups were consistently spaced
throughout the 40 test presentations of competing spondees, with approximately 25% of the errors occurring in each of the four
10-presentation segments of the test. The control group made a much
larger percentage of their errors in the first quarter or half of the test. In
the control group, 95% of the subjects *who were going to make an error*
made at least one in the first five presentations; 100% of those who experienced an error made it in the first 10 presentations. In other words,
if a normal child is going to make an error, he makes it at the beginning
of the test when he is not too sure what he is supposed to do—or he
makes it as a result of inattention when the test becomes boring for him.
The test never becomes boring from being too easy for the LD children;
they start making errors at the beginning of the test and continue to
make errors throughout the test.

Discussion

The following conclusions seem appropriate within the limits of the
population sampled and the audiometric methods described:

(1) There are significant and readily identifiable performance differences on the SSW Test between children with specific learning
disabilities and children achieving normally in academic studies. The
t-test indicated signficance well beyond the .01 level.

(2) All children in the normally achieving control group scored at
or below the standardized limits in all categories of the SSW Test.

(3) The incidence of reversal-type errors appears to be a valid indicator of central auditory dysfunction in younger children, although it diminishes in occurrence as the child grows older and possibly learns to compensate more efficiently and consistently for his perceived reversals. No reversal-type errors were scored by any child in the comparison group.

TABLE 3.
Mean C-SSW scores: condition, ear, and total (% of error), for learning disabled group and comparison group.*

Age	LD Subjects N = 20 Condition Scores					Comparison Subjects (N = 18) Condition Scores				
	RNC	RC	LC	LNC	C-SSW Total	RNC	RC	LC	LNC	C-SSW Total
7 years	3.25	34.5	30.5	5.5		0.0	0.0	0.0	0.0	
		RE = 18.87	LE = 18.0		18.43		RE = 0.0	LE = 0.0		0.0
8 years	1.66	21.66	41.66	8.33		0.0	0.0	0.0	0.0	
		RE = 12.0	LE = 25.0		18.33		RE = 0.0	LE = 0.0		0.0
9 years	4.16	25.83	26.66	3.58		-1.0	2.41	7.33	-.33	
		RE = 15.0	LE = 15.12		15.06		RE = .71	LE = 3.5		2.10
10 years	.25	4.25	28.37	1.87		0.0	1.25	4.62	.25	
		RE = 2.25	LE = 15.12		8.59		RE = .62	LE = 2.42		1.53
11 years	4.2	14.2	30.2	3.6		0.0	2.0	3.0	0.0	
		RE = 9.2	LE = 16.95		13.18		RE = 1.0	LE = 1.5		1.25
Entire Group		RE = 10.88	LE = 17.35		14.14		RE = .65	LE = 2.12		1.39
SD of Scores		RE = 2.91	LE = 2.90		1.70		RE = 1.07	LE = 3.12		1.84

* t-test results show $t \geq .01$ level of significance (see Table 4)

TABLE 4.

Means, standard deviations, and values of t (critical ratio) for C-SSW scores and number of errors experienced.

Corrected Scores (SSW Test)	LD Group (N=20) x̄. SD		Comparison Group (N=18) x̄. SD		t value*
C-SSW Total Scores	14.14	1.70	1.39	1.84	22.21
C-SSW Right Ear Scores	10.88	2.91	.65	1.07	9.98
C-SSW Left Ear Scores	17.35	2.90	2.12	3.12	15.55
Number of errors	23.45	4.24	2.00	2.96	18.09

* To be significant at the .01 level, the t values must be larger than 2.75.

(4) Growing familiarity with the task (as the test progresses) tends to decrease the rate of errors made by children with normal central auditory function while LD children continue to experience the same relative error rate throughout all 40 presentations of spondaic word pairs in the test.

(5) It appears reasonable to consider judging the performance of children 7 years old and older by the criterion of standardized limits for normal performance presently used for the 11- through 60-year-old range.

(6) Any child 7 years or older scoring above the standardized norms (for 11 through 60 years) should be given serious consideration for the possibility of specific learning disabilities being present or potentially present.

(7) There appears to be a possibility that a screening version of the SSW Test could be developed utilizing 5 or 10 presentations of spondaic words (as opposed to the present 40 presentation test). Possible criteria could be that children scoring no errors in the first 5 presentations would be considered as having passed the screening while any child scoring 1 or more errors in the first 5 presentations or 3 or more errors in the first 10 presentations would be considered suspect of central auditory dysfunction and should be administered the entire list of test presentations.

A current challenge for audiologists and others in the communications field certainly includes early identification of children with language and learning disabilities, but after identification must come specific services to remedy their poor performance (Richardson 1974). Certainly, not all children who perform poorly on the SSW Test should be thought of as displaying neurological problems, but a significantly high error score can be indicative of the need for medical evaluation, and the appropriate referrals must be made. Problems in auditory figure-ground-differentiation, which are commonly exhibited by the children who perform poorly on the SSW Test, can often be helped significantly by auditory training procedures to improve their perception of speech in competing backgrounds. Self-teaching programs are available commercially in cassette form which progress in a series of lessons of ascending difficulty (the competing background becomes more and more complex), or a series may always be homemade by anyone interested enough to determine the principles involved. The SSW Test is successful in identifying certain children with learning disabilities and auditory figure-ground-differentiation training quite often can be of benefit to these children.

References

Balas, R. F., and Simon, G. R. The articulation function of a staggered spondaic word list for a normal hearing population. J. Aud. Res., 1964, 4, 285–289.

Boshes, B., and Myklebust, H. R. A neurological and behavioral study of children with learning disorders. Neurology (Minneap.), 1964, 14, 7–12.

Brunt, M. Auditory sequelae of diabetes. Unpublished doctoral dissertation, Univ. of Kansas, 1969.

Brunt, M. The staggered spondaic word test. In J. Katz (Ed.), Handbook of Clinical Audiology. Baltimore, MD.: Williams & Williams, 1972.

Goldman, S., and Katz, J. A comparison of the performance of normal hearing subjects on the staggered spondaic word test given under four conditions—dichotic, diotic, monaural (dominant ear) and monaural (nondominant ear). Paper presented at Amer. Speech and Hearing Ass. Convention, Chicago, 1966.

Hodgson, W. Speech discrimination with children who have central nervous system impairment. Paper presented at the Annual Hearing and Speech Seminar, Kansas Univ. Med. Center, 1966.

Kass, C. and Myklebust, H. Learning disability: an educational definition. J. Learning Disabil., 1969, 2, 38–40.

Katz, J. The use of staggered spondaic words for assessing the integrity of the central auditory nervous system. J. Aud. Res., 1962, 2, 327–337.

Katz, J. The SSW Test: an interim report. J. Speech Hearing Dis., 1968, 33, 132, 132–45.

Katz, J., Basil, R. A., and Smith, J. M. A staggered spondaic word test for detecting central auditory lesions. Ann. Otol., 1963, 72, 908–918.

Katz, J. and Burge, C. Auditory perception training for children with learning disabilities. Menoral Med. J., 1971, 2, 18–29.

Katz, J. and Fishman, P. The use of the detecting spondaic word test as a means of detecting differences between age groups. Unpublished study, 1964.

Katz, J. and Illmer, R. Auditory perception in children with learning disabilities. In J. Katz (Ed.), Handbook of Clinical Audiology. Baltimore, Md.: Williams & Williams, 1972.

Katz, J. and Myrick, D. K. A normative study to assess performance of a group of children, aged seven through eleven, on the staggered spondaic word (SSW) test. Unpublished study, 1965.

Kimura, D. Some effects of temporal lobe damage on auditory perception, Canad. J. Psychol., 1961, 15, 156–165.

Kimura, D. Speech lateralization in an auditory test, J. Comp. Physiol. Psychol., 1963, 56, 899–902.

Masland, R. L. Children with minimal brain dysfunction. In: L. Tarnopol (Ed.), Learning Disabilities: Introduction to Educational and Medical Management. Springfield, Ill.: Charles C. Thomas, 1969.

Myrick, D. K. A normative study to assess performance of a group of children ages seven through eleven on the staggered spondaic word test. Unpublished master's thesis, Tulane University, 1965.

Richardson, S. O. Accountability to the child with a disorder of communication, Presidential Address, 1973 National Convention of Amer. Speech and Hearing Assn., J. Amer. Speech Hearing Assn., 1974, 16, 1, 3–6.

Use of SSW/CES Tests for Identifying Children With Learning Disabilities

Kushner, D., Johnson, D., and Stevens, J.

Thousands of normal and pathological subjects have been evaluated with the Staggered Spondaic Word (SSW) Test, a measure of central auditory function. Recently, a second test, the Competing Environmental Sound (CES) Test was developed. A study (Katz, Kushner and Pack, 1975) was conducted to determine whether a test designed for the identification of left hemisphere functioning (SSW) combined with a test designed to provide information regarding the functioning of the right hemisphere (CES) could be used to identify the involved hemisphere in adults with brain lesions. Results of the study indicated that combined SSW and CES test results provided localization information for adults.

A great number of children with diagnosed learning disabilities reportedly have difficulty processing auditory information. The present experiment was conducted to attempt to determine whether the SSW/CES battery could be used to differentiate normal learners from those children who had been diagnosed as learning disabled.

ASHA Convention, Chicago, Illinois, 1977.

The SSW/CES Battery

The SSW Test is a binaural competing speech test. A detailed description of the test can be found elsewhere (Brunt, 1972). The CES Test will be described here.

The CES Test is a binaural competing sound test in which 14 different recorded sounds are presented simultaneously, one to each ear, through earphones at 50 dB SL. The sounds are: *coughing, dog barking, sneezing, sawing, music, crumpling paper, door slamming, children playing, honking horn, walking in snow,* and *humming.* Four pictures are provided for each test item; two correct responses and two foils. If a subject is not able to name the sounds, he can be instructed to point to the pictures of the sounds he hears.

Subjects

Twenty normal learners and 20 learning disabled children served as subjects. The normal learners had no history of learning disability or skull trauma. I.Q. for these children was reported to be within the normal range, as measured by standard intelligence tests. All learning disabled children had been enrolled for at least one year in a class for the learning disabled, and, when tested, were receiving instruction in a summer school program. I.Q. was reported to be within the normal range for these children, also.

Normal learners and learning disabled subjects were matched for sex and age. Fourteen boys and six girls from each of the two groups participated in the study. In Table 1, the number of subjects is shown by sex and age.

TABLE 1. ▬▬▬▬▬▬▬▬▬▬▬▬▬▬▬▬▬▬▬▬▬▬▬▬▬▬▬▬▬
Number of Subjects x Age and Sex (Total Population = 40)

Age in Years	Number of M/F	Total
6	1 M	1
7	1 M	1
8	3 M, 1 F	4
9	2 F	2
10	4 M, 2 F	6
11	3 M, 1 F	4
12	2 M	2
	14 M, 6 F	20

Procedures

All subjects passed a pure tone screening examination at .5K, 1K, and 4K Hz at 15 dB re: ANSI. Speech Reception Thresholds (SRTs) were obtained via live voice and Word Discrimination Scores (WDSs) were obtained via recorded lists of the CID W-22 Auditory Tests for all subjects. The SSW (List E) and CES tests were administered.

Results and Discussion

Figure 1 shows the percentage of errors for the right and left ear performances on all tests for both groups. SRTs and WDSs were within normal limits and were similar for both groups of children. Thus, the two groups could not be differentiated on the basis of SRTs and WDSs. As shown in Figure 1, the percentage of errors was greater for the learning disabled children than for the normal learners on the SSW Test. Results of a t-test for independent samples indicated a significant difference ($p \leq 0.01$) between the percentage of errors for the two groups in favor of the normal learners. This finding indicates that learning disabled children can be differentiated from normal learners by their performance on the SSW Test.

Examination of Figure 1 for CES test performance revealed a greater percentage of errors for the learning disabled group than for the normal learners. Results of a t-test for independent samples indicated a significant difference between the two groups ($p \leq 0.05$). Thus, the CES Test was found to be useful in differentiating the learning disabled subjects from the normal learners.

FIGURE 1. ━━━━━━━━━━━━━━━━━━━━━━━━━━━━━
Percentage of errors on all tests for both groups of learners.

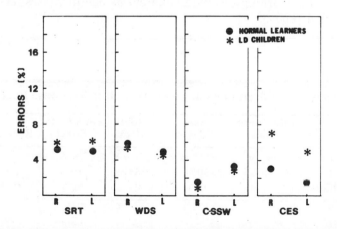

Three different types of response bias—ear effect, order effect, and reversal—can be noted in SSW Test performance (Brunt, 1972). A significant ear effect is identified when there is a difference of five or-more errors between test items beginning in the right ear first and test items presented to the left ear first. A significant order effect occurs with a difference of five or more errors between the first and second spondees. Reversals are defined as a change in word order; that is, words that are repeatead in any order other than the order in which they were presented.

Table 2 shows the response bias for the normal and the learning disabled groups. Forty percent of the normal learners and 85% of the learning disabled subjects showed some type of response bias. A higher percentage of ear and order effect was noted for the learning disabled than for the normal learning subjects. The normal learners made a greater number of errors on the first spondee, while the learning disabled subjects made more errors on the second spondee presented.

Brookshire (1972) wrote that the individual with an auditory system experiencing "noise buildup" tends to process the initial portion of the auditory message accurately, but misses the later portions of the message. The results of this study suggest that learning disabled children were experiencing an auditory system noise buildup—responding appropriately to the initial but inappropriately to the subsequent portion of the auditory message. Reversals were noted for 20% of each population and thus, were not signficant diagnostically.

Pearson correlations were computed between age and test scores for the normal learners and the learning disabled group. For the normal learners, the correlations between SSW test scores and age and CES test scores and ages were not significant. However, a significant difference was found ($p \leqslant 0.05$) between SSW test scores and age and between CES test scores and age for the learning disabled group. This finding suggests that for learning disabled children, as age increases, errors on both tests decrease.

TABLE 2.
Percentage of children in each group exhibiting Response Bias

	Response Bias	Ear Effect	Order Effect	Ear & Order Effect	Reversals
Normal Learners	40%	30%	25%	15%	20%
L.D. Children	85%	55%	60%	30%	20%

Twenty-five percent of the normal learners demonstrated more errors on the SSW than on the CES Test. Eighty-five percent of the learning disabled children demonstrated more errors on the SSW than on the CES Test. These findings indicate that both populations have more difficulty with the processing of verbal stimuli than with the processing of environmental sounds; and that learning disabled children have more difficulty than do normal learners with the processing of both types of stimuli.

In summary, the following conclusions are drawn:

1. It is not possible to use measures of peripheral hearing loss to identify children with learning disabilities.
2. Learning disabled children can be differentiated from normal learners by their performance on both the SSW and CES tests.
3. Ear and order effect on the SSW Test may be used to indicate learning disability.
4. For learning disabled children, the number of errors on both tests decreases as a function of age.
5. Learning disabled children have more difficulty with processing of verbal information and competing environmental sounds than do normal learners.

References

Brookshire, R. H. The role of auditory functions in the rehabilitation of aphasic individuals. In Wertz, R. T. and Collins, M. (eds.), *Clinical Aphasiology Conference Proceedings.* Albuquerque, N.M. (1972).

Brunt, M. The staggered spondaic word (SSW) test. In Katz, J. (ed.), *Handbook of Clinical Audiology.* Baltimore: Williams and Wilkins (1972).

Katz, J., Kushner, D., and Pack, G. The use of competing speech (SSW) and environmental sound (CES) tests for localizing brain lesions. ASHA Convention, 1975.

Performance of Learning Disabled Children and Language Handicapped Children on Central Auditory Tests

Julie Lukas and Ora Eschenheimer

The Staggered Spondaic Word Test (SSW) and Willeford's Central Auditory Processing (CAP) battery were administered to 42 children, divided into three groups of learning-disabled (LD), language-handicapped (LH), and normal subjects, to evaluate any differences in overall patterns of performance among the three groups and to assess which test(s) are most sensitive in identifying LD and LH children. All subjects had peripheral hearing sensitivity within normal limits. A multivariate profile analysis indicated that the relationship of scores across tests (overall pattern) was similar for all three groups, but that the relationship of scores across groups (pattern heights) was significantly different. Children in the normal group scored consistently better than LD and LH children, while LH children scored consistently poorer than children in the normal and LD groups. However, much overlap in CAP scores among the three groups occurred when

ASHA Convention, San Francisco, CA, 1978.

Use of the SSW and CES Tests with Children

standard deviations were utilized. Analysis of the SSW Test, including significant response biases and abnormal total-ear-condition (TEC) category, proved to be the most sensitive measure, providing the clearest delineation among the three groups.

Audiologists now recognize that the peripheral test battery is insufficient for comprehensive auditory evaluation. The assessment of central auditory processors has necessitated the development of specialized tests. A variety of tests attempting to evaluate central auditory functioning has been introduced. As indicated by Willeford and Billger (1978), the diversity of the central auditory tests may be representative of the complexity of the auditory processors and not a reflection of overall test weakness. Hence, different speech test materials and tasks may be necessary for complete assessment of auditory processing. Just as a battery of tests is needed to evaluate function of the peripheral hearing mechanism, it is reasonable to assume that the same is true for the assessment of the central auditory mechanism.

Research has established a relationship between auditory skills and the learning process (Ormson and Williams, 1975; Stubblefield and Young, 175; Orchik, Oeschlager, 1974). Interest is now being focused on the sensitivity of several central auditory tests in identifying the learning-disabled child, as well as his specific deficiency, e.g., binaural synthesis, figure ground, memory, discrimination, and closure (Willeford and Billger, 1978; Pinheiro, 1977; Katz and Medol, 1972). An urgent need exists for appropriate remediation measures. However, current identification and assessment procedures do not provide sufficient diagnostic information to the clinician to confidently recommend specific theraputic intervention. Hence, further refinement of diagnostic tests is essential to the advent of effective remediation procedures. Unfortunately, the efficacy of such tests in identifying learning disabled children is still open to question.

Purpose

The purpose of this study was to evaluate overall patterns of performance on the SSW (Staggered Spondaic Word Test, Katz and Illmer, 1972), and CAP (Central Auditory Processing battery, Willeford, 1978) tests by learning-disabled, language-handicapped, and normal children. The following questions were addressed:

1. Is there a typical pattern of scores across tests that will identify a subject as a member of one particular group?
2. Which test(s) most clearly delineate among the three groups?

Method

Subjects

Forty-two students—14 language-handicapped (LH) and 14 learning-disabled (LD) enrolled in the Diagnostic School for the Neurologically Handicapped, and 14 normal students—were tested. *Language-handicapped* children are those having severe language delay associated with normal intelligence, resulting from central nervous system involvement. *Learning-disabled* children are those who have failed academically at the expected level in several subjects (e.g., spelling and mathematics) despite a history of normal speech and language development and normal intelligence. *Normal* is defined as no known history of language or learning deficiency. (Identification and diagnosis of "language-handicapped" and "learning-disabled" children are routinely performed by the Diagnostic School for the Neurologically Handicapped staff.)

Table 1 shows the mean ages and standard deviations for the three groups. The mean ages for the normal, LD, and LH groups are 14.1, 13.5, and 14.1 years, respectively. All subjects had peripheral hearing sensitivity within normal limits (pure-tone thresholds of at least 10 dB HTL at octave frequencies 500–2000 Hz and 15 dB HTL at 4000 Hz re: ANSI 1969) and a Word Discrimination (W-22) score of at least 88%. Also, all learning-disabled and language-handicapped subjects included in this study scored 90 or better on the performance scale of the Revised Wechsler Intelligence Scale for children (WISC-R) (administered by the school psychologist within one year of the study).

Instrumentation

A Bell and Howell two-channel solid state stereo tape recorder routed through a Maico MA-24 two-channel audiometer (calibrated to ANSI S3.6 1969 specifications) to TDH 39 earphones with MX41AR cushions was used in testing. All subjects were tested in an IAC sound-treated

TABLE 1.

Mean age and standard deviation for each group

Group	Mean	Standard Deviation
Normals	14.1	2.3
LD	13.5	1.7
LH	14.1	2.5

room. The tapes used were the SSW List EC and a high quality duplication of the CAP recorded at the Audio-Visual Laboratory at San Francisco State University.

Procedure

A peripheral test battery consisting of speech reception thresholds, pure-tone thresholds, and a word discrimination (W-22) test was administered. Each child whose results met the criteria for inclusion was administered the Staggered Spondaic Word (SSW) Test and the Central Auditory Processing (CAP) battery, including competing sentences (CS),* filtered speech (FS), and binaural fusion (BF). As found by Willeford (1977), the subjects in this study who took the alternating speech (AS) subtest obtained high scores of 90% or better. Therefore, the AS subtest was eliminated from the test battery in order to reduce test time. To minimize any learning effects, the presentation order of the central auditory tests, including the three subtests within the CAP battery, were randomized. Sensation levels for presentation of the tests were in accordance with those specified by the tests' authors.

Results

The data were analyzed using a multivariate design (Selhorst and Berger, 1978). For purposes of statistical comparisons across tests, raw scores were converted to standard scores (z-scores). The z-score indicates how many standard deviations a score is above or below the mean score for a particular test. Since several types of tests with different number of items, scoring procedures, and standard deviations were used in this study, the z-score conversion allowed more direct comparisons among tests.

Figure 1 shows the multivariate profile analysis (Morrison, 1976) of the standardized mean values for each group. The tests and ear conditions are written horizontally. The SSW Test is represented by right competing (RC) and left competing (LC) conditions only. The 0 line represents the grand mean, which is simply the mean value of all three groups per test per ear. The points above the 0 line are the mean scores which were above the grand mean and similarly, the points below the line are the mean scores which were below the grand mean. This analysis indicates that the pattern of performance across tests for all three groups is similar. That is, the majority of subjects, regardless of group assignment, obtained high scores on the same tests and similarly obtained low scores on the same tests. Any differences in overall pat-

---

* Competing sentences test consisted of repetition of the 30 dB SL sentence only.

FIGURE 1.
Multivariate profile analysis showing the standardized mean values above and below the grand mean (0 line) for each group per test and ear.

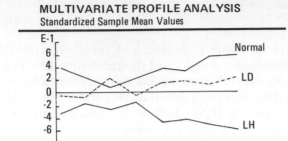

MULTIVARIATE PROFILE ANALYSIS
Standardized Sample Mean Values

tern apparent upon visual inspection of Figure 1 were not found to be statistically significant. For example, the majority of subjects obtained a lower score on the FS test than on the CS test.

Although there was no distinct scoring pattern across *tests* to differentiate one group from another, there were statistically significant differences among the test scores across *groups*. The actual standardized mean scores for each group were significantly different at the $p < .01$ level, $F = 7.53$ (2,39). More specifically, significant statistical differences in scores at the $p < .01$ level were found between the LH and LS groups, $F = 13.37$ (1,39), the LD and normal groups, $F = 8.73$ (1,39), and the LH and normal groups, $F = 14.57$ (1,39). In summary, the multivariate analysis indicates that the relationship of scores across tests was similar for all three groups, but that the relationship of scores across groups was significantly different. The results of the multivariate profile analysis precluded use of this design for evaluating which tests account best for the variance among groups.

If mean scores (percent correct) and standard deviations for all tests and groups (Table 2) are studied at face value, several observations can be made. Right ear scores are consistently better than left ear scores, although the multivariate profile analysis did not show the differences in standard mean values to be statistically significant. Since it is believed that fusion is mediated at the brainstem level (Matzker, 1959), it is not surprising that BF scores do not follow this pattern. It should be noted that the range of scores for the CAP subtests within the normal group was greater than the range for the revised norms (Willeford, 1978). In addition, the mean scores for the filtered speech test were 15% below that of the revised norms. This reinforces the importance of establishing one's own normative data relative to equipment used and the population involved (White, 1977).

TABLE 2. ▬▬▬▬▬▬▬▬

Mean scores (percent correct) and Standard Deviations (   ) for all three groups per test per ear.

	Competing Sentences		Filtered Speech		Binaural Fusion		SSW*	
	Right	Left	Right	Left	Right	Left	Right	Left
N	100%	95%	59%	54%	92%	91%	99%	96%
	(0)	(6.5)	(7.1)	(8.4)	(8.2)	(9.9)	(1.4)	(2.5)
LD	98%	92%	60%	52%	88%	89%	97%	94%
	(4.3)	(10.5)	(7.7)	(8.4)	(10.3)	(9.9)	(3.6)	(4.4)
LH	96%	91%	56%	51%	78%	81%	92%	87%
	(7.4)	(12.3)	(10.7)	(10.4)	(21.4)	(17.9)	(5.8)	(7.3)

* SSW scores represented by Right Competing and Left Competing conditions only.

Abnormal results on the SSW test include an abnormal TEC category or any response bias (ear effect, order effect, reversal, and Type A pattern).* Table 3 shows the percentage of subjects within each group identified as having abnormal results on the SSW Test. Analysis of the SSW Test must progress beyond simply reporting percent correct in order to derive full value from this test. Only two subjects (14%) in the normal group had any abnormal SSW results (5 reversals for one subject and a Type A pattern for the other subject) whereas 79% of the subjects in the LD group and 86% of the subjects in the LH group were identified as having abnormal results in more than one category. That is, when an LH subject's TEC category was significantly depressed, he was more likely to also have significant response bias. An LD subject's results were more often depressed in only one of these three areas.

The left-hand column in Table 4 shows the types and magnitudes of the ear effects for each subject according to groups. An asterisk indicates that the effect is significant according to the test author's criterion. The table clearly shows that none of the subjects in the normal group had significant ear effects. Three subjects in the LD group

---

* TEC category is a descriptor based on the averaged right-left scores, the poorest ear score, and the poorest condition (right ear noncompeting, right ear competing, left ear competing, left ear noncompeting) score.
Ear effect is a significant (5 or greater) difference between the scores for the right ear first (REF) items and the left ear first (LEF) items.
Order effect is a significant (5 or greater) difference between the scores for the first spondee words and the second spondee words.
Reversal is a change in the sequence of the words to that given on the test presentation.
Type A pattern refers to a significantly greater number of errors made in either the right competing condition for REF items or the left competing condition for LEF items.

and over one-half of the subjects in the LH group had significant ear effects. The predominating type of ear effect for all subjects, regardless of significance, was the low/high (L/H) effect. An L/H ear effect indicates that a greater number of errors are made when the items are presented to the left ear first (LEF) than when the items are presented to the right ear first (REF). This is consistent with a right ear-left hemisphere dominance theory. That is, if the contralateral auditory pathway is the primary route for transmitting auditory information, and if the left hemisphere is dominant for speech and language processing, then we would anticipate that speech would be most efficiently processed when transmitted via the right ear.

The right-hand columns in Table 4 show the types and magnitude of the order effects for each subject according to group. Once again, none of the subjects in the normal group have significant order effects. Two subjects in the LD group and one-half of the subjects in the LH group have significant order effects. The predominating type of order effect for LD and LH subjects, regardless of significance, is the high/low (H/L) effect. An H/L order effect indicates that a greater number of errors are made on the first spondee than on the second spondee. Hence, the LD and LH subjects remembered best what they heard last, suggesting a possible memory problem. There is much greater variability in the types of order effects for subjects in the normal group (four L/H and six H/L). This suggests almost a chance occurrence of either H/L or L/H effects, rather than pointing toward a consistent memory problem.

Table 5 shows the percentage of subjects within each group identified as having depressed scores on each test. (Depressed scores are defined as two standard deviations from the normal group mean scores.) The SSW Test had the highest true positive and true negative identification rates, while the CS test had the lowest false positive rate. The BF test had the highest false positive rate. In general, less than one-half of the LD and LH subjects were identified as having depressed scores on each CAP subtest.

TABLE 3.
Percent of subjects within each group identified as having abnormal results on the SSW Test

	TEC Category	ANY Response Bias (excluding Type A pattern)	Type A Pattern	Abnormal Results (in any category)
N	0%	7%	7%	14%
LD	21%	64%	21%	79%
LH	50%	86%	43%	86%

TABLE 4.

Magnitude of ear and order effects on the SSW Test for all subjects in each group.

	EAR	No.	ORDER	No.
	L/H	2	L/H	1
	H/L	1	L/H	1
	L/H	1	H/L	1
	L/H	2	H/L	2
	L/H	2	L/H	2
		0		0
Normals	L/H	3	H/L	4
(N = 14)	L/H	3	L/H	1
	L/H	1	H/L	3
		0		0
	L/H	1	H/L	1
	L/H	3	H/L	3
		0		0
		0		0
	L/H	4	L/H	2
	L/H	3	H/L	3
	L/H	1	H/L*	5
	L/H*	11		0
	L/H	3	H/L	1
	L/H	1	H/L	1
LD	L/H	1	II/L	1
(N = 14)	L/H	2		0
	L/H*	7	L/H	1
		0	H/L	3
	L/H	2	H/L	2
	L/H*	6	H/L	2
	L/II	1	L/H	1
	H/L	1	H/L*	11
	H/L	2	H/L*	6
	L/H*	9	H/L	3
	L/H	3	H/L	1
	L/H*	10	H/L	2
	L/H*	10	H/L	2
	H/L*	5	H/L	3
LH	L/H	1	L/H*	5
(N = 14)	L/H	1	H/L*	13
	L/H*	10	H/L*	7
	H/L	1	L/H	3
	L/H*	5	H/L	3
	L/H*	7		0
	L/H	2	H/L	2
	II/L	3	II/L*	11

---

* Significant according to test author's criterion; i.e., a minimal difference of 5.

TABLE 5.

Percent (N) of subjects within each group identified as having abnormal* results on each test

	LD	LH	N
SSW	79% (11)	86% (12)	14% (2)
CS	50% (6)	43% (6)	7% (1)
FS	7% (1)	14% (2)	14% (2)
BF	22% (3)	43% (6)	29% (4)

* Two standard deviations from the normal group mean scores.

Discussion

The following conclusion may be drawn from the data presented. The pattern of performance across tests for all groups was the same, hence, a typical pattern identifying the LD or LH child did not emerge. However, there were some significant differences in scores among the groups per test. Most noticeable of these differences was on the SSW Test, where the abnormal test results were most frequently apparent in the LH and LD groups. A possible interpretation of these results follows. The LD child may be handicapped by deficiencies in one, many, or all auditory skills. For purposes of identifying such a child, either one test must be broad enough to encompass numerous auditory abilities, or the correct test taxing the deficient auditory ability must be administered. Therefore, we need to take a closer look at the actual tasks involved and auditory skills required by each test. If the SSW Test taxes a greater variety of auditory skills, then it is not surprising that the SSW Test was the most sensitive (high true positives) of the tests. This sensitivity, however, was not based on a single score (TEC category), but rather on a complete and more extensive interpretation of the response biases as described by the test's author. In fact, when using TEC categories as the sole measure, the sensitivity of the SSW Test is dramatically reduced. As can be seen in Table 3, only 21% of the LD and 50% of the LH subjects had depressed TEC categories. When the entire scoring strengths of the test are used (including response bias), 79% of the subjects in the LD group and 86% of the subjects in the LH group are identified as having abnormal SSW results. Perhaps expanding the tasks, refining the tests, and broadening the interpretation of the CAP test would enhance the specificity and sensitivity of this battery as well. For example, repeating both sentences for CS (Willeford, 1977), raising the low pass cutoff frequency for FS (Keith, 1979), and analyzing the syntactic and phonetic errors made on the BF would be of value.

Although the LH subjects scored consistently below the LD subjects, interpretation of test scores for LH children should be carefully considered. Poor scores on a central auditory test employing language stimuli do not necessarily mean a central auditory deficit is present. It is, therefore, important to add to the central auditory battery currently in use some central tests employing stimuli other than language in order to circumvent the language handicap. Tests such as Masking Level Differences (Sweetow and Reddell, 1978) and Pitch Pattern Perception (Pinheiro, 1977) should be further explored.

There are basically three major questions which need further investigation. First, are there any correlations between certain auditory skill deficiencies and *specific* learning disabilities? A clearer delineation of the auditory-visual skills necessary for a good reader, for example, would provide a basic understanding of this complex task. It is important to remember that for purposes of testing and analysis, it is convenient to separate auditory skills, visual skills, etc. However, the interplay of many modalities must ultimately be the focus for a true understanding of each learning disability. Second, are there any correlations between abnormal test performance and certain deficient auditory skills? Katz and Illmer (1972) have found a relationship between a Type A pattern on the SSW Test and learning disabilities in general. Is it possible that this Type A pattern is specific to binaural separation deficiencies? And third, of what significance are these skill deficiencies to the overall resolution of the learning disability? Can improvement in language and academic performance be demonstrated when therapy focuses on these skill deficiencies identified via certain tests?

In conclusion, this study shows that children in the normal group score consistently better than LD and LH children, while LH children score consistently poorer than children in the normal and LD groups. However, much overlap in CAP scores among the three groups occurs when standard deviations are utilized. The SSW Test, with complete interpretation, proved the most sensitive measure, providing the clearest delineation of the three groups. A replication of this study using a larger N would provide valuable information.

Acknowledgements

The authors gratefully acknowledge the valuable comments of Dr. Diane Barrager during the writing of this manuscript. Also, the authors wish to thank John Donaldson for his assistance during the data analysis, and the staff at the Diagnostic School for the Neurologically Handicapped for their cooperation.

References

Katz, J. and Burge, C. Auditory perception training for children with learning disabilities. *Menorah Medical J.*, 2, 18–29 (1971).

Katz, J. and Illmer, R. Auditory perception in children with learning disabilities. In J. Katz (ed.), *Handbook of Clinical Audiology*, Baltimore: Williams and Wilkins (1972).

Katz, J., and Medol, E. the use of phonemic synthesis in speech therapy. *Menorah Medical J.*, 3. 10–18 (1972).

Keith, R. Personal communication (1979).

Matzker, J. Two methods for the assessment of central auditory functions in cases of brain disease. *Ann. Otol.*, 68, 1185–1197 (1959).

Morrison, D. *Multivariate Statistical Methods*, New York: McGraw-Hill (1976).

Orchik, D. and Oeschlager, M. Time-compressed speech discrimination in children: its relationship to articulation ability. Paper presented at the meeting of the American Speech and Hearing Association, Las Vegas (1974).

Ormson, K. and Williams, D. Central auditory function as assessed by time-compressed speech with elementary school age children having articulation and reading problems. Paper presented at the meeting of the American Speech and Hearing Association, Washington, D.C. (1975).

Pinheiro, M. Tests of central auditory function in children with learning disabilities. In R. Keith (Ed.), *Central Auditory Dysfunction*, Cincinnati: University of Cincinnati Medical Center (1977).

Stubblefied, J. and Young, E. Central auditory dysfunction in learning disabled children. *J. Learn. Disabilities*, 8, 89–94 (1975).

Sweetow, R. and Reddell, R. Masking level differences for children with auditory perceptual problems. *J. of the American Auditory Society*, 4, 52–56 (1978).

White, E. Children's performance on the SSW test and Willeford Battery: interim clinical data. In R. Keith (ed.), *Central Dysfunction*, Cincinnati: University of Cincinnati Medical Center (1977).

Willeford, J. Evaluation of central auditory disorders in learning disabled children: differential diagnosis of central auditory dysfunction. *Audiology: An Audio-Journal for Continuing Education*, II, No. 4 (1977).

Willeford, J. Central Auditory processing (CAP) test norms. *Procedures for Tests of Central Auditory Function, Test Manual* (1978).

Willeford, J. and Billger, J. Auditory perception in children with learning disabilities. In J. Katz (ed.), *Handbook of Clinical Audiology*, Baltimore: Williams and Wilkins (1978).

The Effects of Practice on 8–10 Year Old Children Using the Staggered Spondaic Word Test

Stephanie Bryant Minetti and James H. McCartney

Introduction

Katz (1962) introduced the Staggered Spondaic Word (SSW) Test based on concepts of binaural competing messages. The SSW Test is a dichotic procedure using nondistorted English spondee words. These spondee words are presented in a partially overlapping sequence, thus incorporating common words with a difficult competing message presentation. Groen and Hellema (1963) state that the cooperation between ears can be studied as well as the discrimination ability of each ear when test stimuli are presented in this manner.

Katz (1962) explained his rationale for the use of spondee words by stating that spondee words are common, familiar words and are, therefore, applicable to a large population. Spondee words are also intelligible at levels just slightly above pure-tone thresholds. The stability of spondee words remains essentially the same regardless of performance on speech-discrimination tests using monosyllabic words.

The Journal of Auditory Research, 1979, 19, 293–298

Katz et al (1963) found that people with probable central auditory lesions due to head trauma performed poorer on the SSW Test in the ear contralateral to the lesion. They also found a high correlation between the percentage of error on the SSW Test and the percentage of error on the W-22 speech-discrimination test on people with peripheral hearing losses (r = 0.93). The SSW Test score is obtained by subtracting the word discrimination score from the raw SSW Test score.

Balas and Simon (1965) studied the SSW Test in order to establish the most efficient presentation level. They presented SSW Test lists from 0 db SL to 50 db SL to normal-hearing Ss. Results showed that 50 db SL produced the fewest errors. Ss also made few errors at 30 and 40 db SL, indicating the flexibility of presentation level for those persons with reduced dynamic range.

Katz (1968) employed a variety of lengths of the SSW Test to determine which would be most useful. Ss responded to the test at 50 db SL. Lists administered varied from 20 to 80 items; the lists with 40–53 items gave the most reliable information. Ss with conductive losses performed the same as normal-hearing Ss; these made fewer than 15% errors for any of the lengths. Ss with peripheral disorders fell within normal limits when the SSW Test scores were corrected for word discrimination errors. Ss scoring 25% or more errors were felt to have central auditory disorders. Table 1 shows Katz's limits for normal performance.

Although the SSW Test is an excellent test for central auditory nervous system disorders, its application to children under 11 yrs of age is limited. Turner (1966), in a normative study, found performance on the test was poor and inconsistent for Ss under 12 yrs of age. A 20-item children's list was developed by Katz (1968), but performance on this list was still inconsistent. In a review of two unpublished studies, Katz (1968) stated that each author reported a possible ear laterality effect but a consistent correction factor could not be obtained.

TABLE 1
Upper Limit for Corrected SSW Scores*

C-SSW	Normal	Mildly Abnormal	Moderately Abnormal	Severely Abnormal
Total Score	5	15	35	100
Ear Score	10	20	40	100
Condition Score	15	25	45	100

(*Adapted from Katz, 1968, p. 344)

One reason for the inconsistent performance of children may be the confusing practice items used with the SSW Test. The first four presentations are said to be for practice; however, none of these practice items is presented in the same dichotic fashion as the test items. Several investigators (Denny, 1975; Boswell et al, 1974; Hensley et al, 1974) have shown that when practice is related to the main task, performance significantly improves.

Many investigators have explored the area of auditory practice, with some conflicting conclusions. Tillman and Jerger (1959) and Tsappis (1974) found that practice did not improve speech reception thresholds or auditory discrimination ability. However, other investigators have shown that auditory practice leads to an improvement in various test scores. Egan (1948) explored the articulation functions of monosyllabic and of spondee words, and of sentences over different types of communication equipment; he found that discrimination scores of inexperienced Ss improved with practice. Postman and Rosenzweig (1956) and Ritterman (1970) found with nonsense syllables that discrimination scores improved with practice.

This study investigated the effects of practice on the performance of 8–10-yr-old children on SSW scores, testing the hypothesis that performance improves with practice.

Method

A full account may be found in Minetti (1977).

Subjects

These were 20 children aged 8–10 yrs with HTLs≤15 db from 0.5–4 kc/s, with no known history of neurological problems, head trauma, excessive noise exposure, cerebral vascular problems, hereditary hearing problems, and with no obvious perceptual or learning disorders as reported by the parent. Each S was right-handed as evidenced by consistent responses in (a) picking up a paper trumpet and looking through it, (b) kicking a ball, and (c) picking up a pencil.

Equipment

A Maico MA-24 audiometer meeting ANSI specifications was used in an IAC Series 1200 booth. Calibration was performed with calibrated Bruel & Kjaer equipment.

Procedure

Each S first received an ac pure-tone audiogram, followed by SRT, and a speech discrimination test (W-22 list) administered at 50 db re SRT.

The 40 items of the SSW Test, preceded by the four standard practice items, were then given at 50 db re SRT. Half the Ss heard Items 1–40 in order, half heard Items 21–40 and then 1–20 in that order. For both groups the first 20 items heard were to be considered practice.

Instructions were: "You will hear a group of four words. Wait until you have heard all the words and then repeat the words. If you are not sure of the words, guess. The first four groups are for practice. Remember to wait until you have heard all the words before answering." Instructions were repeated as needed during the practice portion of the test.

Results

SRTs were within 5 db of HTL averages for each S. All discrimination scores were 100%.

On the 4 practice items, 50% of these Ss incorrectly repeated the first item, 40% the second, 20% the third, and 60% the fourth.

Table 2 contains the group data by total test and by section. The Mann-Whitney U test (Siegel, 1965) revealed no significant difference between the groups for the total test ($U = 46$; $n_1 = 10$; $n_2 = 10$; $p<.05$), or for Items 1–20 taken as the first half versus Items 1–20 taken as the second half ($U = 25.5$; $n_1 = 10$; $n_2 = 10$; $p<.05$). Thus the improvement between median errors on Items 1–20 by Group I (7.5 errors) vs Group II after practice on Items 21–40 (3.5 errors) did not reach significance.

TABLE 2.
Median and Q for Both Groups Representing Median Number of Errors for Each Section

Section	Group I		Group II	
	Mdn	Q	Mdn	Q
Total	12.5	4.9	11.5	4.5
Halves				
Items 1–20	7.5	3.9	3.5	2.5
Items 21–40	3.2	1.9	8.5	6.0
Competing Stimuli				
First Half*	6.5	2.8	7.5	4.0
Second Half**	3.0	1.1	3.5	2.1
Noncompeting Stimuli				
First Half	0.5	1.4	0.2	0.6
Second Half	0.3	1.0	0.3	2.0

*Items taken before practice
**Items taken after practice

However, the improvement between median errors on Items 21–40 by Group II (8.5 errors) versus Group I after practice on Items 1–20 (3.2 errors) did reach significance ($U = 22.5$; $n_1 = 10$; $n_2 = 10$; $p<.05$).

Group I did not yield a significant reduction in median errors in the second half of its test (drop from 7.5 on its first 20 items to 3.2 on its second 20 items) but Group II did (drop from 8.5 to 3.5) ($T = 6$; $n = 10$; $p<.05$). However, both groups yielded significant reductions in errors in the second half for competing stimuli. Group I yielded a drop from 6.5 to 3.0 ($T = 6$; $N = 9$; $p<.05$), while Group II yielded a drop from 7.5 to 3.5 ($T = 4$; $N = 10$; $p<.02$).

Discussion

These results lend partial support to the conclusions reported by Egan (1948), Postman and Rosenzweig (1956) and Ritterman (1970) about the effects of practice. While Group II reduced the number of errors on the second half of the test, Group I showed no difference when errors on the two halves of the test were compared. Inspection of the direction of differences for the two parts of the test suggest that a more powerful statistical test might result in a significant difference for Group I also.

Both groups produced fewer errors on items involving competing stimuli following practice. Competing stimuli are considered more difficult than noncompeting stimuli. A significant difference was not expected when comparing errors on tghe noncompeting stimuli, since neither group made many errors on the first half of the test.

Between-group comparisons failed to identify significant differences between Items 1–20 taken as practice and after practice. However, a significant difference was found for Items 21–40 under similar conditions. This finding for Items 1–20 as well as the nonsignificant difference between the two parts of the test for Group I introduce contradictory findings.

The results obtained were conflicting in that significantly fewer errors were made on some parts of the SSW Test but not on other parts. Group I showed no significant improvement in total errors for each half of the test. However, examination of the direction of errors showed that fewer were made on the second half of the test after practice. Group I and Group II showed no improvement when comparing noncompeting stimuli. This result is not surprising since neither group made many errors on the first half of the test and therefore not much improvement was possible. But again, each group made fewer errors on the second half of the test. Both groups made significantly fewer errors on the competing portion of the SSW Test. The competing stimuli are more difficult than noncompeting and are weighted more heavily (Katz, 1962, 1968) when determining the possibility of central auditory problems. Therefore, it is important that practice did influence the performance on the competing stimuli. To determine the test score for children under 11 yrs of age, it may be wise to discard the first 20 items and use only the second 20 items. Scores obtained may be more reliable and valid for determining the presence of central auditory problems.

Another contradictory finding was shown in between-group comparisons of Items 21–40 taken under the same conditions. No significant difference was found for Items 21–40. Again, for Items 1–20, Group I (taking these items as practice) made more errors on these items than did Group II (taking these items *after* practice).

Of the comparisons showing no significant difference, all showed fewer errors on items taken after practice. A possible explanation would be the small N of children used. An N larger than 20 would give the statistics more power and would perhaps lead to signifcant differences for all comparisons between test items taken as practice versus those items taken after practice.

Katz (1968), in a review of two unpublished studies, stated that each author reported a possible ear laterality effect for young children. Comparison of right-ear and left-ear stimuli in this study showed no significant difference. In fact, scores for each ear were very close.

The present authors feel that the practice items supplied with the SSW Test are inconsistent and not representative of the test items. Our observation that 50% of Ss incorrectly repeated the first practice item, 40% the second, 20% the third, and 60% the fourth, suggest that Ss did not understand the task from the practice with the standard practice items. More extensive practice, as given in this study, showed that practice truly representative of the test items did improve performance, although not significantly in all cases. These results would support the studies of Denny (1975), Bosewell et al (1974) and Hensley et al (1974) to the effect that when practice was related to the main task, performance significantly improved.

Summary

Katz' Staggered Spondaic Word (SSW) Test was given at 50 db re SRT to 20 normal right-handed children aged 8–10 yrs. Half the Ss heard Items 1–40 in that order, half heard the order Items 21–40, 1–20. Groups yielded similar total scores. For both groups there were no significant L-R ear differences. Practice on a prior 20 items had a significant effect on later responses to competing stimuli in a later 20-item test. There were too few errors on non-competing stimuli for meaningful analysis. Four practice items as provided by a standard version of this test were determined to be too few with children of this age.

Acknowledgement

This report is based upon a Master's thesis completed under the direction of James H. McCartney (see Minetti, 1977). We wish to express thanks to Drs. Maryjane Rees and Robert Tice for their invaluable assistance and critique.

References

Balas, R. and Simon, G. The articulation function of a staggered spondaic word list for a normal hearing population. J. Aud. Res., 1965, 5, 285–289.

Bosewell, S. L., Sanders, B. and Young, S. J. The effects of exposure duration and practice on the immediate memory spans of children and adults. J. Exper. Child Psychol., 1974, 17, 167–176.

Denny, D. R. The effects of exemplary and cognitive models and self-rehearsal on children's interrogative strategies. J. Exper. Child Psychol., 1975, 19, 476–488.

Egan, J. P. Articulation testing methods. Laryngoscope, 1948, 58, 955–991.

Groen, J. and Hellema, A. On the diagnosis of central deafness in children. Internat'l. Audiol., 1963, 2, 103–107.

Hensley, J. H., Lewenstein, J. and Rabinowitz, F. M. Effects of children's spontaneous verbal rehearsal on learning performance under delay of feedback. Child Devel., 1974, 45, 479–482.

Katz, J. The use of staggered spondaic words for assessing the integrity of the central auditory nervous system. J. Aud. Res., 1962, 2, 327–337.

Katz, J. The SSW test: An interim report. J. Speech Hear. Dis., 1968, 33, 132–146.

Katz, J., Basil, R. and Smith, J. A staggered spondaic word test for detecting central auditory lesions. Ann Otol., Rhinol., Laryngol., 1963, 72, 908.

Minetti, S. B. The effects of practice on 8–10 year old children using the Staggered Spondaic Word Test. Unpubl. Master's thesis, California State University at Sacramento, 1977.

Postman, L. and Rosenzweig, M. R. Practice and transfer in the visual and auditory recognition of verbal stimuli. Am. J. Psychol., 1956, 69, 209–226.

Ritterman, S. The role of practice and the observation of practice in speech sound discrimination learning. J. Speech Hear. Res., 1970, 13, 178–183.

Siegel, S. Nonparametric Statistics for the Behavioral Sciences. N.Y.: McGraw-Hill, 1956.

Tillman, T. W. and Jerger, J. F. Some factors affecting the spondee threshold in normal hearing subjects. J. Speech Hear. Res., 1959, 2, 141–146.

Tsappis, A. The effect of practice in auditory discrimination testing. Unpubl. Master's thesis, California State University at Sacramento, 1974.

Turner, L. K. A normative study on the staggered spondaic word test for various age groups. Unpubl. Master's thesis, University of Kansas, 1966.

Diagnostic Significance of the Type A Pattern

on the Staggered Spondaic Word (SSW) Test

Jay R. Lucker, Ed.D., Educational Audiologist

Introduction

The Staggered Spondaic Word (SSW) Test has been utilized in the assessment of central auditory processing dysfunctions of learning disabled children.[1-4] During his workshops on the SSW Test, Katz discussed how a specific response pattern (Type A) had been found primarily with learning disabled children. When an audiologist obtains a Type A SSW pattern with a child, the conclusion drawn is that the child has a learning disability. However, the audiologist often is faced with the task of relating the test results to expected academic problems. Too often the clinician is able to state only that the test results are consistent with test results obtained with other learning disabled children.

In the course of my clinical experience, I have employed the SSW Test with 90 learning disabled children. I have found that only 26% of the learning disabled children obtain Type A SSW patterns. Many learning disabled children demonstrate other difficulties on the SSW Test. In addition, I have found a small number of normal achieving children with Type A SSW patterns. These unexpected findings led me to carefully investigate the relationship between the Type A SSW pattern and academic problems. The following is a discussion of my findings and conclusions which demonstrate the diagnostic significance of the Type A SSW pattern.

Audiology and Hearing Education, 6, 21–23, 1980.

The Type A SSW Pattern

A child may obtain a Type A pattern whether or not the SSW Test results (CSSW) are within normal limits. The Type A pattern is obtained when the cardinal number in the RC condition for the REF or in the LC condition for the LEF is twice as great as any other cardinal number and is at least three points greater. (For a complete discussion of the SSW Test refer to Brunt[1] and Katz.[5]) The following is an example of a Type A pattern. The subject obtained the following eight cardinal numbers:

REF:	RNC	RC	LC	LNC
	0	0	1	0
LEF:	LNC	LC	RC	RNC
	0	6	1	0

The LC value for the LEF condition is six times greater than any other value, and is five points greater than the next highest number. Therefore, this subject obtained a Type A pattern.

Children With Type A Patterns

My interest in the diagnostic significance of the Type A SSW pattern developed when I evaluated a child functioning above grade level (fifth grade) who had severe spelling problems. I was asked to determine whether a subtle central auditory processing problem was interfering with the child's ability to spell. Her SSW Test results were within normal limits for her age. However, analysis of the eight cardinal numbers revealed a Type A pattern:

REF:	RNC	RC	LC	LNC
	0	2	2	0
LEF:	LNC	LC	RC	RNC
	0	6	0	0

When I discussed these results with the girl's teacher, she requested that I test another child with similar spelling problems who was also achieving at grade level. The second girl also obtained a Type A pattern:

REF:	RNC	RC	LC	LNC
	0	0	0	0
LEF:	LNC	LC	RC	RNC
	2	5	0	0

I began to look at the SSW Test results for other children I had tested. I found that 10 learning disabled children I had previously tested obtained Type A patterns. In addition, I found eight other learning disabled children and five normal-achieving children with Type A SSW patterns. In total, I found 23 children with this pattern. The children ranged in age from seven years five months to 19 years four months, with a mean age of 10 years four months. The means and standard deviations for the eight cardinal numbers for this group were:

REF:	RNC	RC	LC	LNC
	0.6	1.5	2.7	0.4
	(0.8)	(1.6)	(1.8)	(0.6)
LEF:	LNC	LC	RC	RNC
	1.0	8.6	1.4	0.4
	(1.3)	(3.2)	(1.4)	(0.6)

It is interesting to note that all 23 children yielded the poorest score in the LC condition for the LEF regardless of handedness (one child was left-handed). In addition, the smallest value for LC was four and the smallest difference between LC and other values was three.

Diagnostic Significance of the Type A SSW Pattern

Seventeen of the 23 children with Type A patterns were identified as having severe problems with spelling and writing. Only six children were not identified as having spelling problems. However, five of these six children were identified as having severe learning disabilities related to reading and writing. For these five children spelling problems may have been masked by the severe reading and writing problems so that their teachers did not identify them as having severe spelling problems. Only one child was not identified as having a learning disability; he was diagnosed as having severe emotional problems, although it is possible that he also had spelling, reading, or writing problems which could not be accurately diagnosed at this time.

Interestingly, of the 17 children with spelling and writing problems, five were not learning disabled. These five children only demonstrated either severe spelling or writing problems. The pattern of spelling errors for four of these children revealed errors of sequencing (e.g., Decmeber for December; balck for black) and problems in sounding out words. The children often would sound out the words but write the incorrect sequence of letters or letters unrelated to the sounds they made. For example, one child sounded out policeman correctly but wrote *ploceasman*. The problems these normal-achievers were having in spelling were the same for the seven learning disabled children with

Type A patterns. Two of these normal-achievers were identified as having writing problems related to organization and sentence structure. One of these two children was only found to have great difficulties writing. He was not able to write more than a simple sentence without help.

The five learning disabled children with Type A SSW patterns who were not identified as having severe spelling problems were identified as having problems in reading related to phonics—problems correctly identifying the sounds that the letters made. This can be labeled a sound-symbol association problem. The difficulties that the children with spelling problems were demonstrating may also be sound-symbol association problems. In addition, the problems in writing found with these children could also be due to difficulties in putting the language (sound) into the written (symbol) form. Therefore, 22 of the 23 children with Type A SSW patterns were demonstrating sound-symbol association problems which affected spelling (17 of the 22 children), reading (15 of the 22 children) or writing (all children). In addition, these sound-symbol association problems were not always related to a significant learning disability (five children were normal-achievers).

During his workshops on the SSW Test, Katz described two cases of learning disabled children with Type A SSW patterns who were found to have abnormal EEG activity in the temporoparietal region of their cortices. This region, which lies between the occipital center where symbols are received by the brain and the posterior temporal lobe (Wernicke's area) where language processing occurs, would appear to be involved in sound-symbol associative functioning. If a dysfunction occurred in this region, we might find sound-symbol association problems. It is hypothesized that dysfunction in this region shows as a Type A SSW pattern, and that the 22 children under discussion with sound-symbol association problems may have a dysfunction in this area of their brains, which led to problems in spelling, reading, and writing and for many children was associated with other learning disabilities.

Educational Implications

When the audiologist evaluates a child and obtains a Type A SSW pattern, the clinician can conclude that the child may have problems in sound-symbol association which may affect spelling, reading, and writing. Also, since the problem is hypothesized to be due to a neurological dysfunctioning, it would be best to find a means of teaching sound-symbol association skills other than the traditional phonic and sounding out approaches. These traditional approaches appear to require normal neurological functioning in the sound-symbol association region. If alternate approaches were used which utilized strengths in other areas, it would appear that the child would learn to compensate for his disability. I have discovered that children with spelling problems who yield Type A SSW patterns significantly improve their spelling abilities if a visual approach to spelling is used and the auditory sounding out approach is abandoned. I have used and suggested for use an approach which teaches the child to look for little words in big words based purely on sight to improve spelling. This approach appears to be helping some children with their spelling. More research is needed to provide support for this approach. In addition, children with Type A SSW patterns demonstrating writing difficulties have shown great improvement in writing when taught how to organize their writing utilizing an approach called the "Wh" Question Organization. According to this approach, components of sentences and paragraphs are organized into questions similar to the questions a journalist might utilize to organize and write a newspaper article.

Conclusions

I do not wish to mislead the reader into believing that all children with spelling, reading, or writing problems have Type A SSW patterns and dysfunctioning in the temporoparietal region. I have seen a number of children with spelling, reading, and writing problems who had other patterns with the SSW Test. For example, two children with spelling problems similar to those described above had normal C SSW results and did not have Type A patterns. However, both children yielded a large number of reversals (17 and 19, respectively).

It appears that spelling, reading, and writing problems can be caused by numerous factors. However, it appears that the Type A SSW pattern is correlated with sound-symbol association problems which lead to difficulties associating the sounds of the letters to the graphic symbols in reading, spelling, and writing. This conclusion suggests that, when the audiologist finds a child with a Type A SSW pattern, the clinician can state that the child may have sound-symbol association problems requiring remediation using a visual approach, and that this problem may interfere with achievement in spelling, reading, and writing.

References

1. Brunt, M. The staggered spondaic word test: In *Handbook of Clinical Audiology,* 2nd edition, ed. Jack Katz. Baltimore: Williams and Wilkins Co., 1978.

2. Katz, J. Clinical use of central auditory tests. In *Handbook of Clinical Audiology,* 2nd edition, ed. Jack Katz. Baltimore: Williams and Wilkins Co., 1978.

3. Keith, R. W., ed. *Central Auditory Dysfunction.* New York; Grune and Stratton, 1977.

4. Young, E., Tracy, J. M. An experimental short form of the staggered spondaic word list for learning disabled children. *Audiology & Hearing Education* 3:7, December/January 1977.

5. Katz, J. The staggered spondaic word test. In *Central Auditory Dysfunction,* ed. Robert W. Keith, New York: Grune and Stratton, 1977.

The New SSW Test (List EE) and the CES Test

Preliminary Analysis of Central Auditory Function in Children Ages 6 to 12 Years

David Warren Johnson, M.S., M.A., C.C.C.
Robert E. Sherman, Ph.D.

Introduction

The Staggered Spondaic Word Test, a central auditory listening task, was introduced almost 20 years ago[1] and has been evaluated in several versions in various populations.[1-19] Each version has had slightly different performance characteristics for the subjects evaluated, whether adults or children. [5-6]. Recently the author of the SSW Test introduced a new version, List EE.* The new version is relatively clean in the sense that the background hiss of the previous List EC edition is no longer present and the auditory figure/ground problem implicit [15,20,21] with the previous tests is therefore absent. In addition, Jack Katz has constructed another central auditory task[8] called the Competing Environmental Sounds Test[5] which utilizes pictures and nonverbal sounds for a dichotic discrimination task.*

Various researchers have advocated a number of different interpretive techniques for dealing with the data generated in the use of the SSW Test.[1-3,5-19] The basic problem lies in the fact that every test tape has been constructed in a slightly different fashion so that timing of

Audiology & Hearing Education, 6, 5–8, 1980

*Available through Auditec, St. Louis, MO.

Use of the SSW and CES Tests with Children

stimuli, signal-to-noise ratio, and other variables make every new test edition a different listening task.[5,6,15,20,21] Since no normative data for the SSW Test (List EE) and the CES Test have been presented to this point, it was decided to develop preliminary normative-type data which could help a clinician utilize these two tests with children. Our goal was not to identify the lesion site, but to determine what normal central auditory function is for children on these test instruments so that learning-disabled children with auditory problems could potentially be more easily identified without the elaborate manipulation of data (e.g., ear effect, reversal, order effect, etc.) utilized in the past [1,4,6,10-12,15,18,19,22,23] and which may be specific test dependent.[4]

The study discussed below is divided into SSW and CES portions. Data resulted from an evaluation of 93 children ranging in age from 6 to 12 years from normal classroom settings. Selection was made from a large group of children functioning within the middle 50% of academic performance and having intelligence within the normal range as measured by a variety of standard intelligence quotient type measures employed in the schools. From this pool, children were selected on the basis of a number of requisites to be discussed below. A general health and medical history questionnaire was obtained on each youngster and was negative for ear disease, hearing problems, or etiology associated with learning disability or hearing impairment.

Prior to evaluation with the SSW and CES Tests, it was determined that all children studied were within the normal range (APT better than 20 dB HL re: ANSI 1969) for puretone air and bone conduction audiometry and had good performance on standard speech reception and speech discrimination tasks (Lists W-1 and W-22 at 50 dB SL, respectively—tapes obtained from Auditec). Tympanograms were obtained and were negative[24] prior to central auditory testing. All children had symmetrical hearing thresholds, no conductive involvement, and hearing for the speech range of better than 20 dB. Otologic examinations were negative within two weeks of audiometry for those evaluated.

All audiometry was performed with a Qualitone Acoustic Appraiser Audiometer calibrated to ANSI 1969 in a quiet room meeting or exceeding noise levels allowable under ANSI S3.1–1960. A Danplex Model ZA 20 Impedance Audiometer was utilized to establish tympanometric pattern. A Panasonic RS256US Cassette Tape Deck was utilized to deliver prerecorded tapes of the respective speech stimuli and nonverbal stimuli through the audiometer.

The subject sample was selected to give balance by each year of age, by sex, and by handedness. There were either three or four subjects in each of 28 age-sex-handedness cells (Table 1). Though the subjects so chosen did not constitute a random sample of all children and thus had a rather conditional norm group quality, the data produced were cleaner for purposes of examining the interrelationship of the indicated factors to error rates in dichotic word and sound recognition. The matter of handedness effect was important since one study[13] reported significance in dealing with the SSW Test and at least one other study reported handedness effects in some dichotic listening tasks.[22] Two subjects were excluded from our study after testing solely because their error rates were so high for their age group that it was presumed to be an unrecognized abnormality.

TABLE 1
Age, sex, and handedness of normal children serving as the initial study population

Group	Number	Age	Sex	Handedness
1	3	6	m	r
2	3	6	m	l
3	3	6	f	r
4	5	6	f	l
5	4	7	m	r
6	3	7	m	l
7	3	7	f	r
8	4	7	f	l
9	3	8	m	r
10	3	8	m	l
11	4	8	f	r
12	3	8	f	l
13	4	9	m	r
14	3	9	m	l
15	3	9	f	r
16	3	9	f	l
17	3	10	m	r
18	3	10	m	l
19	3	10	f	r
20	3	10	f	l
21	3	11	m	r
22	3	11	m	l
23	3	11	f	r
24	4	11	f	l
25	3	12	m	r
26	3	12	m	l
27	3	12	f	r
28	3	12	f	l

Characteristic Patterns of Errors in the SSW Test (List EE)

The SSW Test (List EE) consists of a series of two two-syllable words which were presented by earphones at 50 dB SL re: SRT,[6] one word to each ear, in such a manner that the second syllable of the first word overlapped the first syllable of the second word. The two-syllable words used in the test were compound words like "downtown," or "outside," so that the subject was asked to repeat the four component words. Two of the four component words were heard simultaneously by the subject in his two ears, and his ability to recognize both words was a dichotic listening test.

List EE consists of several practice items followed by 40 word pairs presented to the ears of the child in the overlapping fashion described above. After each word pair, the subject was asked to repeat the words exactly as he heard them. In 20 of the word pairs, the right ear was presented with the initiating word syllable, and in 20 the left ear received it. Considering the competing words only the subject had an opportunity to make 40 errors in identifying the word heard in each ear—20 when the listening ear led the word pair, and 20 when it lagged. In administration of the test, the ear that led the word pair was alternated.

The Data

The raw data of this analysis consisted of error counts (i.e., failure to correctly identify a word element) by subject for competing words heard in right and left ears, with right and then left ear leading the word pairs. There were thus four error counts for each subject, with each count having a maximum possible value of 20. In fact, the number of errors made was typically quite small for the older children—zero or one—and clearly larger (though still a small proportion) for the younger children—two to four errors. It was the nature of such counts that the variability of the numbers observed was related to the expected value of the count. Because the analytic methods of the data analysis assumed a common error variance (homoscedasticity), an initial square root transformation was applied to the raw error counts.[25]

The Data Analysis

Analysis of the study data was conducted according to the following strategy:

The four error counts of each subject (errors in repeating the competing words heard in the right ear, leading, then lagging, and errors in repeating words heard in the left ear, leading, then lagging) were first transformed by a square root transformation in order to strengthen the homoscedasticity assumption made in later steps of the analysis.

Each subject's four transformed error counts were then further transformed into four new variables:

- a component (m) representing a subject's overall average (square root) error count;

- a component (a) representing a subject's deviation from his overall average error for words heard in his right ear;

- a component (b) representing a subject's deviation from his overall average error count for words heard in an ear which initiated or led the word pair;

- a component (ab) representing a subject's deviation from his overall average error count for words heard (in either ear) when the right ear led the word pair.

Each of the above four components was then analyzed separately for its relationship to the age, sex, and handedness of the subjects. The method used for each component was first to average the value (for the three or four subjects) within each age-sex-handedness cell, and then to conduct a $7 \times 2 \times 2$ factorial analysis of variance on the resultant means. (Within cell variance estimates were also computed, but were not relevant to our discussion here.)

Factors which were significantly related to the error counts were identified, and an appropriate model was created to represent the model error rates in the study population.

Results

The main results of the analysis were as follows:

Sex and handedness had no discernible relationship to any of the variables (m), (a), (b), or (ab).

The overall error rate, (m), was clearly and strongly related to the subject's age, with the younger children making the larger number of errors.

There was a slight, but statistically significant ($P = .05$), reduction in error rate for words heard in the right ear (the [a] component). This effect was not shown to be age-dependent, though the six- and seven-year-olds had the largest effects.

Six- and seven-year-olds displayed significantly ($P = .05$) higher error rates for competing words heard in the ear which initiated the word pair.

There was a highly significant ($P = .01$) and consistent reduction in errors for competing words heard in either ear when the right ear initiated the word pair (the [ab] effect).

Since the analyses of variance found no significant relationship of the study variables to sex or handedness, we represented the estimated effects (m), (a), (b), and (ab) a they relate to age alone (*Table 2*).

The components estimated in the Table 2 data related to the square root of the number of errors made in 20 opportunities. Error variances associated with these estimated components were not presented but could be extracted from the ANOVA tables.[26]

The data of Table 2 were used to form estimates of the expected percentage of competing word errors. The clearest effects that should be included in such estimates were the overall age effect (m) and effect due to the right or left ear leading the word pair (ab). Confidence intervals for the estimated values were established utilizing error residuals from the ANOVAs. Table 3 presents such constructed estimates along with the 95% confidence interval estimates.

Two comments would appear appropriate. First, the observed age effect was quite consistent, yet no attempt was made to extend our methods to include a regression function for the age effect. This would almost surely have permitted us to tighten our confidence intervals on the expected percentage errors for the various age levels, but at the ex-

TABLE 2
Summary of SSW Model Variables and Age

Age (years)	(m)	(a)	(b)	(ab)
6	2.11	−.35	.21	−.06
7	1.53	−.18	.23	−.30
8	1.21	.00	.00	−.16
9	.91	−.15	.03	−.12
10	.80	.10	−.05	−.14
11	.80	−.16	.06	−.19
12	.75	−.06	−.06	−.27
Average	1.15	−.12	.06	−.18

TABLE 3. ▬▬▬▬▬▬▬▬▬▬▬▬▬▬▬▬▬▬▬▬▬▬▬▬▬▬

Estimated expected percentage of competing word errors by age and the ear that leads the word pair (with 95% confidence interval on the estimate)

Age (years)	Words missed when right ear is leading	Words missed when left ear is leading
6	18.6 (13.8 to 24.2)	26.1 (20.3 to 32.6)
7	9.1 (5.9 to 13.1)	14.5 (10.3 to 19.5)
8	5.3 (2.9 to 8.4)	9.6 (6.2 to 13.6)
9	2.7 (1.1 to 5.0)	5.9 (3.4 to 9.2)
10	2.0 (.6 to 4.0)	4.8 (2.5 to 7.8)
11	1.9 (.6 to 4.0)	4.8 (2.5 to 7.7)
12	1.7 (.5 to 3.6)	4.3 (2.2 to 7.2)

pense of some new assumptions regarding the nature (or shape) of the curve of the age effect. As things stand, each age effect was independently estimated.

Second, the reduction in errors observed for words heard when the right ear was leading the word pair conceivably was due to a differential degree of difficulty in the words that happen to have been chosen for that portion of the test. By inspection of the test and previous test instruments using the SSW technique,[4,7,14,15,18,22] such a problem seemed unlikely.

Characteristic Patterns of Errors in the Competing Environmental Sounds (CES) Test.

The Competing Environmental Sounds (CES) Test, after several practice items, required the subject to identify pictures of two nonverbal sounds (e.g., a dog barking, or a man sneezing) when sounds were presented simultaneously, one to each ear, 20 times. This test was simpler than the SSW listening task since there was no staggering or sequence to the sound pairs. The same subjects were tested and the error counts were analyzed in much the same manner as with the competing word test.

Results

The main results of the analysis were as follows:

The sex or handedness of a subject showed no signficant relationship to his error count.

Age was clearly related to a subject's error count ($P = .01$), with the younger subjects making the greater number of errors.

Errors occurred significantly more often among sounds heard in the right ear ($P = .01$).

CES-expected percentage errors for sounds presented to the right and left ears of children ages 6 through 12 are presented in Table 4.

As with the SSW, there was a possibility that the competing sounds presented to the right ear chanced to be more difficult to interpret than those presented to the left ear. This seemed unlkely, since this ear effect was consistent with previous reports of subject performance on competing sounds stimuli.[8,9]

Discussion

Our analysis showed that sex and handedness had no clear relationship to error rate for the SSW Test (List EE) or the CES Test and was consistent with most previous studies of the SSW listening task,[5,6] but perhaps in disagreement with some dichotic listening studies.[14,22] Age did show a relationship to error rate, the younger children having the higher error rate. This was consistent with previous studies. [1-19] For the SSW Test, the error rate in the right ear was statistically less than in the left ear. On the other hand, for the CES Test, the error rate in the left ear was statistically less than in the right ear. These findings were predictable. [4,5,15,18,22]

Children younger than eight years did have more errors than one might anticipate. Although this has been observed before,[14,22] two factors might account for this finding. First, in the middle 50% of academic performance in the lower grades are children who are found

TABLE 4. ═══════════════════════════════════
Estimated expected percentage of competing sounds errors for the competing environmental sounds (CES) test (with approximate 95% confidence interval)

Age (years)	Sounds missed in right ear	Sounds missed in left ear
6	8.1 (4.7 to 12.4)	5.1 (2.5 to 8.6)
7	4.6 (2.2 to 8.0)	2.5 (.8 to 5.0)
8	3.5 (1.4 to 6.5)	1.7 (.4 to 3.9)
9	3.1 (1.2 to 6.0)	1.4 (.3 to 3.5)
10	.7 (0 to 2.2)	.1 (0. to .8)
11	.6 (0 to 2.1)	.1 (0 to .7)
12	1.3 (.2 to 3.3)	.3 (0 to 1.5)

to have learning disability several years later when the academic performance process more clearly delineates them. Therefore, the relatively large error rate may reflect non-normal children being present in the younger test groups of "normals." The finding that six- and seven-year-olds on the SSW Test displayed higher error rates for competing words heard in the ear which initiated the word pair may suggest actual word memeory storage differences between the younger children and the older children, or it may reflect true central auditory maturation processes in the six- and seven-year-old normal population. Order effects may compound our interpretation difficulties, then, since they were noted here in our study as well as in previous studies.[5,6,9,15,18]

This study does support previous work, generally, and does provide tentative normative data for the SSW Test (List EE) and the CES Test for children ages 6 to 12. If the data for 11- and 12-year-olds were considered similar to adult performance as the literature would likely suggest, these data may be extended for adults through 60 years of age.[5,14,17] Table 5 could be considered possible "normal" performance for adults on these two tests, but would of course require verifying study.

Are these tests practical when scored in this manner? If the goal is identification of children with auditory processing problems, this type of scoring would be highly desirable, since people unfamiliar with "pattern considerations" could use the test for identification given these normtive data for performance. As for the use of this scoring in adults, there would likely be much lost if pattern considerations were not considered by the clinician; however, for identification purposes, this simplified scoring system would not be inappropriate for clinicians not trained in the niceties of the respective tests. Unusual error rates may be anticipated to stick out like the proverbial sore thumb; preliminary studies using learning disabled youngsters now under way tend to confirm this.

TABLE 5.
Hypothesized expected percentage of errors for the SSW Test and the CES Test for normal adults (with approximate 95%) confidence interval)

SSW Test List EE	Words missed when right ear is leading	Words missed when left ear is leading
Adults to age 60	1.8 (.55 to 3.8)	4.55 (2.35 to 7.45)
CES Test	Sounds missed in right ear	Sounds missed in left ear
Adults to age 60	.85 (.1 to 2.7)	.2 (0 to .6)

Acknowledgement

The authors thank the Bloomington, Minnesota, Public School System for its cooperation in this study. In addition, gratitude is expressed for the instrumentation for this study which was calibrated and loaned to the investigators by Electro Medic Inc. (General Radio 1933 Sound Level Meter), Maico Hearing Instruments, Inc. (Danplex Model ZA 20 Impedance Audiometer), and Qualitone, Inc. (Qualitone Acoustic Appraiser Audiometer). Special thanks are extended to Michael Reder, M.D., for his otological evaluations of children inolved in this study.

References

1. Katz, J. The use of spondaic staggered words for assessing the integrity of the central auditory nervous system. *J. Aud. Res.* 2:327–337, 1962.

2. Balas, R. Staggered spondaic word test: Support. *Ann. Otol. Rhinol. Laryngol.* 80:132–134, 1971.

3. Berlin, C., Chase, R., Dill, A., et al. Auditory Findings in Patients with Temporal Lobectomies. Paper presented at the annual meeting of the American Speech and Hearing Association, 1965.

4. Brunt, M. Performance on Three Auditory Tests by Children with Functional Articulation Disorders. Master's thesis at the University of Pittsburgh, 1962.

5. Katz, J. The Staggered Spondaic Word Test. In *Central Auditory Dysfunction*, ed. R. W. Keith, pp. 103–127. New York: Grune & Stratton, 1977.

6. Katz, J. The SSW Test: An interim report. *J. Speech Hear. Disord.* 33:132–146, 1968.

7. Katz, J., Basil, R. A., Smith, M. A. A staggered spondaic word test for detecting central auditory lesions. *Ann. Otol. Rhinol. Laryngol.* 72: 908–917, 1963.

8. Katz, J., Kushner, D., Pack, G. The Use of Competing Speech (SSW) and Environmental Sound (CES) Test for Localizing Brain Lesions. Paper presented at the annual meeting of the American Speech and Hearing Association, 1975.

9. Kushner, D., Johnson, D., Stevens, J. Use of SSW/CES Tests for Identifying Children with Learning Disabilities. Paper presented at the annual meeting of the American Speech and Hearing Association, 1977.

10. Lynn, G. E., Gilroy, J. Evaluation of central auditory dysfunction in patients with neurological disorders. In *Central Auditory Dysfunction*, ed. R. W. Keith, pp. 177–218. New York: Grune & Stratton, 1977.

11. Lynn, G., Gilroy, J. Neuro-audiological abnormalities in patients with temporal lobe tumors. *J. Neurol. Sci.* 17:167–184. 1972.

12. Lynn, G., Benitez, J., Eisenbrey, A., et al. Neuro-audiological correlates in cerebral hemisphere lesions: Temporal and parietal lobe tumors. *Audiology* 11:115–134, 1972.

13. Morrill, J. C. A Staggered Spondaic Word Test as an Indicator of Minimal Brain Dysfunction in Children. Master's thesis at Texas Technological College, 1969.

14. Myrick, D. K. A Normative Study to Assess Performance of a Group of Children Ages Seven through Eleven on the Staggered Spondaic Word Test. Master's thesis at Tulane University, 1965.

15. Pinheiro, M. L. Tests of central auditory function in children with learning disabilities. In *Central Auditory Dysfunction*, ed. R. W. Keith, pp. 223–254. New York: Grune & Stratton, 1977.

16. Stephens, S. D. G., Thornton, A. R. D. Subjective and electrophysiologic tests in brainstem lesions. *Arch. Otolaryngol.* 102:608–613, 1976.

17. Turner, L. A Normative Study on the SSW Test for Various Age Groups. Master's thesis at the University of Kansas, 1966.

18. White, E. J. Children's performance on the SSW Test and Willeford battery: Interim clinical data. In *Central Auditory Dysfunction*, ed. R. W. Keith, pp. 319–340. New York: Grune & Stratton, 1977.

19. Young, E., Tracy III, J. M. An experimental short form of the staggered spondaic word list for learning-disabled children. *Audiology & Hearing Education* (3):7, December/January 1977.

20. Berlin, C., Lowe-Bell, S., Cullen, J., et al. Dichotic speech perception: An interpretation of right ear advantage and temporal offset effects. *J. Acoust. Soc. Amer.* 53:699–709, 1973.

21. Brotsky, S. Auditory figure-ground perception in neurologically impaired children. *J. Aud. Res.* 10:5–10, 1970.

22. Bryden, M. P. Laterality effects in dichotic listening: Relations with handedness and reading ability in children. *Neuropsychologia* 8:443–450, 1970.

23. Emmerich, D. S., Goldenbraum, D. M., Hayden, D. L., et al. Meaningfulness as a variable in dichotic hearing. *J. Exp. Psychol.* 69:433–436, 1965.

24. Jerger, J. Clinical experience with impedance audiometry. *Arch. Otolaryngol.* 92:311–324, 1970.

25. Ostle, B. *Statistics and Research.* p. 340. Ames, IA: Iowa State University Press, 1963.

26. Searle, S. R. *Linear Models.* pp. 365–369. New York: John Wiley & Sons, 1971.

27. Speaks, C. Dichotic listening: A clinical or research tool? In *Central Auditory Processing Disorders*, ed. M. D. Sullivan, pp. 1–25. Omaha: University of Nebraska Biomedical Communications, 1974.

The Use of the **Staggered Spondaic Word** and the **Competing Environmental Sounds Tests** in the Evaluation of Central Auditory Function of Learning Disabled Children

David Warren Johnson, Mary Lee Enfield, and Robert E. Sherman

Children aged 6 to 12 years with intelligence and pure-tone hearing within the normal range (91 functioning academically within the middle 50% and having uneventful hearing health histories and 76 demonstrating learning disabilities) were evaluated with dichotic central auditory listening tasks. Auditory response patterns were established and analyzed for normal and learning disability-specific performance. Children with learning disabilities performed more poorly than "normal" peers on verbal and nonverbal listening tasks, suggesting learning disabled children may be identified by auditory performance on dichotic listening skills.

Ear and Hearing, 2, 70–77, 1981.

Children with learning disabilities are those who fail to learn despite normal intelligence. Minimal brain dysfunction, inability to understand or listen, poor balance, clumsiness, and incoordination have been noted in these children, among a myriad of problems (9, 13, 14, 16–18). It has been reported that peripheral auditory dysfunction occurs in about one-third of these youngsters (8), but many more basic auditory problems have been reported, including reduced auditory learning (13), decreased ability to sequence auditory information (8, 13), reduced ability to discriminate same/difference sound variations (8), difficulty in separating auditory stimuli from background noise (9), and the general decreased ability process auditory information on a central basis. "Processing" includes such things as auditory memory, auditory blending skills, auditory comprehension, and audition as a function of simultaneous visual input, timing, and rhythm (4, 8, 9, 13, 14).

Resulting behavior may manifest as speech and language delay, hyperactivity, poor motor coordination, lack of responsiveness, uncontrolled temper, school failure, developmental irregularity, behavioral deviation, and general communication difficulties in speech, language, reading, writing, and the like. Often, confusion and moodiness reflect the child's inability to deal with his basic problem and his recognition of his failure (13).

Central Auditory Function

There has been interest in the central auditory functioning of children for some time, particularly as to how central auditory pathway function and auditory processing relate to minimal brain dysfunction and learning disabilities observed in the classroom (3, 4, 8, 9, 14, 15, 17, 19, 20). A number of auditory tests in current use relating to listening skills like selective listening (5), listening to unrelated words (2), listening to sentences or directions (2, 12, 18), and other similar testing instruments (15, 16) have been utilized in the evaluation of central auditory problems in children. Essentially, strings of morphemes are presented to children so that the strings are heard simultaneously binaurally. The child's task is to reproduce the string by repeating or following the directions implicit in the string.

These measures are not dichotic in the sense that a different stimulus is heard in each ear. Dichotic listening tests potentially can be used to evaluate auditory functioning when the ears are hearing different stimuli (6).

The Staggered Spondaic Word Test (SSW) was developed almost 20 years ago and continues to be a useful tool for the study of both hearing ability and auditory processing ability (3, 7–9, 14–16, 20). Essentially, the test is constructed of a pair of 2-syllable words which are presented with syllables overlapping independently to each ear. The effect is to hear the first syllable of one word in the first ear, the second syllable of that word in that ear simultaneously with the first syllable of a second word in the opposing ear, and the second syllable of the second word in the second ear. The subject is forced to interpret the dichotic competing stimuli, a central nervous system task (4, 7). This task requires the subject to repeat the actual words (4, 7), maintain the correct order of the words (7), and repeat the words when the right ear and then the left ear is the ear initiating the spondaic word pairs (7). The test has been used with a broad variety of populations with normally developed nervous systems (above 10 years of age) demonstrating ability repeat all words in the proper order (3, 14, 20). Some normative data on adults for the SSW test have been reported (3, 8, 20). Reported norms on children show an "age effect," presumably reflecting maturation of the nervous system (9, 14, 15).

The Competing Environmental Sounds Test (CES) has been recently developed as a complementary central auditory test. Although the SSW test is sensitive to verbal processing problems (3, 7, 14, 15) the CES test is in theory sensitive to nonverbal auditory processing problems (all music and common sounds).

The logic in the use of the SSW test assumes that the central nervous system tends to process auditory information in a specific fashion. Verbal stimuli are received and encoded in the cochlea. This information is then transmitted through the VIIIth nerve to the ipsilateral lower brainstem and proceeds through the contralateral upper brainstem to the cortex level auditory reception area contralateral to the ear originally receiving the information. Verbal information in the right ear is thus processed in the left hemisphere. Information received in the left ear is transmitted to the right hemisphere auditory reception area which then relays the data by means of the corpus callosum to the left hemisphere for processing (10). This method of auditory processing is not invariable in all people, but is considered the dominant method of auditory processing of verbal information in approximately 85 % of the population (21).

The logic in the use of the CES test is based upon a similar model. For nonverbal stimuli, the data are assumed to be encoded in the cochlea and transmitted through the VIIIth nerve to the ipsilateral lower brainstem. It is then relayed to the contralateral upper brainstem where it continues to the cerebral hemisphere contralateral to the ear initially receiving the data. Nonverbal data received at the left ear are ultimately received in the right hemisphere and processed there. Nonverbal data received in the right ear proceed to the left hemisphere auditory reception area but are then relayed to the right hemisphere by the corpus callosum for processing (10, 11).

The models discussed here do not consider the complete anatomy or physiology of the central auditory nervous system. Certainly ipsilateral pathways exist, for instance, which allow for direct relaying of information from the ear receiving information to its ipsilateral hemisphere on the cortex level. That method of hemisphere access to auditory information, however, does not appear to be dominant in most people. In addition, the left hemisphere may not be dominant for language as suggested by this model for all people, but this model does describe reasonably well the primary auditory pathway systems in at least 85% of the normal hearing population (21). Indeed, it was this hemisphere dominance issue for language which caused us to seek a correlation of auditory functioning with handedness to be discussed below.

If the models presented represent actual auditory processing, then, theoretically, the SSW test relates to the left hemisphere problems because it is verbal whereas the CES test relates to the right hemisphere auditory reception difficulties because it is nonverbal. Taken together, the 2 tests may then allow evaluation of auditory-based problems related to hemisphere involvement.

Method

A study was constructed to form an age-specific normative base for central auditory function in normal children with the SSW and CES tests. Simultaneously, data were collected in a similar manner for children with learning disabilities for comparison purposes. Specifically, we sought:

1. to determine "normal" response patterns in children for the dichotic hearing tests, the newly available SSW test (list EE), and the CES test;
2. to determine characteristic response patterns for the dichotic hearing tests in children with severe learning disabilities;
3. to determine how children with learning disabilities deviate from normals in central auditory function;
4. to determine which auditory test factors correlate with which specific disabilities.

Subjects

Ninety-one children ranging in age from 6 to 12 years were selected from normal classroom settings to establish normal central auditory function parameters. Subjects were randomly selected from those children functioning within the middle 50% of academic achievement with the constraint that the sample would be balanced across age, sex, and handedness. Balancing was done to enable the examination of the relationship of these factors to auditory test results. Subjects were further limited to those demonstrating no unusual health history, e.g., head trauma, birth complication, unusual prenatal disease, or early childhood disease history. Three potential subjects were eliminated on the basis of health events potentially related to auditory performance.

Seventy-six learning disabled subjects included essentially all children aged 6 to 12 identified as having learning disabilities in 4 suburban schools. These schools had special education resources and accepted referrals for learning disabilities from other schools within the district. Identified learning disabilities included a wide variety of learning difficulties (Table 1).

All children had been evaluated by age-appropriate intelligence tests and were considered by their teachers to be of normal intelligence. Both normal and learning disabled youngsters were drawn from the same four schools.

Testing Protocol and Equipment

Air and bone conduction audiometry at 0.5, 1, 2, and 4 kHz (1) and immitance audiometry were performed on the children who were functioning within the normal academic range. Children with hearing poorer than 20 dB HL at these frequencies, children with air/bone gaps of 10 dB or more at any frequency tested, and children with tympanograms suggestive of conductive involvement were rejected from the normal group.

Children receiving special education services were given an abbreviated protocol to minimize fatigue during the central testing. Hearing thresholds at 1 kHz were determined for the learning-disabled children. Those with thresholds poorer than 20 dB at this frequency were rejected from the study. All children (the academically normal as well as the learning disabled) were regularly screened for hearing thresholds at 1, 2, and 4 kHz in grades 1, 3, and 5 for hearing loss greater than 15 dB as part of a regular school-based hearing conservation program. Children failing such screening or children with a history of conductive involvement resulting from serous otitis or the like were regularly monitored for hearing function on a monthly basis in this school system. None of the children in the learning disabled group had failed any screening and hence high-tone hearing loss below 4 kHz was unlikely. In light of attending behavior problems encountered in some learning disabled children and in light of the historical passing of screening measures for the mid and higher frequency range, the threshold at 1 kHz was judged an acceptable reference level for administration of the SSW and CES tests. Although no learning disabled

TABLE 1.
Types of learning disabilities noted in learning disability child group[a]

Age	Subjects	Sequencing (%)	Reversals (%)	Coordination (%)	Oral Reading (%)	Sound Blending (%)	Concrete Learning (%)	Spatial Relations (%)	Auditory Discrimination (%)	Auditory Memory (%)	Visual Discrimination (%)	Visual Memory (%)	Behavioral Inconsistencies (%)	Mathematics (%)	Reading (%)
6	4 males 2 females	50	83	67	100	50	67	17	33	67	50	83	67	33	67
7	7 males 3 females	50	70	40	90	80	40	70	30	70	60	80	30	0	70
8	6 males 5 females	54	64	18	82	45	18	0	73	27	73	64	64	0	82
9	7 males 5 females	33	42	33	83	50	42	42	58	42	67	58	33	0	92
10	14 males 4 females	61	61	28	94	72	44	44	39	39	83	72	61	0	100
11	13 males 4 females	47	76	47	88	71	100	75	59	65	76	65	41	0	94
12	3 males 3 females	33	33	17	67	33	17	50	33	17	67	67	33	0	50

(All problem columns grouped under "Problem.")

[a] Judgment of learning disability was based on performance on elements of the Illinois Test of Psycholinguistic Abilities, the Wechsler Intelligence Scale for Children, the Slingerland Screening Test for Language Disabilities, the Stanford Diagnostic Reading Test, the Stanford Diagnostic Mathematics Test, the Wide Range Achievement Test, and the Gates-McGinite Vocabulary and Comprehension Test.

Use of the SSW and CES Tests with Children

child failed the 1 kHz test intensity criterion, some children were ill when the testing was being done and thus were not included in this study.

Children who passed the pure-tone portion of the testing protocol were familiarized with the listening task with a routine taped word list (W-22 half-list per ear). Each child was then administered the SSW Test (list EE) at a 50 dB level about 1 kHz threshold. The CES Test was administered at the same level while the child had pictures which accompany this test on his or her lap.

Analysis

Data consisted of subject errors made in repeating words correctly and in repeating the words in the proper order for the SSW test. CES data consisted of subject errors made in picture identification. Data for normals were initially grouped by age, sex, and handedness categories. Data for children with learning disabilities, lacking balance by sex and handedness, were examined for age effect.

Mean performance and standard deviation calculations were performed for the respective groups by age. Differences between the normal and learning-disabled groups were examined with t-tests. Interaction of special learning disability with auditory perception performance of the SSW test (list EE) and on the CES test was explored.

Findings

Neither sex nor handedness displayed a significant relationship to the children's performance on either the SSW test (list EE) or the CES test in the normal group.

Figures 1 through 4 present the mean and standard deviation data for the various error categories of the SSW test (list EE) and the CES test for the 2 study groups. Generally, the number of errors lessens with age for each study group (Figure 1). Figure 2 presents similar data for the CES test. Reversal behavior (where the subject repeats the test words in an inappropriate order) showed no demonstrable age trend (Figure 3).

Figure 4 presents error data by error category for summed errors for the noncompeting and competing modes. Generally, children performed with fewer errors as they matured. The higher error rates for each age category did occur in the left competing stimulus mode.

The various stimulus modes were examined for the SSW test and CES test with a t-test to determine whether the 2 groups were significantly different from one another. Table 2 presents t-tests computed for each test parameter where the degrees of freedom used in computation were limited to one less than the N of the smaller of the 2

FIGURE 1.
Number of errors by age on the Staggered Spondaic Word Test

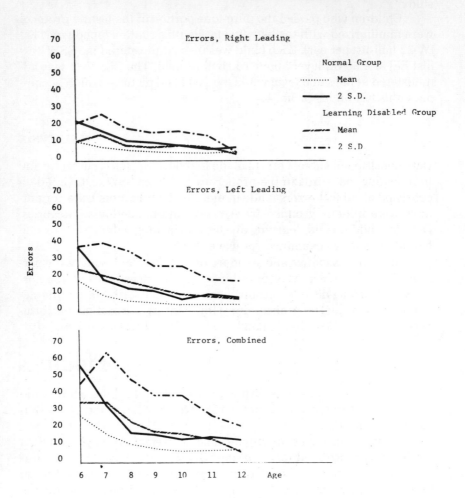

study groups, in effect causing the *t* values in Table 2 to be more conservative than had a compromise *N of both the normal and the learning disabled children been formed. Many of the t* values demonstrated a statistically significant difference between the error rates of the normal and learning-disabled children, the learning-disabled youngsters generally making more errors, in essence supporting the graphic presentation of data in Figures 1 through 4.

From Table 2, it can be seen that the most consistent significantly different error rates occurred in the left leading conditions of the SSW test. Learning disabled children performed more poorly that the normal youngsters on the CES test, but differences were smaller.

Use of the SSW and CES Tests with Children

FIGURE 2.
Number of errors by age on the Competing Environmental Sounds Test

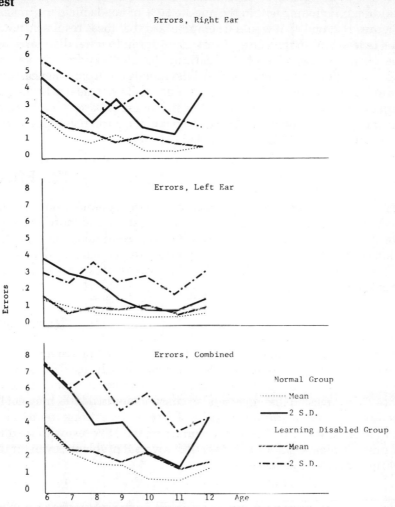

Error rates were compared for children with different types of learning disability. There was no clear association of errors with specific disability.

Discussion

Central Auditory Function and Specific Learning Disability

Children with learning disabilities evaluated in this study incorporated many different types of learning problems (Table 1). In this broad group, both the SSW test and the CES test methodology show some promise in being able to differentiate learning disabled children from children functioning within the middle 50% of academic performance (Figures 1, 2, and 4). It would be emphasized that these results do not at this time establish the value of these tests for individual diagnosis, but the mean performance of the learning disabled children on several tasks lay approximately 2 standard deviations out from the mean performance of normal children. Data for age 6 did not clearly fit the pattern of ages 7 to 12, perhaps reflecting that many children with learning disability are not identified by age 6, so that the normal group for age 6 may have included learning disabled children.

Ear Effect

Error rates for words heard in each ear were examined. Both groups make fewer errors for word stimuli in the right ear and more errors for word stimuli in the left ear in the dichotic condition. The CES test showed that there were slightly more errors in the right ear than in the left ear for both groups. These data are consistent with the auditory process models discussed here.

Reversals

The reordering of stimuli by the subject when the words are repeated to the examiner (Figure 3) did not appear to be strongly age dependent or strongly related to learning disability versus normal academic function. This suggested that reversals, so conspicuous in adults, may not be greatly related to learning disability. There was no strong trend in our data to suggest a correlation of reversals on the SSW test with reading or other academic skills likely to reflect reversal problems, even for the learning-disabled youngsters.

FIGURE 3.
Number of reversals by age on the Staggered Spondaic Word Test

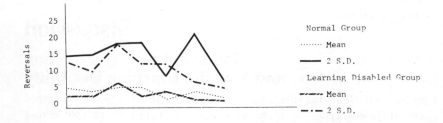

Use of the SSW and CES Tests with Children

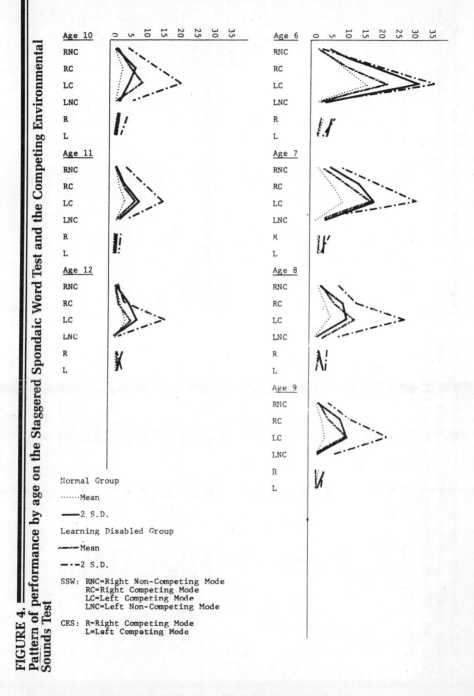

FIGURE 4.
Pattern of performance by age on the Staggered Spondaic Word Test and the Competing Environmental Sounds Test

Normal Group

.... Mean

—— 2 S.D.

Learning Disabled Group

⸺⸺ Mean

— · — 2 S.D.

SSW: RNC=Right Non-Competing Mode
       RC=Right Competing Mode
       LC=Left Competing Mode
       LNC=Left Non-Competing Mode

CES: R=Right Competing Mode
       L=Left Competing Mode

TABLE 2.
t values computed for the difference in mean error rates between normal and learning-disabled children on the SSW and CES tests (actual mean error rates in Figures 3 to 6)

Age	Right Non-competing Right Leading	Right Competing Right Leading	Left Competing Right Leading	Left Non-competing Right Leading	Left Non-competing Left Leading	Left Competing Left Leading	Right Competing Left Leading	Right Non-competing Left Leading	# Normal Children/Learning Disabled
6	2.10[1]	1.28	-0.41	-0.48	-0.49	-2.45[2]	-1.20	0.26	14/6
7	-1.11	-1.63	0.57	-2.26[1]	-2.37[2]	-5.84[3]	-2.43[2]	-1.64	14/10
8	-0.61	-1.24	-1.66	-1.63	-1.68	-3.97[4]	-0.81	-1.78	13/9
9	-2.07[1]	-0.87	-0.87	-1.69	-1.90[1]	-3.97[4]	-1.81[1]	-2.49[5]	13/12
10	-1.20	-1.59	-1.15	-2.42[2]	-1.06	-4.31[3]	-1.75[1]	-2.18[2]	12/16
11	-1.01	-1.69	0.42	-0.97	-2.27[2]	-3.15[4]	-1.67	-1.40	13/17
12	1.00	-0.65	1.59	-1.75	0.00	-1.43	2.67[2]	1.00	12/6

Age	Reversals Right Leading	Reversals Left Leading	CES Right Errors	CES Left Errors	Right Non-competing Total	Right Competing Total	Left Competing Total	Left Non-competing Total	#Normal Children/Learning Disabled
6	0.19	0.30	-0.06	-0.25	1.65	-0.37	-1.86	-0.71	14/6
7	0.07	0.61	-0.82	0.87	-2.00[1]	-2.62[2]	-3.34[4]	-2.73[2]	14/10
8	-0.11	-0.63	-0.97	-0.02	-1.94[1]	-1.25	-3.36[4]	-1.79	13/9
9	1.03	0.29	1.03	-1.06	-2.93[5]	-1.53	-3.01[5]	-2.21[2]	13/12
10	-0.94	-1.94[1]	-1.81[1]	-3.01[4]	-2.29[2]	-1.87[3]	-3.45[4]	-2.94[1]	12/16
11	0.61	0.55[1]	-1.87[1]	-1.66	-1.40	-1.92[1]	-1.90[1]	-1.93[1]	13/17
12	-0.79	-0.14	0.34	-1.17	1.48	1.33	-0.98	-1.75	12/6

[1] p = 0.10, where df was computed with the smaller of the 2 groups (normals and learning disabled) as N-1.
[2] p = 0.05 where df was computed with the smaller of the 2 groups (normals and learning disabled) as N-1.
[3] p = 0.001 where df was computed with the smaller of the 2 groups (normals and learning disabled) as N-1.
[4] p = 0.01 where df was computed with the smaller of the 2 groups (normals and learning disabled) as N-1.
[5] p = 0.02 where df was computed with the smaller of the 2 groups (normals and learning disabled) as N-1.

Age-Specific Performance and Identification of Learning-Disabled Youngsters

Overall, performance on both the CES and SSW tests improves with age. Mean performance of learning-disabled children was almost uniformly poorer than that of the normal group for all test modes. For the 6-year-old children, the differences were proportionately smaller and the variability greater, so that the distinction between groups was slight (Figure 4). Error rates of the 11- and 12-year-old children were only slightly different, again promising less value for discrimination. The best discrimination for the normal and learning disabled groups would seem to be for the 7- to 10-year-old children. The CES data followed a similar though perhaps less clear pattern.

Figure 1 displays a slight tendency for subjects to make fewer errors in the right leading condition than in the left leading condition whereas Figure 2 shows a slight tendency for errors to be more in the left condition than in the right ear condition. This is consistent with the auditory hemisphere laterality effect discussed above.

Children with learning disabilities fail to learn despite normal intelligence. It has been suggested that their nervous systems are unable to shut down or inhibit nonmeaningful "noise" stimuli introduced into the system (6). In addition, there seems to be some time constant for each type of stimuli at which the sequential stimuli cease to be perceived separately but are perceived as one. Simply put, children with learning difficulties require more time to process incoming data.

It may be hypothesized that the SSW and CES tests listening tasks overload the response systems of children with learning problems so that the speed of the incoming sensory stimuli "blur" the data, whether they be simultaneous words or sounds. Certainly, studies on the rate of sound presentation (8, 17, 19), and the present study would tend to support this concept that the learning disabled have reduced auditory processing/perception skills.

Classroom Significance

These data suggest specific classroom intervention strategies for learning-disabled younsters who perform poorly on the SSW test. Even when peripheral function is normal, central problems need to be addressed. If one ear stops understanding when the other ear is busy, the classroom setting must seek to minimize such competition. It is especially important to note that the problem is not that the child does not hear, but rather that he cannot understand well when the noise is present. The "naughty child" who does not follow directions may not be responding to the teacher because he cannot understand when noise is present. Reverberation problems for a child sitting next to a hard, reflecting surface may be as much a noise problem for the learning disabled youngster as is an air conditioner, air vent, window, door, or whatever.

Directions for Research

The staggered spondaic word listening task would seem to be a useful strategy for development of a general learning disability test. Competing environmental sounds seem less sensitive to the disabilities we encountered. It may be that specific learning disabilities may be distinguished by error patterns in competing spondaic word listening tasks, but our limited data could not identify such relationships.

What about prosthetic management of these children with central auditory disabilities? Perhaps some children may benefit from earplug or earmuff intervention strategy to mask out background noise in selective listening situations. Selective use of amplification (e.g., CROS type, classroom auditory trainer, etc.) may be a strategy to allow a child to better use hearing for understanding in noisy settings by allowing the better understanding ear to receive additional phonemic information. Educational research in these areas is needed to determine the efficiacy of such intervention schema.

References

1. American National Standards Institute. 1969. American National Standard Specification for Audiometers. ANSI 3.6–1969. New York.

2. Baker, H. J. 1967. Detroit Tests of Learning Aptitude. Bobbs-Merrill Co., Inc., Indianapolis, IN.

3. Brunt, M., and C. P. Goetzinger, 1968. A study of three tests of central function with normal hearing subjects. Cortex 4, 288–297.

4. Conners, C. K., K. Kramer, and F. Guerra. 1969. Auditory synthesis and dichotic listening in children with learning disabilities. J. Special Ed. 3, 163–169.

5. Goldman, G., M. Fristoe, and R. W. Woodcock. 1974. Auditory Skills Battery. American Guidance Service, Circle Pines, MN.

6. Hebb, D. O. 1976. Physiological learning theory. J. Abnorm. Psychol. 4, 309–314.

7. Katz, J. 1962. The use of the staggered spondaic words for assessing the integrity of the central auditory system. J. Aud. Res. 2, 327–337.

8. Katz, J., and C. Burge. 1971. Auditory perception training for children with learning disabilities. Menorah Med. J. 2, 18–29.

9. Katz, J., and R. Illmer. 1972. Auditory perception in children with learning disabilities, in J. Katz, ed. Handbook of Clinical Audiology. The Williams & Wilkins Co., Baltimore, MD.

10. Kimura, D. 1975. Cerebral dominance for speech. pp. 365–371. in D. B. Tower, ed. The Nervous System. Vol. 3, Raven Press, New York.

11. Knox, C., and D. Kimura. 1970. Cerebral processing of nonverbal sounds in boys and girls. Neuropsychologia 8, 277–287.

12. MacGrady, H. 1964. Verbal and Non-verbal Functions in School Children with Speech and Language Disorders. Ph.D. Thesis, Northwestern University, Evanston, IL.

13. Minimal Brain Dysfunction. 1969. National Project in Learning Disabilities in Children. Public Health Service Publication Number 2015, 5–20, 54–60. United States Government Printing Office, Washington, D.C.

14. Morrill, J. C. 1969. A staggered spondaic word test as an indicator of minimal brain dysfunction in children. Master's Thesis, Texas Technological College, Lubbock, TX.

15. Myrick, D. K. 1965. A normative study to assess performance of a group of children ages seven through eleven on the staggered spondaic word test. Master's Thesis, Tulane University, New Orleans, LA.

16. Pinheiro, M. L. 1977. Tests of central auditory function in children with learning disabilities. pp. 223–254, in R. W. Keith, ed. Central Auditory Dysfunction. Grune and Stratton, New York.

17. Sommers, R. K., W. H. Moore, Jr., W. Brady, and P. Jackson. 1976. Performances of articulatory defective, minimal brain dysfunctioning, and normal children on dichotic ear preference, laterality, and fine-motor skills tasks. J. Spec. Ed. 10, 1, 5–14.

18. Spencer, E. M. 1958. An investigation of the maturation of various factors of auditory perception in preschool children. Ph.D. Thesis, Northwestern University, Evanston, IL.

19. Tallal, P., and M. Piercy. 1974. Developmental aphasia: Rate of auditory processing and selective impairment of consonant perception. Neuropsychologia 12, 83–93.

20. Turner, L. 1966. A normative study on the SSW test for various age groups. Master's Thesis, University of Kansas, Lawrence, KS.

21. Willeford, J. A., and J. M. Billger. 1978., Auditory perception in children with learning disabilities. pp. 410–425, in J. Katz, ed. Handbook of Clinical Audiology, Ed. 2. The Williams & Wilkins Co., Baltimore.

Acknowledgements

The authors thank the Bloomington, Minnesota, Public School System for its cooperation in this study. In addition, gratitude is expressed for the instrumentation for this study which was calibrated and loaned to the investigators by Electro-Medic Incorporated (General Radio 1933 Sound Level Meter), Maico Hearing Instruments Incorporated (Danplex Model ZA 20 Impedance Audiometer), and Qualitone Incorporated (Qualitone Acoustic Appraiser Audiometer). Special thanks are extended to Michael Reder, M.D., for his otological evaluations of children involved in this study and to John Lindgren, M.A., Speech-Language Pathologist responsible for evaluation of our learning disabled youngster's hearing function.

Preliminary Analysis of SSW Test and CES Test Data in 7 Normal and 13 Learning Disabled School Children 6–9 Years Old*

David Johnson

Twenty children with normal intelligence, aged six to nine, were arbitrarily selected from normal classrooms, seven functioning in the middle 50% of academic performance (Group I) and 13 receiving special education services for part of the school day for learning disability (Group II). All children were evaluated neurologically and audiologically, including testing with the SSW Test (List EE) and the CES Test. SSW and CES scores were compared to normative data developed from previous studies within the same school system.

Preliminary data analysis of initial data suggested that many neurologically abnormal youngsters function normally in the classroom for educational purposes (five of our normal children were neurologically abnormal). Learning disability was not automatically associated with neurological dysfunction (five learning disabled youngsters were neurologically normal). (See Table 1.)

*Initial Analysis of Data: David Johnson, M.S., M.A., C.C.C., Audiologist, Department of Otolaryngology, University of Minnesota Medical School and Hennepin County Medical Center, 701 Park Avenue South, Minneapolis, MN 55423

Use of the SSW and CES Tests with Children

TABLE 1.
Neurological Profiles of Study Subjects

Neurological/Coordination Features — values: 1 = Mild/Soft Sign, 2 = Strong/Hard Sign, — = absent

Subject	Age	Muscle tone	Upper reflexes	Lower reflexes	Ankle clonus	Toe problems	Chorea	R(ight) hand	L(eft) hand	R. finger/thumb	L. finger/thumb	R. alternate digit	L. alternate digit	R.→L. mirroring	L.→R. mirroring	Finger→nose	Romberg	R. foot stand	L. foot stand	R. hop	L. hop	Tandem stand	Tandem gait	Graphesia	Speech problems	R. proprioception	L. propioception	Tongue	Thumb width	Eye & foot laterality	Hand & foot laterality	Eye & hand laterality	Diagnosis
Group I — Normals																																
1	7	—	—	—	—	—	1	1	1	1	1	1	1	2	2	—	—	—	—	1	1	1	1	1	1	—	—	1	—	1	1	1	MBD
2	8	—	2	2	—	—	1	2	2	2	2	1	1	1	2	—	—	—	—	1	1	—	—	—	1	—	—	1	—	1	1	1	MBD
3	7	2	2	2	—	—	1	—	—	—	—	—	—	2	—	—	—	—	—	—	—	—	—	—	1	—	—	—	—	—	—	—	WNL
4	8	2	2	2	2	2	2	1	1	1	1	2	2	1	1	—	—	—	—	2	2	—	—	—	—	—	—	—	—	—	—	—	OTHER
5	8	2	2	2	—	—	1	1	1	1	1	1	1	1	1	—	—	—	—	1	1	—	1	—	—	—	—	1	—	—	—	—	MBD
6	7	2	—	2	3	—	1	—	—	—	—	2	—	1	1	—	—	—	—	1	1	—	1	1	—	—	—	1	—	—	—	—	OTHER
7	8	—	—	—	—	—	—	—	—	—	—	—	—	1	2	—	—	—	—	—	—	—	—	—	—	—	—	—	—	—	—	—	WNL
Group II — Learning Disabled																																
8	7	2	2	2	2	—	1	—	—	1	1	1	1	—	1	—	—	—	—	1	1	—	—	1	—	—	—	1	—	—	—	—	STATIC ENCEPHALOPATHY
9	7	—	—	—	—	—	—	—	—	—	—	—	—	1	—	—	—	—	—	1	1	—	—	—	—	—	—	—	—	1-1	1-1	—	WNL
10	7	2	2	2	2	—	1	1	1	1	1	1	1	2	2	—	—	—	—	1	1	—	—	1	—	—	—	1	—	—	—	—	OTHER
11	9	2	2	2	2	—	1	1	1	1	1	1	1	1	1	—	—	—	—	1	1	—	—	2	—	—	—	1	2	1	1	—	MBD
12	8	—	—	—	—	—	—	—	—	—	—	—	—	—	—	1	—	—	—	—	—	—	—	—	—	—	—	—	—	—	—	—	WNL
13	6	2	2	2	2	2	2	—	—	—	—	—	—	—	—	—	—	—	—	—	—	—	—	—	—	—	—	—	—	—	—	—	STATIC ENCEPHALOPATHY
14	7	2	2	2	2	—	—	—	1	—	1	—	—	1	—	—	—	—	—	—	—	—	—	—	—	—	—	—	—	1	1	—	WNL
15	7	2	2	2	2	—	—	1	1	1	1	1	1	—	—	—	—	—	—	—	—	—	—	1	—	—	—	—	—	1	1	—	WNL
16	8	—	2	2	2	—	1	2	1	1	2	1	2	—	—	—	—	—	—	1	1	—	—	1	—	—	—	1	—	1	1	1	STATIC ENCEPHALOPATHY
17	7	—	2	2	—	—	—	1	2	1	1	2	1	—	—	—	—	1	—	2	1	—	—	1	—	—	—	1	—	1	1	1	STATIC ENCEPHALOPATHY
18	7	—	—	—	—	1	—	1	1	1	1	1	1	—	—	—	—	—	—	—	—	—	—	1	—	—	—	—	1	1	—	1	OTHER
19	7	2	2	—	2	2	2	1	1	1	1	1	1	—	—	—	—	—	—	—	—	—	—	1	—	—	—	1	—	—	—	—	STATIC ENCEOPHALOPATHY
20	7	—	—	—	—	—	—	—	—	—	—	—	—	—	—	—	—	—	—	—	—	—	—	—	—	—	—	—	—	1-1	—	—	WNL

1 Mild/Soft Sign
2 Strong/Hard Sign

Preliminary Analysis of SSW and CES Test Data in School Children

TABLE 2.
Central Auditory Profile of Study Subjects: SSW Data/CES Data

Subjects	Age	Right Leading				Left Leading					Totals					R. CES	L. CES
		RNC	RC	LC	LNC	LNC	LC	RC	RNC	Type A	RNC	RC	LC	LNC	Reversals		
1	7	—	—	—	*	—	—	—	—	—	—	—	—	—	—	—	*
2	8	—	—	—	—	—	**	—	—	—	—	—	—	—	—	—	—
3	7	—	—	—	—	—	*	—	*	—	*	*	—	—	—	—	—
4	8	—	—	—	—	—	*	—	—	—	—	—	—	—	—	—	—
5	8	—	—	—	—	—	—	—	—	—	—	—	—	—	—	—	—
6	7	—	*	—	—	—	**	—	—	—	—	**	—	—	—	*	—
7	8	—	—	—	—	—	**	—	—	—	—	—	—	—	—	—	—
8	7	—	—	—	—	—	*	—	—	**	—	—	**	**	—	—	—
9	7	—	—	—	*	—	—	—	—	—	—	—	**	—	—	—	—
10	7	—	—	*	—	—	*	—	—	**	—	—	**	—	—	—	—
11	9	—	—	—	—	—	*	—	—	—	—	—	—	—	**	—	—
12	8	—	—	—	—	—	**	—	—	—	—	—	—	—	—	—	—
13	6	—	—	—	—	—	*	—	—	—	—	—	—	—	—	—	—
14	7	—	—	—	—	—	*	—	—	**	—	—	—	—	—	—	—
15	7	—	—	—	—	—	—	—	—	—	—	—	—	—	—	—	—
16	8	—	—	—	—	—	**	—	—	**	—	—	**	—	**	—	—
17	7	*	*	—	—	—	*	—	—	**	*	—	**	—	—	—	—
18	7	—	—	—	*	*	—	—	—	**	—	—	—	—	—	—	—
19	7	—	—	—	—	**	**	—	—	—	—	—	**	—	—	—	—
20	7	**	—	—	**	**	**	—	—	—	**	—	**	**	—	—	—

*Outside 2 SD
**Outside 3 SD

Normative Data Source: Johnson DW, Enfield ML, Sherman RE: The Use of the Staggered Spondaic Word and the Competing Environmental Sounds Tests in the Evaluation of Central Auditory Function of Learning Disabled Children. *Ear and Hearing* 2:70–77, 1981.

Use of the SSW and CES Tests with Children

Auditory performance as measured with the "usual" audio-metrics did not differentiate the two groups. Group II youngsters did perform more poorly than did the normal Group I youngsters. The learning disabled children of Group II demonstrated Type A patterns, poorer discrimination in the total left competing discrimination mode, or performed poorly on reversal measures of the SSW Test. The CES Test did not prove very useful in differentiating the groups. Type A patterns, total left competing discrimination function, and reversal function differentiated 69% of the children who were learning disabled in Group II, but none of the children functioning in the academically normal Group I were identified (Table 2).

Additional analysis of these and other data are in the early stages of evaluation and preparation for publication. These preliminary data do suggest that the SSW Test has elements useful in differentiating some of the learning-disabled population from children functioning within the middle 50% of academic performance. It is noteworthy that the test performance appears sensitive to educational performance rather than to neurological status alone.

Acknowledgement:

Support of the General Mills Foundation and the Bloomington Public Schools (Minnesota) to complete these central auditory studies is acknowledged. Child selection and audiometrics (Mary Lee Enfield, Ph.D., Director of Special Education, Bloomington Schools, and Jack Lindgren, M.A., Clinical Speech Coordinator, Bloomington Schools) and neurological assessment (Stephen Smith, M.D., Pediatric Neurologist) are gratefully noted. Acoustic Appraiser Audiometer calibration was provided by Qualitone Hearing Instruments.

Performance on Measures of Central Auditory Function by Learning Disabled Children:
A Report of Clinical Data

Michael E. Dybka, Ph.D.   Frank E. Sansone, Ph.D.

In the past few years interest in the evaluation of central auditory function in children has increased dramatically. Two measures of central auditory function in children are the Staggered Spondaic Word (SSW) Test (Stubblefield and Young, 1975; Katz and Illmer, 1972; Katz, 1962, 1968) and the Central Auditory Processing Battery (CAP), a series of four tasks utilized by Willeford (1974, 1976, 1978).

The SSW is a dichotic task in which each test item consists of two spondee words presented in an overlapping manner. A different spondee is presented to each ear with the last half of the first spondee overlapping with the first half of the second. The leading ear changes with each item, creating an equal number of right and left ear stimulations. The conditions of right noncompeting (RNC), right competing (RC), left competing (LC) and left noncompeting (LNC) allow for each ear to receive stimulation in isolation as well as in competition (Brunt, 1972). (For a complete description of the SSW the reader is referred to Brunt [1972, 1978].)

The CAP utilized by Willeford (1974, 1976, 1978a) consists of four tasks—competing sentences, filtered speech, binaural fusion, and alternating speech. (For a complete description of these tasks the reader is referred to Willeford [1978a].)

The SSW and the CAP both represent distorted speech measures and were originally developed for the evaluation of central auditory function in adults. Recently, however, it has been demonstrated that these measures may also be useful in identifying central auditory dysfunction in children classified as learning disabled (White, 1977; Stubblefield and Young, 1975; Willeford, 1974, 1976, 1978a).

The utilization of distorted speech measures with children requires a different perspective than their use with adults. The focus of a central auditory evaluation with adults is usually to determine a site of lesion in relationship to some pathological insult which impairs central auditory function. With children, although a site of lesion orientation exists, the focus is not to determine the area of presumed pathological insult. Rather, the focus is an attempt to describe the child's ability to interpret auditory information when the extrinsic redundancy is reduced and the central auditory system is stressed to its critical listening limits. Analysis of performance on these measures leads to a description of central auditory function based upon the listening tasks presented.

This change in perspective when employing distorted speech measures with children may produce different patterns of performance than expected from adults. The SSW and CAP have been suggested as determiners of brainstem or temporal lobe involvement with an adult population. On the SSW, ipsilateral depressions in performance are thought to reveal brainstem involvement; contralateral depressions in performance are thought to reveal temporal lobe involvement (Brunt, 1972; Katz, 1962, 1968, 1970, 1977). The CAP tasks are also thought to differentiate between brainstem and temporal lobe involvement. Depressed performance on the binaural fusion and alternating speech tasks are thought to reveal ipsilateral brainstem involvement, while depressed performance on competing sentences and filtered speech are felt to indicate contralateral temporal lobe involvement (Willeford, 1974, 1976, 1978a).

Lynn and Gilroy (1975) have demonstrated patterns of response performance consistent with site of lesion in adults. The SSW and CAP were administered to a sample of adults with tumors in the posterior region of the temporal lobe. Mean scores for competing sentences, filtered speech, and a modified SSW task were all depressed in the ear contralateral to the site of lesion.

The work of Lynn and Gilroy (1975) confirmed that patterns of performance consistent with brainstem versus temporal lobe involvement in adults can be identified through the SSW and CAP. Of interest to the present investigation was whether or not similar patterns of performance occur when the SSW and CAP are employed with learning disabled children.

The purpose of this investigation was to determine patterns of performance for a group of learning disabled children when the SSW and CAP were combined into a test battery. An additional purpose was to compare performance on these measures to the most recent norms for children. The suggested normative data of Stubblefield and Young (1975) was used for the SSW. Willeford's revised norms were employed for the CAP (Willeford, 1978b).

The employment of the SSW and the CAP as a battery for central auditory evaluations with a learning disabled population may provide additional diagnostic information through emerging patterns of performance. Such information may contribute to a more complete description of central auditory functioning in the learning disabled child.

Methods and Procedures

The subjects employed in this investigation consisted of 16 children (14 males and 2 females) between the ages of 8 and 10. Subjects were classified as learning disabled through evaluation by a local school district. The evaluation consistsed of educational testing, psychological testing, and staff consultations. All subjects demonstrated intellectual functioning within normal limits as determined by standardized intelligence measures. Each subject was placed in a learning disability classroom and had demonstrated at least a one-year delay in academic achievement as measured by standardized educational measures.

Procedures

Data for this investigation were obtained in a single testing session for each subject. Initially, each subject's pure tone sensitivity, middle ear function, speech reception threshold, and word discrimination was assessed. Criteria for acceptance as a subject included:

Use of the SSW and CES Tests with Children

1. Air conduction thresholds of 10 dB HL or better (ANSI 1969).
2. Type A tympanogram (Jerger, 1970).
3. Speech reception thresholds within 5 dB of the pure tone average at 500 Hz, 1000 Hz, and 2000 Hz.
4. Word discrimination scores of 90% or better for CID W-22 word lists presented at 40 dB above the SRT via live voice.

The SSW and the four tasks of the CAP were then administered to each child using standardized instructions and procedures (Willeford, 1978b; Katz, 1977). The order of test administration was counterbalanced. Raw scores on the SSW were converted to C-SSW scores (Katz, 1973). The CAP scores were computed in terms of percent correct on each of the four tasks (Willeford, 1978). Performance on these measures was compared to the most recent normative data for eight-year-old children. The normative data of Katz (1968) was utilized for the SSW. This choice was based on the suggestion of Stubblefield and Young (1975). Their data supported the contention that Katz's norms of 1968 were appropriate for normal, academically achieving children down to age seven. Willeford's revised normative data of 1978 was employed for the CAP (Willeford, 1978b).

Equipment

All testing was completed in a 401 Industrial Acoustics Corporation sound booth. The tympanograms were obtained utilizing an American Electromedics 83 Impedance Bridge. Pure tone and speech audiometric measures were obtained from a Grason Stadler 1704 audiometer calibrated to ANSI (1969) standards. The SSW and CAP were presented via taped stimuli from a CD Superscope cassette tape recorder routed through the Grason Stadler 1704 audiometer.

Results

Mean scores were computed across subjects for the SSW and CAP tasks.
Table 1 represents mean C-SSW scores (percent error scores) for each condition; right noncompeting (RNC), right competing (RC), left competing (LC), and left noncompeting (LNC). The two noncompeting conditions revealed error scores within the suggested norms of Stubblefield and Young (1975). The two competing conditions (RC, LC) demonstrated error scores well above the suggested norms—22.6 for the right ear and 36.06 for the left ear. The mean error score for the left ear was found to be significantly ($p<.05$) greater than the right ear. In addition a wide range of reversals, 0 to 23, was noted. Fewer reversals were seen as error scores increased.

TABLE 1

Mean C-SSW scores for a group of learning disabled children (N = 16) as compared to suggested norms (Katz, 1968) for children 7 and older[a]

	RNC[b]	RC	LC	LNC
C–SSW (LD group)	5.25	22.6	36.06	8.56
C–SSW (Katz, 1968)	−9–15	−9–15	−9–15	−9–15

[a]Norms suggested by Stubblefield and Young, 1975.

[b]RNC–right noncompeting; RC–right competing; LC–left competing; LNC–left noncompeting.

TABLE 2

Mean CAP scores for a group of learning disabled children (N = 16) as compared to Willeford's (1978b) norms for 8-year-old children.

	CS[a]	FS	BF	AS
LD group (N=16)				
Right ear	73.12	60.25	49.06	94.37
Left ear	58.75	58.00	50.62	93.12
Willeford's (1978b) norms for eight-year-old children				
Right ear	98.00	65.70	76.80	99.50
Left ear	83.00	65.80	76.80	98.80

[a]CS–competing sentences; FS–filtered speech; BF–binaural fusion; AS–alternating speech.

Table 2 illustrates mean percent correct scores for the four tasks of the CAP. Performance on the competing sentence task and the binaural fusion task was well below the revised 1978 norms of Willeford (Willeford, 1978b). Mean scores for the filtered speech task were slightly below the suggested norms, while the alternating speech task produced a mean percent correct score within the normal range. Significant ear differences were noted only for the competing sentence task. This task revealed a significantly ($p<.05$) lower mean percent correct score (58.75) when the primary message was presented to the left ear.

In order to compare the mean percent error scores from the SSW with the mean percent correct scores from the CAP, error scores on the SSW were converted to percentage correct scores, thus making the data from the two measures compatible. Table 3 represents Spearman Rank Order correlations for percent correct scores on the right and left competing conditions of the SSW and the right and left competing sentences, filtered speech, and binaural fusion from the CAP. The two noncompeting conditions from the SSW and the alternating speech

TABLE 3

Spearman rank order correlations between C–SSW scores and the CAP

C–SSW Condition	CAP-task	rho
right competing	right competing sentences	.73
right competing	right filtered speech	.43
right competing	right binaural fusion	.49
left competing	left competing sentences	.79
left competing	left filtered speech	.14
left competing	left binaural fusion	.52

task of the CAP were eliminated from the correlation analysis, since performance on these tasks was within the norms utilized for this investigation. A statistically significant correlation ($p<.01$) was observed between the SSW scores and the competing sentence task—0.73 for the right ear and 0.79 for the left ear. The slightly higher correlation for the left ear was consistent with poorer performance for the left ear on both of these measures.

The correlation between SSW scores and binaural fusion was also significant ($p<.05$)—0.49 for the right and 0.52 for the left ear. However, the correlation was not as high as that observed for the SSW and competing sentence task.

The SSW and the filtered speech task demonstrated nonsignificant and divergent correlations—0.43 for the right and 0.14 for the left ear.

Discussion

The results of this investigation revealed mean error scores on the SSW for a group of learning disabled children which were similar to those previously reported (Stubblefield and Young, 1975). Such data supports the sensitivity of the SSW as a measure of central auditory function for learning disabled children.

Three of the four tasks of the CAP also demonstrated results indicative of a sensitive measure of central auditory function in learning disabled children. The alternating speech task produced mean scores within the normal range. Additionally, all subjects within our sample achieved a score on this task which was within the normal range. Based upon these results, the alternating speech task did not appear to be a sensitive measure and might be eliminated when employing the CAP with learning disabled children.

The correlation analysis demonstrated a definite relationship between performance of the SSW and the CAP. The SSW and the competing sentence task showed the strongest related performance.

Related performance was also noted between the SSW and the binaural fusion task; however, this relationship was not as strong as between the SSW and competing sentence task. No significant relationship between performance on the SSW and the filtered speech task was observed. Thus, there appeared to be a decreasing relationship between performance on the SSW and the CAP. The strongest relationship was between the SSW and the competing sentence task, followed by binaural fusion, with filtered speech showing the weakest relationship.

These patterns of related performance on the SSW and the CAP tasks are dissimilar from those observed in adults. Lynn and Gilroy (1975) reported poorer scores on the SSW, competing sentence task, and the filtered speech task for the ear contralateral to the lesion for a sample of adults with tumors in the posterior region of the temporal lobe. The present investigation revealed related performance between the SSW, competing sentence, and binaural fusion tasks.

If similar patterns between adults and children with learning disabilities existed on these measures, one would expect to see one of two patterns of related performance. One pattern would include related performance between the SSW, competing sentences, and filtered speech. This pattern would be consistent with the results of Lynn and Gilroy (1975) and indicative of temporal lobe involvement. The other possible pattern would be related performance on the SSW, binaural fusion, and alternating speech tasks. Such a pattern would indicate brainstem involvement. The patterns of related performance seen in this investigation are different than either one of the patterns suggested for adults. Therefore, the listening tasks employed in these measures seem to produce different effects on the auditory system when used with children as opposed to adults.

One basis for the related performance seen in this investigation may lie in the dichotic competing stimuli employed. The SSW, competing sentence task, and the binaural fusion task all involve a dichotic task with varying degrees of competition. However, the filtered speech task is presented monaurally without competing stimuli. Based upon our data, as the degree of dichotic competing stimuli became less, the relationship between the SSW and the CAP tasks also became less. The SSW and competing sentence task both involve a dichotic competing stimulus. Related performance was seen whether the competing stimulus was to be processed, as on the SSW, or discarded, as on the competing sentence task. The binaural fusion task also involves a dichotic task, however, the degree of competition is less than that of the SSW or competing sentence task. Thus, the relationship between the SSW and binaural fusion was not as strong. These relationships were slightly stronger for left ear stimulation, with the competing stimulus presented to the right ear. The filtered speech task does not include a competing stimulus and is a monaural task. Therefore, when compared to the dichotic competing stimuli of the SSW, no significant relationship was observed.

An additional basis for the relationships seen in this investigation may be related to the type of competing stimuli. Selective attention to a desired message during a dichotic task has been shown to be influenced by the transitional probabilities between words (Treisman, 1964). Treisman demonstrated that an irrelevant message delivered by the same speaker involving similar content was a more difficult task than that presented by two different speakers. The dichotic competing stimuli found on the SSW, competing sentence task, and the binaural fusion task met the descriptions of Treisman, thereby producing an affect on selective attentional abilities and subsequent performance on these tasks.

The relationships seen in this investigation appear then to be based not only on the dichotic task and the degree of competition, but on the type of competition as well.

Conclusions

The results of this investigation demonstrated that both the SSW and the CAP, excluding alternating speech, are sensitive measures for the identification of central auditory dysfunction in learning disabled children. Furthermore, by combining the SSW and the CAP tasks, patterns of performance emerged related to the degree of competition found in a dichotic task and also to the type of competition. Competing messages delivered by the same speaker and of a similar nature provided the most difficulty for this sample of learning disabled children. The relationship between the listening tasks involved and their effect on selective attention warrants further investigation.

Although the results from this investigation are seen as providing additional diagnostic information regarding central auditory function in learning disabled children, they may also provide information concerning rehabilitative planning. The relationships seen in this investigation point to the need for rehabilitative planning centered around the child's ability to handle competing messages and enhance his selective attentional abilities. It would appear that rehabilitative techniques which reduce the degree and nature of competing stimuli would enhance selective attention and appropriate interpretation of the message.

References

American National Standards Institute, *Specifications for Audiometers, ANSI S3.6–1969.* New York: American National Standards Institute, 1969.

Brunt, M. A. The staggered spondaic word test. *Handbook of Clinical Audiology,* Katz, J. (ed.), Baltimore: Williams and Wilkins (1972).

Brunt, M.A The staggered spondaic word test. *Handbook of Clinical Audiology,* Katz, J. (ed.), 2nd edition, Baltimore: Williams and Wilkins (1978).

Jerger, J. Clinical experience with impedance audiometry. *Arch. Otolaryngol.,* 92, 311–324, 1970.

Katz, J. The use of staggered spondee words for assessing the integrity of the central auditory nervous system. *Journal of Auditory Research,* 2, 327–337, 1962.

Katz, J. The SSW test—an interim report. *Journal of Speech and Hearing Dis.,* 33, 132–146, 1968.

Katz, J. Audiological diagnosis: cochlea to cortex. *Menorah Med. Journal,* 1, 25–38, 1970.

Katz, J. *The SSW Test Manual,* Auditec of St. Louis, Brentwood Mo., 1977.

Katz, J. and Illmer, R. Auditory perception in children with learning disabilities. *Handbook of Clinical Audiology,* Katz J. (ed.), Baltimore: Williams and Wilkins (1972).

Lynn, G. E. and Gilroy, J. Effects of brain lesions on the perception of monotic and dichotic speech stimuli. *Central Auditory Processing Disorders,* Sullivan, M. (ed.), Omaha: University of Nebraska Press (1975).

Stubblefield, J. and Young, E. Central auditory dysfunction in learning disabled children. *Journal Learning Disab.,* 8, 89–94, 1975.

Treisman, A. M. The effect of irrelevant material on the efficiency of selective listening. *American Journal Psychol.,* 77, 533–546, 1964.

White, E. Children's performance on the SSW test and Willeford battery: Interim clinical data. *Central Auditory Dysfunction,* Kieth, R. (ed.), New York: Grune and Stratton, Inc., 1977.

Willeford, J. Central auditory function in children with learning disabilities. Paper presented at the meeting of the American Speech and Hearing Association, Las Vegas, 1974.

Willeford, J. Central auditory function in children with learning disabilities. *Journal Audiology and Hearing Education,* 2, 12–20 (1976).

Willeford, J. and Bilger, J. Auditory perceptual dysfunction in learning disabled children. *Handbook of Clinical Audiology,* Katz, J. (ed.), 2nd edition, Baltimore: Williams and Wilkins (1978a).

Willeford, J. Procedures for Central Auditory Processing Battery and expanded norms. Supplement contained in Central Auditory Processing Battery Tape, 1978b.

Identification of Central Auditory Dysfunction in Chidren With Learning Disabilities

Terry K. Lewis, M.A., Richard G. Winkelaar, M.A.

Evaluation of central auditory function in children with learning disabilities is discussed. Audiological-neurological results on four children, aged 7-12 years, are presented with special emphasis on the relationship between the central auditory and neurological findings. Results suggest central auditory dysfunction in these children can be identified, but diagnostic and interpretative caution is essential because of the inherent limitations of central testing with this population.

Learning disabilities can cause severe educational difficulties for school aged children. The wide variety of symptoms may include specific difficulty in auditory perception, psychological function, understanding, integrating, and utilizing information. Symptom severity ranges from mild to severe, and it is generally accepted that some type of central nervous system dysfunction not related to sensory, motor, intellectual, or emotional handicap causes the disability. Incidence figures vary, ranging from 10–20%, although only 1–3% of these children are usually in special classes (Chalfant and Scheffelin;[1] Myklebust and Boshes;[2] Silverman and Metz;[3] Katz and Illmer[4]).

Central auditory perceptual processing difficulties have been recognized by numerous investigators (Myklebust;[5] Katz and Illmer;[6] Dermody;[7] Witkin[8]), and recently there has been a greatly heightened interest in audiological assessment of nonperipheral auditory perceptual problems related to learning disabilities (Keith;[9] Willeford and Billger;[10] Willeford;[11],[12] Pinheiro;[13] Costello;[14] Katz[15]).

Conventional speech audiometric tests are not sensitive enough to identify central auditory deficiencies, and normal performance is often exhibited on standard word discrimination tasks. Audiological tests of central auditory function therefore utilize speech stimuli which have been electronically modified in a variety of ways to decrease signal redundancy. These signal decrements make the listening task more difficult and stress the auditory system, often permitting identification of subtle abnormalities missed by the easier conventional tests.

The Staggered Spondaic Word (SSW) Test is one test which has been successfully used to identify central auditory dysfunction in older children and adults (Katz;[16] Jerger;[17] Winkelaar and Lewis[18]). It appears to be relatively uncontaminated by the effects of peripheral hearing loss and is standardized for patients 11–60 years of age (Katz;[19] Brunt[20]). It may be used for children 5–11 years in age if test scores are considered in terms of the relatively greater number of errors and increased variability due to the age factor. The scores can be based on the upper limits of normal performance for each age group, with scores outside these limits for a particular age considered abnormal (Myrick;[21] Katz[22]).

Briefly, the test consists of 40 spondaic words. One is presented to the right ear and the other to the left, with the lead ear alternating. The second syllable of the first word overlaps the first syllable of the second word (Figure 1) creating four stimulus conditions: right ear noncompeting (RNC), right ear competing (RC), left ear competing (LC), and left ear noncompeting (LNC). The words typically are presented at a 50 dB sensation level. Patients with intact auditory reception areas have no difficulty repeating competing items (e.g., "light" and "lunch"), and have errors scores of less than 10%. Patients with lesions affecting auditory reception have difficulty repeating competing syllables in the ear contralateral to the affected hemisphere. They obtain corrected (C-SSW) error scores in excess of 15%.

In addition to the quantitative scoring, Katz[23] suggests qualitative scoring procedures, including analysis of ear effects, order effects, and

Use of the SSW and CES Tests with Children

reversals. A significant ear effect is an error score of +5 or greater in one ear for competing and noncompeting items, and suggests more diffuse areas of dysfunction involving the anterior temporal and parietal areas. A significant order effect occurs when the first spondee is correctly identified +5 or more times than the second or vice versa, and suggest diffuse areas of dysfunction involving the frontal lobes. These effects are analyzed with the adjusted (A-SSW) scoring procedure. Reversal of item order ("day-light-lunch-time" becomes "light-time-lunch-day") is regarded as potentially significant when reversals exceed four. These may be related to dysfunction in the pre-post central gyrii [fronto parietal region] (Katz and Pack[24]).

The purpose of this paper is to discuss identification of central auditory abnormalities in children with learning disabilities using the SSW Test. Audiological results on four children will be presented, and the central auditory test results will be related to the neurologial findings.

Case Reports

Patient 1 Age 10, exhibited delayed language development, misarticulations, and reading difficulties. Conventional audiological test results (Figure 2A) indicated normal hearing sensitivity, word discrimination, and middle ear function. The C-SSW test results (Figure 2B) suggested central auditory dysfunction. The 40% error score for left ear competing items and the less than 15% error scores for all the others would be consistent with dysfunction in the right temporal area. EEG results (Figure 2C) indicated focal abnormality in the right temporal lobe.

FIGURE 1. ▬▬▬▬▬▬▬▬▬▬▬▬▬▬▬▬▬▬▬▬▬▬▬▬▬▬
Sample items from the Staggered Spondaic Word Test.

TIME SEQUENCE

	1 ⟶	2 ⟶	3
RE	DAY	LIGHT	
LE		LUNCH	TIME

LE	FOR	GIVE	
RE		MILK	MAN

FIGURE 2.
Audiological and Neurological findings on patient 1.
A-Audiogram, speech audiometry, impedance
B-SSW
C-Neurological report

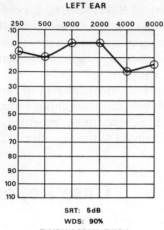

A

LEFT EAR	RIGHT EAR

SRT: 5dB
WDS: 90%
TYMPANOGRAM: TYPE A
ACOUSTIC REFLEXES: NORMAL SENSATION LEVELS

SRT: 5dB
WDS: 90%
TYMPANOGRAM: TYPE A
ACOUSTIC REFLEXES: NORMAL SENSATION LEVELS

B

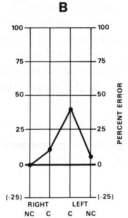

RIGHT   LEFT
NC   C   C   NC

C

Impression of some degree of focal abnormality persistently seen on the right side, particularly in low temporal and posterior locations.

Patient 2   Age 7, exhibited delayed language development and reading difficulties. Conventional audiological results (Figure 3A) were again normal in all respects. The C-SSW results (Figure 3B) indicated a 76% error score for right competing items and 70% for left competing items, with noncompeting items being 26% or less. These results, when considered in light of the normative score ranges for children that age,

FIGURE 3.

Audiological and Neurological findings on patient 2.
A–Audiogram, speech audiometry, impedance
B–SSW
C–Neurological report

A

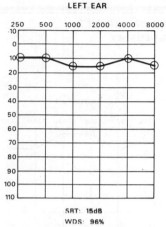

LEFT EAR

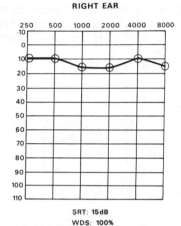

RIGHT EAR

SRT: 15dB
WDS: 96%
TYMPANOGRAM: TYPE A
ACOUSTIC REFLEXES: NORMAL SENSATION LEVELS

SRT: 15dB
WDS: 100%
TYMPANOGRAM: TYPE A
ACOUSTIC REFLEXES: NORMAL SENSATION LEVELS

B

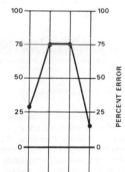

C

Waking spontaneous recording exhibits
moderately irregular alpha activity in
the occipital, parietal, and posterior
temporal regions bilaterally. A small
amount of random sharp activity arises
out of the theta activity in the right
posterior temporal region.

suggested either an immature listening pattern or central auditory dysfunction in both temporal lobes. EEG results (Figure 3C) indicated focal abnormality in both temporal lobe areas.

Patient 3 Age 12, exhibited reading difficulties and letter reversals in writing. Normal results were obtained on all conventional audiological tests (Figure 4A). The C-SSW results (Figure 4B) were normal, suggesting no auditory reception area dysfunction. However, in qualitative scoring, 16 response items were reversed (e.g., "black-board-air-mail" would become "black-mail-air-board"). The EEG report (Figure 4C) indicated no specific lesion site, but did suggest mildly abnormal activity with no focal abnormality.

FIGURE 4.
Audiological and Neurological findings on patient 3.
A-Audiogram, speech audiometry, impedance
B-SSW
C-Neurological report

A

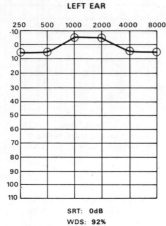

SRT: 0dB
WDS: 92%
TYMPANOGRAM: TYPE A
ACOUSTIC REFLEXES: NORMAL SENSATION LEVELS

SRT: 0dB
WDS: 100%
TYMPANOGRAM: TYPE A
ACOUSTIC REFLEXES: NORMAL SENSATION LEVELS

B   **C**

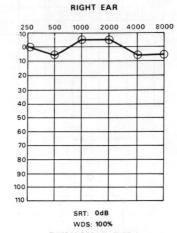

Diffuse mildly abnormal EEG because of excessive amount of fast activity. This activity suggests abnormality of a non-specific nature but is not diagnostic. Excessive amount of mild irregularity noted also to be considered abnormal. Some random sharper activities seen occasionally. The tracing is mostly irregular with occasional regularity low to medium in amplitude, fair to poorly modulated. No definite focal abnormality noted.

REVERSALS: 16

Patient 4   Age 11, displayed very delayed language development and specific linguistic problems involving syntax and vocabulary. All standard audiological test results were normal (Figure 5A). C-SSW results (Figure 5B) indicated 91% and 79% error for the right and left ear competing items, with 46% error for the noncompeting items. These results again suggest dysfunction in the temporal lobe area. Unfortunately, a neurological report was not available for this child. The

FIGURE 5.
Audiological and Neurological results on patient 4.
A-Audiogram, speech audiometry, impedance
B-SSW
C-Neurological report

A

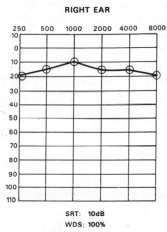

SRT: 10dB   SRT: 10dB
WDS: 92%   WDS: 100%
TYMPANOGRAM: TYPE A   TYMPANOGRAM: TYPE A
ACOUSTIC REFLEXES: NORMAL SENSATION LEVELS   ACOUSTIC REFLEXES: NORMAL SENSATION LEVELS

B   **C**

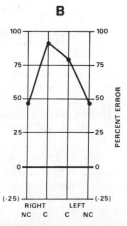

Neurological report not available.

tests results and the indicated language difficulties would, however, be consistent with central auditory dysfunction in the temporal lobe area (Luria;[25] Chalfant and Scheffelin;[26] Katz and Illmer[27]).

The presented clinical findings demonstrate the usefulness of evaluating central auditory function in children. Conventional audiological results including monaural word discrimination indicated abnormality, but the central auditory evaluations suggested each child had certain dysfunctional auditory skills. These appeared to have certain neurological correlates and were reasonably consistent with findings obtained in adult populations. It is, however, a very signficant step from the site of lesion concept in adults to the same concept in children, even with supporting neurological evidence. This is due in part to the inherent limitations of central auditory testing for any population. In addition, the greater variability in pediatric test results and possible ear effects caused only by normal maturation pose additional restrictions. Interpretation of test data, at least at this point in time, often must be limited to a description of the child's performance on the central auditory tests. This is a reasonable approach and begins to focus attention appropriately on remediation of the suspected problem. Effective remedial programs are urgently needed, and although progress is being made (Willeford;[28] Pinheiro;[29] Katz[30]) much remains to be done. While continued healthy skepticism about the board implications and applications of the tests is necessary (Duane[31]), further judicious use of the SSW and other central auditory tests should do much to facilitate development of more accurate and reliable tests and even better remedial programs.

Acknowledgement

The authors wish to express appreciation to L. Zachary for her assistance in manuscript preparation. This study was supported in part by Foothills Hospital, Calgary, Alberta.

References

1. Chalfant, J. and Scheffelin, M. Central processing dysfunction in children. U.S. Dept. of Health, Education & Welfare. Bethesda, Maryland. 1969.

2. Myklebust, H. and Boshes, B. Final report, minimal brain damage in children. U.S. Dept. of Health, Education and Welfare. Washington, D.C. 1969.

3. Silverman, L. and Metz, A. Number of pupils with specific learning disabilities in local public schools in the United States. Spring, 1970. *Ann. N.Y. Acad. Sci.*, 205:146–57. 1973.

4. Katz, J. and Illmer, R. Auditory perception in children with learning disabilities. In Katz, J. (ed.), *Handbook of Clinical Audiology.* Baltimore: Williams & Wilkins (1972).

Use of the SSW and CES Tests with Children

5. Myklebust, H. *Auditory Disorders in Children.* New York: Grune & Stratton (1954).

6. Katz, J. and Illmer, R., *op. cit.* 1972.

7. Dermody, P., Noffsinger, P. D., Hawkins, C. P. *et al.* Auditory processing difficulties in children with learning disabilities. Paper presented at the annual ASHA convention, Washington, D.C. 1975.

8. Witkin, B. R. Auditory perception—implications for language development. *Lang. Spch. Hear. Services in Schools,* 31:52. 1970.

9. Keith, R. (ed.). *General Auditory Dysfunction.* New York: Grune & Stratton (1977).

10. Willeford, J. and Billger, J. Auditory perceptual dysfunction in learning disabled children. In Katz, J. (ed.): *Handbook of Clinical Audiology,* 2nd edition. Baltimore: Williams & Wilkins (1978).

11. Willeford, J. Central auditory function in children with learning disabilities. *Audiology & Hearing Education,* 12–20 Feb.–Mar., 1976.

12. Willeford, J. Differential diagnosis of central auditory dysfunction. In Bradford, L. (ed.), *Audiology: An Audio Journal for Continuing Edcucation,* II:4. New York: Grune & Stratton (1977).

13. Pinheiro, M. Tests of central auditory function in children with learning disabilities. In Keith, R. (ed.), *Central Auditory Dysfunction,* Cincinnati: Grune & Stratton (1977).

14. Costello, M. Evaluation of auditory behavior of children using the Flowers-Costello Test of central auditory abilities. In Keith, R. (ed.). *Central Auditory Dysfunction.* Cincinnati: Grune & Stratton (1977).

15. Katz, J. The staggered spondaic word test. In Keith, R. (ed.): *Central Auditory Dysfunction.* Cincinnati: Grune & Stratton (1977).

16. Katz, J., Basil, R. and Smith, J. A staggered spondaic word test for detecting central auditory lesions. *Ann. Oto. Rhino. Laryng.,* 72:908. 1963.

17. Jerger, J. and Jerger, S. Clinical validity of central auditory tests. *Scand. Audiol.,* 4: 147–163. 1975.

18. Winkelaar, R. and Lewis, T. Audiological tests for evaluation of central auditory disorders. *J. Otolyng. (Can.),* 6:2, 127–134, 1977.

19. Katz, J., *op. cit.,* 1963.

20. Brunt, M. The staggered spondaic word test. In Katz, J. (ed.), *Handbook of Clinical Audiology.* Baltimore: Williams & Wilkins (1972).

21. Myrick, D. A normative study to assess performance of a group of children ages seven through eleven on the SSW test. Unpub. Master's Thesis, Tulane University, 1965.

22. Katz, J. Staggered Spondaic Word Test Workshop, Menorah Medical Center, Kansas City, MO, 1974.

23. Katz, J. Clinical use of central auditory tests. In Katz, J. (ed.), *Handbook of Clinical Audiology,* Baltimore: Williams & Wilkins. 1978.

24. Katz, J. and Pack, G. New developments in differential diagnosis using the SSW Test. In Sullivan, M. (ed.), *Central Auditory Processing Disorders,* University of Nebraska Press, Lincoln. 1975.

25. Luria, A. Higher Cortical Function in Man. Consultants Bureau, New York. 1966.

26. Chalfant, J. and Scheffelin, M., *op. cit.* 1969.

27. Katz, J. and Illmer, R., *op. cit.* 1972.

28. Willeford, J. Assessing central auditory behavior in children: A test battery approach. In Keith, R. (ed.): *Central Auditory Dysfunction,* Cincinnati: Grune & Stratton. 1977.

29. Pinheiro, M., *op. cit.* 1977.

30. Katz, J. and Illmer, R., *op. cit.* 1972.

31. Duane, D. Summary remarks at symposium on central auditory dysfunction. In Keith, R. (ed.). *Central Auditory Dysfunction,* Cincinnati: Grune & Stratton. 1977.

Central Auditory Nervous System Dysfunction in Echolalic Autistic Individuals

Amy Miller Wetherby, Robert L. Koegel, and Maurice Mendel

Accumulating evidence suggests either a primary or secondary cortical dysfunction in the language-dominant hemisphere of autistic children. In this study, the central auditory function of six autistic subjects was assessed experimentally using a battery of tests which included the Staggered Spondaic Word Test, the Competing Environmental Sound test, and monaural hearing tests, as well as supplementary measures of language and handedness. The autistic subjects ranged in age from 8–24 years and displayed a wide range of language abilities and severity of echolalia. The results showed that although all of the subjects had normal hearing on the monaural speech tests, there was indication of central auditory nervous system dysfunction in the language-dominant hemisphere inferred from the dichotic tests for those subjects displaying echolalia; and essentially normal dichotic test results for those subjects who were previously diagnosed autistic, but were no longer echolalic. One subject who received a year of intensive language treatment was assessed periodically over the course of the year to chart

Journal Speech and Hearing Research, 24, 420–429, 1981.

changes in performance on the test of central auditory function for dichotic stimuli. This subject showed changes in the dichotic test of central auditory function which were consistent with the language improvement shown during the course of the year. For each subject, the locus of central auditory dysfunction indicated by the assessment measures was consistent with the characterized language deficits. The results are discussed from a neurolinguistic framework in an effort to delineate a neurogenic etiology of autistic language deficits.

Central Auditory Nervous System Dysfunction in Echolalic Autistic Individuals

The syndrome of autism is defined behaviorally as including: (a) disturbances of developmental rate; (b) inconsistent responses to sensory stimuli; (c) abnormal speech, language, and cognitive capacities; and (d) abnormal relations to people, events, and objects (Ritvo and Freeman, 1978). Many theories of the etiology of autism have been posited to account for these features. Recent theories postulate an underlying neurological basis (Ornitz and Ritvo, 1976), although there has been little direct evidence, and the exact nature of a dysfunction is as yet unknown (Ritvo and Freeman, 1978). Most of the speculations and data implicate either a primary cortical dysfunction (e.g., Damasio and Maurer, 1978; Tanguay, 1976; Hauser, DeLong and Rosman, 1975), or a possible cortical dysfunction secondary to abnormalities in the brainstem (Simon, 1975; Ornitz, 1974) or thalamus (Coleman, 1979; Damasio and Maurer, 1978).

A neurogenic etiology of autism has been supported by long-term follow-up studies. Even in autistic children with no abnormalities on neurological examinations in early childhood, about 30% developed epileptic seizures during adolescence (Rutter and Bartak, 1971). EEG findings have been variable (Ornitz and Ritvo, 1976), but a consistent suppression of vestibular nystagmus has been evidenced in autistic children (Ornitz, 1974). Previous studies of the late components of the auditory evoked potentials in autistic children have found minimal and variable differences when compared to normal children (Ornitz and Ritvo, 1976). However, Student and Sohmer (1978) have recently found atypical auditory nerve and brainstem evoked potentials in a group of 15 children with autistic traits. Although this evidence is far from conclusive, these findings suggest a central nervous system dysfunction in vestibular and/or auditory brainstem nuclei associated with autism.

Damasio and Maurer (1978) have proposed a neurological model of the etiology of autism. From an analysis of patterns of behavioral disturbances exhibited by autistic children, they have suggested that the underlying dysfunction is located in the mesial frontal and temporal lobes, basal ganglia and thalamic nuclei. Coleman (1979) theorized that the thalamus is the location of dysfunction underlying the symptoms of autism. Although there is currently no anatomical evidence from clinical or autopsy studies to verify these sites of lesion, these authors agree that multiple etiologies manifest a relatively consistent symptomatology of autism.

With regard to cortical loci of dysfunction, speculation of an underlying neuropathology of the left hemisphere (see Tanguay, 1976) has been formulated to explain receptive and expressive language deficiency in autistic children in marked contrast to proficiency in various nonverbal and musical abilities (Applebaum, Egel, Koegel, and Imhoff, 1979; Lockyer and Rutter, 1970). This speculation has evolved from evidence that, in the majority of the normal population, certain linguistic functions are lateralized to the left hemisphere, while the right hemisphere appears to be specialized for visuospatial and musical functions (Searleman, 1977, Krashen, 1976; Kimura, 1973; Bogen, 1969; Penfield and Roberts, 1966). Evidence suggestive of a left hemisphere abnormality in autistic children has been reported by Hauser et al., (1975). In an examination of pneumoencephalograms, they found an enlargement of the left temporal horn of the lateral ventricle in 15 out of 17 cases exhibiting the syndrome of autism. Five of these 15 cases also showed some dilation of the right ventricular system. Hauser et al. attributed the ventricular enlargement to medial temporal lobe dysfunction. Although these findings are striking, they must be regarded with caution, in view of evidence of gross structural asymmetries of the normal brain (Geschwind, 1974).

Consistent with the notion of a left hemisphere impairment, Blackstock (1978) recently proposed that autistic children process information predominantly with the right hemisphere. In support of this theory he found that autistic children showed a left ear preference for verbal and musical stimuli. Heir, LeMay, and Rosenberger (1979) examined computerized brain tomograms in 16 autistic patients for left–right structural asymmetries of the posterior language region. In only five of the autistic patients was the left region wider than the right, and nine had a reversed cerebral asymmetry. In contrast, a majority of the mentally retarded and neurological control patients exhibited a wider left posterior language region.

The aforementioned studies suggest evidence of an abnormality in the structural and functional asymmetry of the brain associated with autism. A disruption in or a deviation from the normal process of cerebral lateralization (Moscovitch, 1977) may explain the occurrence of some autistic features such as abnormal language development and inconsistent responses to sensory stimuli.

Central Auditory Assessment

Inconsistent and inappropriate responses to auditory stimuli and delayed language development often lead to an early suspicion of hearing loss prior to a diagnosis of autism (Ornitz, 1973; Kanner, 1943). However, in general, autistic children do not show primary perceptual deficits (Damasio and Maurer, 1978). Therefore, an assessment of the integrity of the central auditory nervous system in autistic children seems warranted to aid in delineating a possible cause of their inconsistent responding. In this investigation the Staggered Spondaic Word (SSW) and Competing Environmental Sound (CES) test battery was used experimentally to assess central auditory function for competing stimuli. The SSW Test was chosen because it is an easy listening task and provides both quantitative and qualitative measures of central dysfunction. The SSW Test was developed by Katz in 1960, and to date, over 10,000 patients with various disorders have been evaluated with this procedure (Katz, 1977b). However, use of the SSW Test with the autistic population has not been reported in the literature. Therefore, our investigation should be viewed as preliminary and speculative in nature.

The SSW Test has been shown to be an effective standardized test in examining central auditory nervous system disorders for individuals 11 to 60 years of age (Brunt, 1972). Normal limits have been strictly defined and there is little variability among normal listeners within this age group. Normative results for children are poorer and more variable than for adults. SSW norms have, however, been obtained on children from 11 down to 5 years (White, 1977; Katz and Illmer, 1972). The typical error pattern for normal children is a poorer score in the left ear and response bias, suggesting incomplete maturation in anterior auditory processing areas of the brain and possibly that cerebral lateralization is not yet complete (Brunt, 1978; White, 1977). Adjusting the SSW scores in a standard manner helps to eliminate processing errors and provides a purer measure of the integrity of the auditory reception area. White (1977) found that, at all ages, the SSW adjusted scores were normal or close to normal by adult standards. She suggested that "the SSW Test may be used in the future to evaluate not only the auditory reception center in children, but related cortical auditory processing areas as well" (White, 1977, p. 332).

Analysis of SSW results may indicate the location of a lesion (i.e., either anatomical damage or physiological dysfunction) within auditory pathways of the brainstem and cerebral hemispheres. Confidence in predicting the location of lesions has developed from data on patients with medically and surgically confirmed sites of lesion (Brunt, 1972, 1978). Specific criteria for categorizing the SSW scores have been devised and established by Katz (1968, 1977a), based on normal subjects and patients with peripheral and/or central problems. Each SSW scores falls into a category of normal, mild, moderate or severe which facilitates the differential diagnosis of auditory dysfunction.

Performance difficulty is partly determined by onset-time differences of each test item (Katz, Harder, and Lohnes, 1977). Severe or moderate SSW scores suggest a central distortion arising from an auditory reception involvement in the contralateral hemisphere, involvement of the interhemispheric pathway (corpus callosum/anterior commissure), or a brainstem involvement ipsilaterally. Patients with cortical dysfunction sparing the auditory reception area show normal or mild SSW scores. Since test items are counterbalanced for each ear receiving the first spondee, response biases should not normally contaminate the SSW scores. When evident, response biases have diagnostic significance in localizing brain dysfunction in specific auditory processing areas of the brain [e.g., fronto-temporal, fronto-parietal, temporo-parietal, and temporo-occipital regions] (Brunt, 1978).

The Competing Environmental Sound test, also devised by Katz (1976), is based on the SSW and serves as a companion procedure to it. It may be effective in supplementing the SSW results in the differential diagnosis of auditory reception versus corpus callosum/anterior commissure dysfunction. It may also be effective in identifying the impaired hemisphere when compared to the SSW Test (Katz, 1976). Although the CES test is still in the preliminary stages of clinical application, it does provide supplementary information to the SSW Test.

The specific purpose of the present study was to determine whether empirical measures of central auditory processing for dichotic stimuli might be indicative of problems underlying deviant auditory responses and deviant linguistic systems of echolalic autistic children. The SSW test battery was used as an experimental research tool with a small group of autistic individuls in a preliminary study in which the following questions were asked:

1) Is there empirical evidence indicative of an underlying central auditory dysfunction, despite normal hearing on monaural speech tests, in these echolalic autistic individuals?

2) If so, does the indicated locus of central auditory dysfunction inferred from the dichotic tests for each subject relate to the receptive/expressive language deficit?

Method

Subjects

Six autistic subjects, ranging in age from 8–24 years, participated in this study. Descriptions of each are provided below. Subjects selected for this investigation were those who were: (1) diagnosed autistic according to the U.S. National Society for Autistic Children criteria (Ritvo and Freeman, 1978) by both ourselves and at least one independent source; (2) able to repeat intelligibly at least four syllables for the purposes of administering the SSW Test; (3) eight years of age and older, because of the clearer normative data on the SSW Test for these age groups. Additionally, subjects were selected to exemplify a range of linguistic abilities and severity of echolalic behavior as often exhibited by autistic children.

Subject 1, a 24-year-old male, lived in a foster home and attended a training center for disabled adults. His expressive language was limited to extensive and frequent immediate and delayed echolalia, short one- and two-word labeling, and one-word responses to questions. He had a tendency to perseverate on a few particular delayed echolalic utterances (e.g., "want some coffee," "that's disgusting"). Although he had very little comprehension of written material, he could read and write most words. Given a pencil, he would incessantly write words until the pencil was removed from his hand; this was analogous to his verbal behavior, which consisted of incessant delayed echolalia. His intonation patterns were bizarre, giving his voice a high pitched, shrill quality. He exhibited self-stimulatory behavior (e.g., finger manipulation, bizaare vocalizations), toe walking, disruptive behavior (e.g., slapping), and was excessively active and easily distracted.

Subject 2, an 18-year-old male, lived at home and attended a class for autistic children. He did not initiate speech and his language consisted of one-word utterances and moderately frequent (approximately 15–20% of total utterances) immediate echolalic responses. His receptive abilities were better than his expressive abilities in that he could follow commands and respond appropriately to questions, but he had a tendency to give the minimum possible response. He could read and write with some elementary comprehension. His voice was monotonic and he tended to whisper. His self-stimulatory behavior was extensive and included rocking, hand flapping, and swishing saliva.

Subject 3, a 14-year-old male, lived at home and attended a special education class in a junior high school. His language was characterized by a lack of spontaneity (he did not initiate speech) and by the presence of occasion (less that 10% of total utterances) immediate and delayed echolalia. He could follow commands requiring nonverbal responses, but generally responded inappropriately to questions requiring verbal responses (e.g., inappropriate use of yes/no; echoed phrases; pronoun reversals; confused word orders). He could read and write at the third-grade level. His voice quality was characterized by a monotonous inflection. He often covered his ears with his hands in the absence of any loud external sound. He exhibited some self-stimulatory behavior (e.g., finger flicking and hand flapping) and disruptive behavior (e.g., wrist grabbing and slapping).

Subject 4, an 8-year-old male, lived at home and attended a special education class while being mainstreamed into a normal first-grade classroom. At the time of this study, he was participating in a one-year clinic treatment program. At the beginning of treatment (early treatment), his expressive language consisted of moderately frequent (approximately 15–20% of total utterances) immediate and delayed echolalia, perseverative question asking, and responses inappropriate to context. His academic skills were minimal and he did not interact with other children. He occasionally exhibited self-stimulatory behavior (e.g., hand flapping).

Over the course of the past year, this subject learned to read and write at the first grade level and learned basic first-grade math concepts. By the end of treatment (late treatment), he played appropriately at a kindergarten/first-grade level with children he knew at home and school. He initiated elementary conversations and asked appropriate questions, but often perseverated on particular phrases or topics and talked excessively. He rarely exhibited immediate echolalia, although he still evidenced some delayed echolalia. He displayed hand flapping only when he was particularly excited.

Subject 5, an 8-year-old male, lived at home and had been mainstreamed into a normal second-grade classroom. He was *previously* diagnosed as autistic by the same diagnosticians using the same criteria employed for the other subjects. However, his parents had participated in an extensive parent-training treatment program in our laboratory when he was three years of age. Prior to treatment, his language consisted of moderately frequent immediate echolalia. At the time of the present tests, his receptive expressive language abilities and his academic skills were adequate for the second grade. His conversational speech, other than containing some confabulations, was normal.

Subject 6, a 13-year-old female, lived at home and attended regular seventh grade classes in junior high school. Similar to Subject 5, she was *previously* diagnosed as autistic by the same diagnosticians using the same criteria employed for the other subjects. Her parents had participated in an extensive parent-training treatment program in our laboratory beginning when she was five years of age. Prior to treatment, her language consisted of frequent immediate echolalia and perseveration of phrases and questions. At the time of the present tests she carried on normal (but excessive) conversational speech. She would talk on and on about topics of special interest to her (e.g., art and history).

Test Procedures

A battery of four audiological tests was administered to each child. The battery was composed of two monaural hearing tests and two dichotic tests designed to assess central auditory function. Supplementary measures of language and handedness were also taken.

Monaural hearing tests   Hearing for speech presented monaurally was assessed with *speech reception threshold* (SRT) tests and *word discrimination scores* (WDS) separately for each ear. Speech reception thresholds were established with the recorded CID W-1 spondaic word test using a descending method and 5 dB increments. Word discrimination scores were obtained with the recorded CID W-22 monosyllable word test (Lists 1D and 2D) presented at 40 dB above SRT.

Dichotic tests   Central auditory function for competing stimuli was assessed with the *Staggered Spondaic Word* (SSW) *Test* (List EC) and the *Competing Environmental Sound* (CES) *Test* (List E1) presented at 50 dB above SRT. (For a complete description of the SSW Test, the reader is referred to Brunt (1978) and Katz (1977a).) The raw SSW (R-SSW) scores were summed and converted to percent error scores for the right and left ear competing (C) and noncompeting (NC) conditions. The corrected SSW (C-SSW) scores and adjusted SSW (A-SSW) scores were calculated. Additionally, the results were analyzed for ear effect, order effect, reversals, and Type A pattern response biases (see Katz, 1977a). The CES scores (see Katz, 1976) were summed and converted to percent error scores for the right and left ear. The eight equations based on the SSW and CES test comparisons were calculated to suggest the hemisphere involved (Katz, 1976).

Audiological testing procedures   The SRT, WDS, SSW, and CES test stimuli were pre-recorded on commercially available tapes from Auditec of St. Louis. The tapes were presented by earphones

(Telephonics TDH-39) to each child via a high-quality tape player (Viking 433) and diagnostic audiometer (Maico MA-24) and were administered in a sound-treated booth (General Acoustics) meeting ANSI standards. Each testing session lasted between one and two hours, depending on the subject's cooperation. The training procedures and audiological test battery were completed in 1–4 sessions, depending on the subject's level of functioning.

SSW pretraining procedures   Because the severely autistic subjects were unable to follow the relatively lengthy pre-recorded instructions given to normal subjects, it was necessary to provide the following pre-training procedures in place of the instructions. These procedures were designed to accomplish the same end result as the pre-recorded instructions (i.e., to instruct the children to repeat groups of words). The procedures were based upon principles of shaping and stimulus fading as outlined by Lovaas, Schreibman, and Koegel (1974), Schreibman and Koegel (in press), Rincover and Koegel (1977), and Risley and Wolf (1967). Taking advantage of the subjects' echolalic speech, each subject was first asked (live voice) to repeat a one-spondee training item from the CID W-1 Spondaic Word list (i.e., spondees not contained on the SSW Test). Each item was preceded by the carrier phrase, "are you ready." The subject was praised for repeating the training item, and was told "no" for repeating the carrier phrase, or for failing to repeat all of the training item. After the subject would reliably repeat any one- or two-spondee training items, a fading procedure was implemented in order to transfer responding from live voice to the regular pre-recorded SSW training stimuli. The procedure involved beginning with the female experimenter's live voice, followed by the female experimenter's tape recorded voice, presented first in sound field and then binaurally over earphones. This was followed by a male experimenter's tape recorded voice presented binaurally over earphones, then the male pre-recorded voice on the regular SSW training items presented binaurally over headphones. This training procedure was terminated when the subject would repeat five consecutive two-spondee training items presented binaurally over headphones. At this point, the subjects would respond to the standard pre-recorded SSW practice items in the same manner as a person who followed the pre-recorded instructions. Therefore, it was possible to administer all 40 of the SSW Test items under standard conditions.

CES pretraining procedures.   The following pre-training procedure was used instead of the more complicated instructions on the pre-recorded CES tape. The subject was first shown pictures representing each sound from the CES tape, and asked to "point to (name of a sound)." Next, each test sound was presented (in sound field) and the subject was asked to "point to (sound)." The sounds from the CES training items were then presented binaurally over headphones, first one sound at a time and then two sounds sequentially, before the subject was asked to point to the pictures. Finally, the CES test itself was presented in the normal manner, with two competing sounds and the subject pointing to two pictures.

Measures of language comprehension   Two standardized receptive language tests were administered to provide a measure of each subject's language development. The *Carrow Test for Auditory Comprehension of Language* (TACL) was used to measure auditory comprehension of vocabulary, morphology, and syntactic structures (Carrow, 1973). The *Peabody Picture Vocabulary Test* (PPVT) was used to measure receptive vocabulary development (Dunn, 1959). Total raw scores and age-equivalency scores were attained for both tests. Additionally, the TACL raw scores were analyzed for vocabulary, morphology, and syntax subscores, as suggested by Carrow (1973), and percentages were calculated for each to permit relative comparisons.

Measures of handedness   Handedness was assessed using items from the Edinburgh Handedness Inventory (Oldfield, 1971) that were most appropriate for children: writing, drawing, throwing, scissors, comb, toothbrush, knife, spoon, hammer, and screwdriver. Each item was placed in front of the child (at midline), who was then instructed to demonstrate the use of each object. The hand used was recorded. For throwing, the child was instructed to throw a ball three times and the hand used more often was recorded. The number of items performed with each hand was summed and a laterality index was computed using the equation $R - L/R + L \times 100$, as suggested by Oldfield (1971). A positive index $(+1 \rightarrow 100\%)$ indicated the degree of right-handedness, and a negative index $(-1 \rightarrow 100\%)$ indicated the degree of left-handedness. A score near or equal to zero indicated no hand preference.

Experimental Design

Initially, the monaural hearing tests, the SSW Test, and the supplementary measures were administered to all six subjects. Subsequently, the SSW Test was readministered after an interval of 3–4 months to all subjects to check test–retest reliability. The CES Test was administered only once at about the time of the second SSW Test. In the case of Subject 4 (who received a year of language treatment), the SSW Test was administered a total of five times at 2–3 month intervals; twice within the first six months of treatment (Early Treatment), and three times within the last six months of treatment (Late Treatment) as a progress measure of central auditory function.

Reliability of Interpretation of SSW/CES Tests

The SSW and CES test results were analyzed and interpreted independently by Amy Wetherby and Jack Katz. In all instances the two scorers were in agreement as to the interpretation. However, for Subject 3, Katz suggested a more detailed interpretation (see results for Subject 3).

Results

Monaural Hearing Tests

The monaural hearing tests indicated normal hearing sensitivity for speech and word discrimination for all subjects. The poorest SRT obtained was 10 dB (range: 0–10 dB) and the poorest WDS was 96% from any subject.

Dichotic Tests

The results of the tests of central auditory function for dichotic stimuli are reported below for each subject. The test–retest results of the SSW Test were fairly consistent and stable for all subjects (except Subject 4, who received treatment). The reported response biases were the same from test to retest for all subjects, although the percent error scores varied slightly.

Subject 1: The test–retest results on the SSW and the CES scores for Subject 1 are shown at the top of Figure 1. On the SSW Test, Subject 1 demonstrated depressed scores (elevated percent errors) bilaterally, with a greater number of errors in the competing than in the noncompeting conditions. The C-SSW scores for test and retest were in the moderately depressed range and the A-SSW scores were in the mild range. Additional calculations (not shown in the figure) showed significant Ear High/Low (more errors on the items beginning in the right ear) and Order Low/High (more errors on the second spondee) response biases. CES scores were depressed in the right ear. These results are suggestive of a central auditory dysfunction in the posterior temporal region. The involvement may be in the auditory reception area of the left hemisphere, possibly extending deeply to the corpus callosum/anterior commissure. This diagnosis is consistent with the subject's severe language comprehension problem (see Table 1) and incessant echolalia (see subject description).

FIGURE 1. ━━━━━━━━━━━━━━━━━━━

Measures of central auditory function
SSW Test results for the echolalic subjects who did not receive
treatment during the study (Subjects 1, 2, and 3). Corrected SSW
percent error scores for the right- and left-ear competing (C) and
noncompeting (NC) conditions for test and retest. CES percent error
scores are shown for the right ear (RE) and left ear (LE).

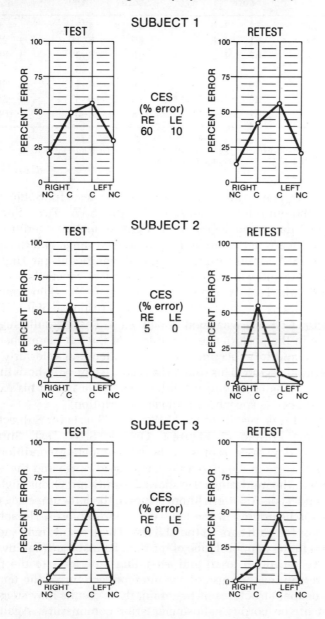

TABLE 1. ▅▅▅▅▅▅▅▅▅▅▅▅
Supplementary Measures of Language Comprehension and Handedness

Subject	Age	TACL		PPVT		Handedness
		Raw Language Score	Age	Raw Language Score	Age	
1	24	52	3–0	46	4–7	0%
2	18	61	3–8	60	6–10	+ 23%
3	14	67	4–1	59	6–8	+ 80%
4 early	8	*	*	25	2–9	*
late		59	3–6	48	4–11	+ 50%
5	8	96	6–11 + **	79	10–5	+ 38%
6	13	97	6–11 + **	118	18–0	+100%

* Score not available from early treatment
** The TACL is standardized for ages 3–0 to 6–11; a child older than 11 would be expected to achieve a score close to 101, as did Subjects 5 and 6.

Subject 2: The results of the SSW and CES tests for Subject 2 are shown in the middle of Figure 1. On the SSW Test, Subject 2 demonstrated depressed scores in the right-competing condition. The C-SSW scores were in the moderately depressed range and the A-SSW scores were in the mild range. He showed significant Ear High/Low, Order High/Low (more errors on the first spondee), reversals (change in word order), and Type A pattern (more errors in the right competing condition for items beginning in the right ear) response biases. Performance on the CES test was good in both ears. These results suggest a dysfunction in the posterior temporal lobe of the left hemisphere (not involving the auditory reception area) and extending anteriorly to the fronto-temporal region. This diagnosis is consistent with both the subject's level of language comprehension (see Table 1) and his extreme lack of spontaneous speech (see subject description).

Subject 3: The results of the SSW and CES tests for Subject 3 are shown at the bottom of Figure 1. On the SSW Test, Subject 3 demonstrated depressed scores in the left-competing condition. The C-SSW scores were in the moderately depressed range and the A-SSW scores were in the mild range. He showed significant Order High/Low, reversals, and Type A pattern (more errors in the left-competing condition for items beginning in the left ear) response biases. He achieved perfect scores for both ears on the CES test. These results may suggest a dysfunction in the temporal lobe of the right hemisphere (not involving the auditory reception area) and extending anteriorly to the fronto-temporal region; or, because of the interconnections of the temporal lobe with deeper structures of the brain, these results may suggest involvement of the corpus callosum/anterior commissure. Again, this diagnosis is consistent with both the subject's level of language comprehension (see Table 1) and his extreme lack of spontaneous speech (see subject description).

Subject 4: The results of the SSW and CES tests for Subject 4, who received treatment during this investigation, are shown in Figure 2. The first two tests, which were administered during early treatment (tests 1 and 2 shown at the top of Figure 2), showed depressed scores in the right competing condition, with some improvement from test 1 to test 2. (These depressed scores were far poorer than the normal children tested by White (1977), who showed errors up to 35% in the

FIGURE 2.
Measures of central auditory function
SSW Test results for Subject 4, who was assessed over a year of intensive treatment. Corrected SSW percent error scores for the right- and left-ear competing (C) and noncompeting (NC) conditions for test 1 and 2 during early treatment and tests 3, 4, and 5 during late treatment. CES percent error scores are shown for the right ear (RE) and left ear (LE).

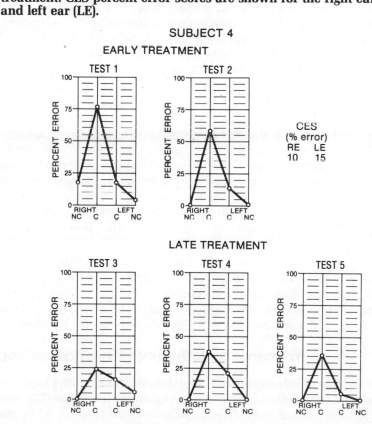

competing condition.) A depressed right ear score is atypical in children and may be suggestive of a problem in the posterior temporal region of the left hemisphere. He showed an Order High/Low response bias on the first two tests, which is commonly found even in children at this age, and may suggest that the anterior part of the brain is not yet fully matured in handling SSW material. During late treatment (when he showed considerable improvement in his functional language ability) he was tested three additional times (tests 3, 4, and 5 shown at the bottom of Figure 2). These tests showed improved central auditory function compared to the early-treatment period. The right-ear scores (the mean of the right competing and noncompeting scores) were well below the early-treatment level (from a right-ear score of 48 on test 1 to 18 on test 5), and there was no response bias on any of these three tests. The late treatment SSW results suggest a persisting but milder problem in the posterior left hemisphere and an improvement in anterior cerebral function. The results of the CES comparison with the SSW were consistent with a left hemisphere problem. The suggested improvement in posterior and anterior functioning might be seen as relating to Subject 4's improved verbal comprehension score (PPVT results) and improved spontaneous speech (see subject description). That is, he improved in only certain areas of language functioning, and is still functioning overall at a severely impaired level.

Subject 5: The results of the SSW and CES tests for Subject 5, who had completed extensive treatment in our laboratory (and who no longer evidenced language abnormality), are shown at the top of Figure 3. Subject 5 demonstrated a typical error pattern for an 8-year-old child with slightly depressed scores in the left competing condition. The A-SSW scores were within the normal range, by adult standards. He showed Order High/Low, reversals, and Type A pattern response biases, which are commonly shown in children and suggest that the fronto-temporal region has not yet fully matured. He achieved perfect scores on the CES Test, in additin to the normal SSW results. Thus, his central auditory diagnosis is consistent with his normal language behavior.

Subject 6: The results of the SSW and CES tests for Subject 6, who also received extensive treatment in our laboratory and who evidenced normal language function, are shown at the bottom of Figure 3. She demonstrated normal central auditory function by adult standards on the SSW Test, no response bias and perfect scores on the CES Test.

Measures of Language Comprehension

The wide range of language functions exhibited by these six subjects is portrayed in the results of the receptive language measures. The raw scores for the TACL and PPVT are given in Table 1, followed by the

FIGURE 3. ▬▬▬▬▬▬▬▬▬▬▬▬▬▬▬▬▬▬▬
Measures of central auditory function
SSW Test results for Subjects 5 and 6, who were previously echolalic
but had received early treatment and had normal language at the
time of these tests. Corrected SSW percent error scores for the right-
and left-ear competing (C) and noncompeting (NC) conditions for test
and retest. CES percent error scores are shown for the right ear (RE)
and left ear (LE).

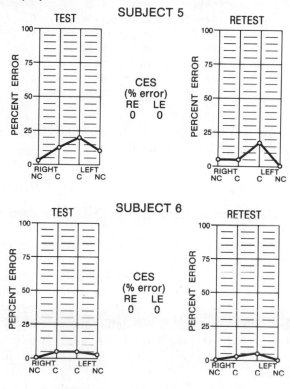

language age-equivalency scores. All subjects showed relatively better
performance on the PPVT compared to the TACL, probably because
the former assesses only vocabulary while the latter also tests syntax
and semantics. Analysis of the TACL raw scores, shown in Table 2, indicates relatively better vocabulary comprehension in comparison to
morphology and syntax for all subjects.

Measure of Handedness

The laterality indices computed for each subject are shown in Table 1.
The scores ranged from 0% (no hand preference) to +100% (right-
handed). Four of the six subjects demonstrated incomplete right-

TABLE 2.
TACL vocabulary, morphology and syntax subscores and percentages of total items answered correctly for that subscore.

Subject	Vocabulary Raw Score	Vocabulary Percent Correct	Morphology Raw Score	Morphology Percent Correct	Syntax Raw Score	Syntax Percent Correct
1	28	68%	20	41%	4	33%
2	34	82%	22	45%	5	41%
3	34	82%	26	54%	7	58%
4 late	30	73%	25	52%	4	33%
5	41	100%	46	95%	9	75%
6	40	97%	46	95%	11	91%

handedness, and one demonstrated a lack of hand preference. Only one demonstrated complete right-handedness.

Discussion

The major findings of this investigation may be summarized as follows:

1. Although all of the subjects had normal hearing on the monaural speech tests, there was reliable indication (from test to retest on the SSW test battery) of central auditory nervous system dysfunction in the language-dominant hemisphere inferred from the dichotic tests for those subjects displaying echolalia, and essentially normal dichotic test results for those subjects who were previously diagnosed autistic but were no longer echolalic.

2. The subject who received a year of intensive language treatment showed improvement in the dichotic test of central auditory function, which appeared to be consistent with the language improvement.

3. The locus of central auditory dysfunction inferred from the assessment measures was consistent with the language deficits for each subject.

Language Abilities and SSW Performance

These results show that performance on the SSW Test appears to be related to language ability. This is consistent with the fact that the performance of normal children improves with age and, thus, with language development, reflecting maturation of the anterior auditory processing area (White, 1977).

The errors made by our subjects were probably not a result of a general inability to take a test of this nature, because all of the subjects repeated two spondees in a binaural mode. For similar reasons, the poor test results probably do not reflect a short-term memory deficit. Rather, poor test performance seems more likely to have been due to cerebral immaturity (probably impaired development) or cerebral dysfunction of the auditory processing areas. These interpretations seem particularly likely in the subjects over 11 years of age (Subjects 1, 2, 3, and 6). Improvement in Subject 4's test performance may reflect cerebral maturation, or the effects of treatment on abnormal brain functioning, suggesting the possibility of an interaction of neural plasticity and treatment. Further support for such an interaction comes from the results of the two subjects (Subjects 5 and 6) evidencing normal central auditory function. These subjects were previously diagnosed as autistic by the same criteria as the other four subjects but had received early treatment and had essentially normal results.

Hemispheric Locus of Dysfunction

Of the other four subjects who evidenced central auditory dysfunction on the dichotic tests, their results were all associated with a disturbance at a locus involving one hemisphere or the corpus callosum/anterior commissure. These interpretations support the speculation that linguistic deficits associated with autism are related to an underlying neuropathology of the language-dominant hemisphere or a disruption in the development of cerebral lateralization. Furthermore, incomplete right-handedness was evident in most of the subjects. This may be a clinical indicator of early brain pathology. This lack of hand preference is consistent with large-scale studies of handedness in autistic children showing a higher frequency of non-righthandedness in autistics as compared to normals (Boucher, 1977; Colby & Parkinson, 1977).[1]

Analysis of the SSW and CES test results may indicate a left hemisphere dysfunction in Subjects 1, 2, and 4. Interpretation of these results as a dysfunction of the language-dominant hemisphere seems warranted in view of the receptive and expressive language deficits. It seems reasonable to assume from his SSW and CES test results that Subject 3 is right-dominant for language. His depressed scores in the left ear on the SSW Test suggest involvement of the right hemisphere.

---

[1] Degree of righthandedness may be influenced by early training in manual skills. For example, the parent of Subject 3 reported that as a young child, the boy preferred his left hand; however, at age 14, his laterality index was +80%.

The SSW Test (a verbal task) was moderately depressed in performance, while the CES Test (a nonverbal task) was performed without error. It therefore seems likely that the right hemisphere was impaired,
and that it was the language-dominant hemisphere for this subject. Additionally, comparing the results of Subjects 2 and 3 reveals that they
are very similar, except the depressed scores are in opposite ears. This
supports the contention that Subject 3's cerebral lateralization is the
reverse of that of Subject 2 and of the more common left lateralization
of language.

Intrahemispheric Locus of Dysfunction

Analysis of the SSW Test results indicates that the cortical dysfunction
is primarily in or near the region of the anterior motor speech area
(Broca's area) in Subjects 2 and 3, and in or near the region of the
posterior auditory association area (Wernicke's area) in Subjects 1 and
4. This is particularly interesting because the predominant
characteristic of both Subject 2 and Subject 3's language behavior is
paucity of spontaneous speech, which is consistent with disturbances
of expressive speech associated with anterior lesions acquired in
adulthood (Brown, 1972; Luria, 1966). In contrast, Subjects 1 and 4
showed a more severe language comprehension problem which is consistent with receptive language problems associated with posterior lesions, as their SSW results might imply (Brown, 1972; Luria, 1966). Furthermore, the lower frequency of echolalia in Subjects 2 and 3 is
similar to the nonfluent character of an aphasic with an anterior lesion,
while the higher frequency of echolalia in Subjects 1 and 4 resembles
the fluent nature of an aphasic with a posterior lesion.

The characterized dysfunction in the anterior versus posterior
region in these subjects shows a striking similarity to the transcortical
aphasias and other pathological conditions manifesting echolalia. As
described by Goldstein (1948), the transcortical aphasias are
characteristized by a preserved ability to repeat despite a loss of spontaneous speech (transcortical motor aphasia), or a severe comprehension problem (transcortical sensory aphasia), or both (mixed transcortical aphasia).

Outside of the autism literature, echolalia is a characteristic of
normal language acquisition as well as a multitude of childhood and
adult neuropathologies, including mental retardation, chronic epilepsy, senile dementia, transcortical aphasia, psychosis, and toxic
states (Whitaker, 1976; Brown, 1975; Quadfasel and Segarra, 1968;
Goldstein, 1948; Stengel, 1947, 1964; Schneider, 1938; Pick, 1924; Barr,
1898). The neurological substrata underlying echolalia have previously
been discussed as an isolation of the speech area in which Broca's and

Wernicke's area and the connecting pathways are at least partially intact and disconnected from higher cortical functions (Geschwind *et al.*, 1968; Goldstein, 1948).

The underlying mechanism of echolalia in autism similarly may be partial damage in the region of Broca's or Wernicke's area, leading to impaired development of higher cortical association areas. In contrast to damage incurred in an adult with a fully developed use of language, damage in early infancy prior to language acquisition has a disruptive effect upon the formation of neural systems underlying language (e.g., Luria, 1973). In children, complete development of higher cortical function is dependent upon the integrity of the lower areas. It is possible that dysfunction in brainstem nuclei, thalamic nuclei, and/or subcortical structures disrupts the development of higher cortical association areas. Therefore, our results are consistent with speculations that lower areas may be involved (Coleman, 1979; Damasio and Maurer, 1978; Ornitz, 1974). A further implication of this line of thought is that the concomitant effect of treatment and neurological maturation may be instrumental in the recovery process of autism, indicating that treatment intervention is most effective before completion of postnatal development of the brain (e.g., early treatment, such as that given to Subjects 5 and 6 in this investigation).

The SSW test battery appears to be sensitive to cerebral dysfunction in these echolalic autistic children. Our preliminary findings support the accumulating evidence of a neurogenic etiology of autism. Future research should be directed at validating the use of this test battery on a larger population of autistic subjects. Measures of central auditory function taken in conjunction with measures of auditory/vestibular brainstem nuclei and thalamic function may help to resolve the question of whether the cortical dysfunction is a primary etiology of the symptoms of autism or a secondary effect of underlying brainstem or thalamic dysfunction. Application of the SSW Test to differentiating subgroups of echolalic autistic children (i.e., anterior versus posterior) may lead to more effective language intervention procedures.

Given the preliminary state of the art pertaining to the identification of specific loci of dysfunction in autism, and the variety of specific theories regarding etiology, we realize our comments pertaining to locus of dysfunction may be seen as controversial by some. Our use of the SSW test battery was intended for research purposes, and interpretations of the test results presented in this paper are speculative in nature. Continued research in this direction, in conjunction with direct neurological measures may ultimately lead to the clinical application of these tests with autistic individuals. We hope that this investigation will serve as a stimulus for the systematic study of this area.

References

Applebaum, E., Egel, A. L., Koegel, R. L., and Imhoff, B. Measuring musical abilities of autistic children. *Journal of Autism and Developmental Disorders*, 9(3), 279–284 (1979).

Barr, M. W. Some notes on echolalia, with the report of an extraordinary case. *Journal of Nervous and Mental Disease*, 25, 20–30 (1898).

Blackstock, E. Cerebral asymmetry and the development of early infantile autism. *Journal of Autism and Childhood Schizophrenia*, 8, 339–353 (1978).

Bogen, J. The other side of the brain II: An appositional mind. *Bulletin of the Los Angeles Neurological Societies*, 34, 135–162 (1969).

Boucher, J. Hand preference in autistic children and their parents. *Journal of Autism and Childhood Schizophrenia*, 7, 177–187 (1977).

Brown, J. *Aphasia, Apraxia and Agnosia*. Springfield, Illinois: Charles C. Thomas (1972).

Brown, J. The problem of repetition: A study of "conduction" aphasia and the "isolation" syndrome. *Cortex*, 11, 37–52 (1975).

Brunt, M. The staggered spondaic word test. In J. Katz (ed.), *Handbook of Clinical Audiology*, 1st edition. Baltimore: Williams & Wilkins (1972).

Brunt, M. The staggered spondaic word test. In J. Katz (ed.), *Handbook of Clinical Audiology*, 2nd edition. Baltimore: Williams & Wilkins (1978).

Carrow, E. *Test for Auditory Comprehension of Language*, 5th edition. Austin: Learning Concepts (1973).

Colby, K., and Parkinson, C. Handedness in autistic children. *Journal of Autism and Childhood Schizophrenia*, 7, 3–9 (1977).

Coleman, M. Studies of the autistic syndromes. In R. Katzman (ed.), *Congenital and Acquired Cognitive Disorders*. New York: Raven Press (1979).

Damasio, A., and Maurer, R. A neurological model for childhood autism. *Archives of Neurology*, 35, 777–786 (1978).

Dunn, L. *Peabody Picture Vocabulary Test*. Circle Pines: American Guidance Services (1959).

Geschwind, N. The anatomical basis of hemispheric differences. In S. Dimond and J. Beaumont (eds.), *Hemispheric Function in the Human Brain*. New York: Halstead Press (1974).

Geschwind, N., Quadfasel, F., and Segarra, J. Isolation of the speech area. *Neuropsychologia*, 6, 327–340 (1968).

Goldstein, K. *Language and Language Disturbances*. New York: Grune & Stratton (1948).

Hauser, S., DeLong, G., and Rosman, N. Pneumographic findings in the infantile autism syndrome. *Brain*, 98, 667–688 (1975).

Hier, D., Lemay, M., and Rosenberger, P. Autism and unfavorable left-right asymmetries of the brain. *Journal of Autism and Developmental Disorders*, 9, 153–159 (1979).

Kanner, L. Autistic disturbances of affective contact. *Nervous Child*, 2, 217–250 (1943).

Katz, J. The SSW test: An interim report. *Journal of Speech and Hearing Disorders*, 33, 132–146 (1968).

Katz, J. *The Competing Environmental Sound Test Instructions*. St. Louis: Auditec (1976).

Katz, J. *The SSW Test Manual*, 2nd edition. St. Louis: Auditec (1977a).

Katz, J. The staggered spondaic word test. In R. Keith (ed.), *Central Auditory Dysfunction*. New York: Grune & Stratton (1977b).

Katz, J., Harder, B., and Lohnes, P. *Lead/Lag Analysis of SSW Test Items*. Paper presented at the American Speech and Hearing Association Convention, Chicago (1977).

Katz, J., and Illmer, R. Auditory perception in children with learning disabilities. In J. Katz (ed.), *Handbook of Clinical Audiology*, 1st edition. Baltimore: Williams & Wilkins (1972).

Kimura, D. The asymmetry of the human brain. *Scientific American*, 228, 70–78 (1973).

Krashen, S. Cerebral asymmetry. In H. Whitaker, and H. Whitaker (eds.), *Studies in Neurolinguistics*, Vol. 2. New York: Academic Press (1976).

Lockyer, L., and Rutter, M. A five to fifteen-year follow-up study of infantile psychosis: 4. Patterns of cognitive ability. *British Journal of Social and Clinical Psychology*, 9, 152–163 (1970).

Lovaas, O. I., Schreibman, L., and Koegel, R. L. A behavior modification approach to the treatment of autistic children. *Journal of Autism and Childhood Schizophrenia*, 4, 111–129 (1974).

Luria, A. *Higher Cortical Functions in Man*. New York: Basic Books (1966).

Luria, A. *The Working Brain*. New York: Basic Books (1973).

Moscovitch, M. The development of lateralization of language functions and its relation to cognitive and linguistic development: A review and some theoretical speculations. In S. Segalowitz and F. Gruber (eds.), *Language Development and Neurological Theory*. New York: Academic Press (1977).

Oldfield, R. The assessment and analysis of handedness: The Edinburgh inventory. *Neuropsychologia*, 9, 97–113 (1971).

Ornitz, E. Childhood autism: A review of the clinical and experimental literature. *California Medicine*, 118, 21–47 (1973).

Ornitz, E. The modulation of sensory input and motor output in autistic children. *Journal of Autism and Childhood Schizophrenia*, 4, 197–215 (1974).

Ornitz, E., and Ritvo, E. The syndrome of autism: A critical review. *The American Journal of Psychiatry*, 133, 609–621 (1976).

Penfield, W., and Roberts, L. *Speech and Brain Mechanisms*. New York: Atheneum (1966).

Pick, A. On the pathology of echographia. *Brain*, 47, 417–429 (1924).

Rincover, A., and Koegel, R. L. Classroom treatment of autistic children: II. Individualized instruction in a group. *Journal of Abnormal Child Psychology*, 5, 113–126 (1977).

Risley, T., and Wolf, M. Establishing functional speech in echolalic children. *Behavior Research and Therapy*, 5, 73–78 (1967).

Ritvo, E., and Freeman, B. National Society for Autistic Children definition of the syndrome of autism. *Journal of Autism and Childhood Schizophrenia*, 8, 162–167 (1978).

Rutter, M., and Bartak, L. Causes of infantile autism: Some considerations from recent research. *Journal of Autism and Childhood Schizophrenia*, 1, 20–32 (1971).

Schneider, D. The clinical syndromes of echolalia, echopraxia, grasping, and sucking. *Journal of Nervous and Mental Disease*, 88, 18–35; 200–216 (1938).

Schreibman, L., and Koegel, R. L. A guideline for planning behavior modification programs for autistic children. In S. Turner, K. Calhoun, and H. Adams (eds.), *Handbook of Clinical Behavior Therapy*, New York: John Wiley & Sons (in press).

Searleman, A. A review of right hemisphere linguistic capabilities. *Psychological Bulletin*, 84, 503–528 (1977).

Simon, N. Echolalic speech in childhood autism: Considerations of possible underlying loci of brain damage. *Archives of General Psychiatry*, 32, 1439–1446 (1975).

Stengel, E. A clinical and psychological study of echo-reactions. *Journal of Mental Science*, 93, 598–612 (1947).

Stengel, E. Speech disorders and mental disorders. In A. DeReuck and M. O'Connor (eds.), *Disorders of Language*. Boston: Little, Brown & Co. (1964).

Student, M. and Sohmer, H. Evidence from auditory nerve and brainstem evoked responses for an organic brain lesion in children with autistic traits. *Journal of Autism and Childhood Schizophrenia*, 8, 13–20 (1978).

Tanguay, P. Clinical and electrophysiological research. In E. Ritvo (ed.), *Autism: Diagnosis, Current Research and Management*. New York: Spectrum Publications (1976).

Whitaker, H. A case of isolation of the language function. In H. Whitaker and H. Whitaker (eds.), *Studies of Neurolinguistics*, Vol. 2. New York: Academic Press (1976).

White, E. Children's performance on the SSW test and Willeford battery: Interim clinical data. In R. Keith (ed.), *Central Auditory Dysfunction*. New York: Grune & Stratton (1977).

Acknowledgements

This research was supported by U.S. Public Health Service Research Grant No. MH 28210 from the National Institute of Mental Health and by U.S. Office of Education Research Grant No. G007802084 from the Bureau of Education for the Handicapped. The authors would like to extend special thanks to Dr. Jack Katz for interpretation of the SSW Test results and for his comments and review of the manuscript. We would also like to thank Dennis Arnst, Enoch Callaway, Janis Costello, Jeffrey Danhauer, Sanford Gerber, Diane Gilchrist, Monica Goller, Roberta Jackson, Jean Johnson, Jody Pyper, and A. Loes Schuler for their comments and review of the manuscript. Special thanks to Glen Dunlap, Andrew Egel, Julie Lozow, and Mary Ann Voorhis for assisting with the pretraining.

Related Readings

J. Katz and R. Illmer. Auditory perception in children with learning disabilities. *Handbook of Clinical Audiology*, 1st edition. Baltimore: Williams & Wilkins (1972), 540–563.

M. L. Pinheiro. Tests of central auditory function in children with learning disabilities. *Central Auditory Dysfunction*, R. Keith (ed.). New York: Grune & Stratton (1977), 223–256.

E. J. White. Children's performance on the SSW Test and Willeford battery: Interim clinical data. *Central Auditory Dysfunction*, R. Keith (ed.). New York: Grune & Stratton (1977), 319–340.

Use of the SSW and CES Tests with Children

Although the SSW Test has been normed for the age group between 10–60, the question remains, "But what about the older patient?" The first five articles in this section examine performance of older adults on the SSW Test. Balas was the first to consider the question, and current work is underway to extend the upper limits of the age range. It stands to reason that a test of central auditory function should be applicable to a population in which CANS dysfunction has been documented.

The next two papers relate SSW results to performance of adult aphasics and various measures used to identify that problem. More work of this type needs to be done.

The application of the SSW Test to measure or assess central auditory function in specific types of CANS disorders extends beyond the older adult. Researchers have used the SSW Test to determine CANS status in stutterers, chronic alcoholics, temporal lobe epilepsy, and multiple sclerosis. These articles and reports are included here to point up the need for continued cross-validation of the test with known problems affecting the CANS.

Finally, Brunt's use of the SSW Test (R-SSW) in the prediction of a hearing handicap is another recent contribution to the long line of research questions being considered throughout the country.

7

Use of the Staggered Spondaic Word Test With Adult Populations

Results of the Staggered Spondaic Word Test With an Old Age Population

Robert F. Balas, M.A.

Twenty young normal listeners, with a mean age of 20, and 20 elderly listeners, with a mean age of 69 and no marked deviation in auditory sensitivity or discrimination, were administered a competing message test. This "distorted speech" technique incorporated partially overlapping spondaic words and is known as the Staggered Spondaic Word (SSW) Test. The old age group had far more incorrect responses compared to the control group. Differences were most divergent in the competing conditions. The subjects 70 years of age or above differed significantly from subjects below 70 years of age. It appears that the total SSW score and/or the particular response pattern of an individual might reflect qualitative differences, which may eventually provide further insight concerning the locus and extent of central nervous system degeneration. Thus, these results tend to confirm the hypothesis upon which this test is based. Nevertheless, the results indicate that the SSW Test is not completely free from peripheral factors.

Master's thesis, Northern Illinois University, DeKalb, Illinois, 1962.

Effects of Age and Sex on Dichotic Listening: The SSW Test

Carolyn McCoy, Myrtice Butler, and Jan Broekhoff

Introduction

Studies on hearing sensitivity with aging have indicated since the early work of Bunch (1929) that hearing progressively diminishes with age, that the greatest loss occurs in high frequencies, that males have a greater loss than females, and that over age 65 (Sataloff and Menduke, 1957) hearing changes are relatively small (Glorig and Nixon, 1962; Hinchcliffe, 1959; Bunch et al, 1929). There are numerous structural and neurological changes that occur in the auditory system with age, including increased pigmentation, deposits within cells, nerve and cellular degeneration, and a buildup of bony cuffs at the basal end of the cochlea which cut off neural exits (Kronigsmark, 1969; Kirikae et al, Kromptic-Nemanic, 1969). These changes were reported to have more effect on speech discrimination than on pure-tone detection.

Since the early work by Bocca et al (1954; 1955) and by Calearo and Lazzaroni (1960) it has been found that pathology within the central auditory nervous system (CANS) can be detected by overloading. Overloading has included speech alterations through low- or high-pass frequency filtering, speed alterations of the signal, signal/noise alterations, or the addition of competing messages.

Journal of Auditory Research, 1977, 17, 263–268

Katz (1962) developed the Staggered Spondaic Word (SSW) Test, a dichotic test for the assessment of the CANS. The SSW tests R and L ear performance under two listening conditions and total dichotic listening. Therefore, scores may be obtained for conditions of R noncompeting, R competing, L noncompeting, L competing (ear effect) and for total dichotic listening.

Several studies have been conducted with the SSW. Katz (1962) reported the results of six case studies on individuals in the categories of normal, cerebral palsied, aged, sensorineural hearing loss, and conductive hearing loss. Katz found that Ss with CANS dysfunction had more difficulty with SSW but that all Ss exhibited some difficulties with competing messages. Balas (1965) indicated that minimal presentation level of the SSW was 30–40 db SL while Turner (1966) noted that the most reliable age range for the SSW was 12–50 yrs.

Brunt reported that the SSW appears to be "sensitive to CANS problems and is highly correlated to the middle posterior portions of the superior temporal gyrus" (in: Katz, 1972, p. 344). However, studies dealing with the aged suggest that using the SSW to differentiate CANS changes from an aging condition or aging changes may be extremely difficult.

Balas (1962) used the SSW to study age effect for two groups (14–28 yrs and 60–80 yrs) of 20 Ss each (18F and 2M in the younger group and 5F and 15 M in the older group). The results indicated (1) a significant difference between older and younger groups for SSW performances; (2) no significant difference between R and L ear per age group for SSW performance; and (3) a high correlation (.70) between age and SSW performances. The data from the older Ss were divided into five groups by the total number of response errors noted and their distribution across the four listening conditions of the SSW. A small but significant correlation of .38 was obtained for the above groups. Due to small sample size, generalizations were guarded.

It appears then that hearing changes occur with age, but that these changes may or may not impair auditory processing. It is the purpose of this paper to present a preliminary report of auditory processing in the aged of both sexes as measured by the SSW. This paper also intends to assess the performance of older males and females on the SSW when differences in pure-tone sensitivity are statistically eliminated.

Method

Subjects

These were randomly selected from a younger and older group so that 15 M and 15 F comprised each group. Mean age for Group I was 23 yrs, for Group II, 66 yrs. Pure-tone thresholds were obtained by the ASHA standard method, in the order: 1, 2, 4, 6, 8, 1, .5, .25 kc/s. Ear order per S was alternated unless an S indicated a "better" ear in which case that ear was always tested first.

Apparatus

For testing peripheral hearing and for obtaining SSW scores, a Grason-Stadler Model 162 speech audiometer was used, a Beltone Model CX-CW pure-tone audiometer, and an Ar-Tic Model 414 dual-channel tape recorder. Listening was by AP 20 earphones, Audiometry was done in an IAC hearing suite while the SSW was presented under earphones in a quiet room adjacent to the hearing suite.

Procedure

The SSW was presented at the MCL level for each ear. Ss were instructed to listen to the directions and to indicate when the taped male's voice reached MCL level. Once the MCL level for each ear was established, Ss were instructed to listen to the directions and to respond as directed. Forty items of the test were administered. Twenty words were initiated in the R ear and 20 in the L. The earphones were alternated with every other S so that the same word pairs would not be initiated in the R or L ear. All errors of addition, articulation, omission, reversals, and substitutions were then recorded.

To assess the effects of age for both sexes on dichotic listening at each ear, the SSW data were first analyzed by a two × two factorial analysis of variance. Prior to analysis, the SSW error percentages were transformed to arc sines. Since dichotic listening might be affected by hearing sensitivity, a further analysis was performed in which pure tone scores were used as a co-variate, thus in effect eliminating the influence of hearing sensitivity as measured by pure tones at the speech frequencies plus 4 kc/s. All effects were tested at the .05 level of significance.

Results

The results of the ANOVA at the R ear are in Table 1. The F-ratio for the main effect of age (29.78) indicated that older Ss performed significantly poorer than young Ss well beyond the .05 level. Males tended to perform significantly poorer than females. The significant age × sex interaction effect ($F - 10.01$), however, indicated that a large part of the differences could be accounted for by the poorer performances of the older males. Post-hoc analysis of the results revealed that the differences between young males and females, and between young and old females were not significant. The disordinal interaction is presented in Figure 1.

The results at the L ear were nearly identical to those at the R, although the *F* ratios for sex (4.27; *p* = .043) and age × sex (4.93; *p* = .030) were slightly lower.

The results of the Analysis of Covariance for the SSW at the R ear are reported in Table 2, first with pure-tone sensitivity at the speech frequencies as covariate, and next with the speech frequencies plus 4 kc/s controlled. Results indicated that when the pure tones at the speech frequencies were statistically controlled, the main effect of age and the age × sex interaction were reduced but were still significant at the .05 level. When 4 kc/s was included in the covariate, no significant main effect or interaction was present. The analysis at the L ear revealed a similar trend in performance. Here, control of the pure tones at the three speech frequencies as well as the addition of 4 kc/s eliminated all significant effects. These results indicated some asymmetry in ear performance.

FIGURE 1. ━━━━━━━━━━━━━━━━━━━━━━━━━━━━━
Mean SSW performance at the R ear by age and sex

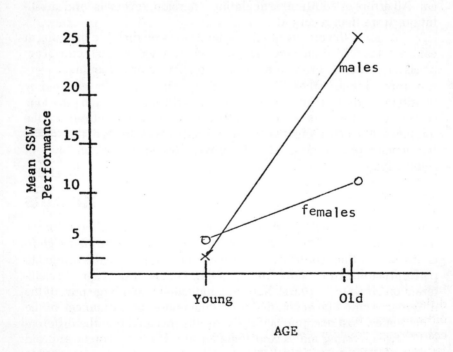

Use of the Staggered Spondaic Word Test with Adult Populations

TABLE 1. ▬▬▬▬▬▬
Analysis of Variance of SSW Scores for the R Ear

Source	SS	DF	MS	F	Probability
Age	2656.78	1	2656.78	29.78	0.000
Sex	648.52	1	648.52	7.27	0.009
Age × Sex	892.58	1	892.58	10.01	0.003
Error	4995.38	56			

Discussion

The results of the ANOVA indicated that the main effects of age and sex and the interaction effect were significant bilaterally. The main effects suggest that older Ss and males had more difficulty with dichotic listening tasks. The fact that older Ss had more difficulties is supported by the Balas (1962) study. Katz (1962) also noted that older Ss had difficulty with dichotic listening. However, post-hoc analysis of the interaction indicated that the differences noted could be accounted for by the poorer performances of the older males.

One possible reason for older male subjects having difficulties with dichotic listening may be the greater loss in hearing sensitivity that appears with advancing age in males (Corso, 1963). To test the effect of the peripheral ear on dichotic listening, an analysis of covariance was conducted to eliminate statistically the influence of the peripheral ear.

TABLE 2. ▬▬▬▬▬▬
Analysis of Covariance of SSW Scores for the R Ear

Source	SS	SS DF	MS	F	Probability
Three Frequencies					
Age	173.28	1	173.28	4.06	0.049
Sex	16.28	1	16.28	0.38	0.539
Age × Sex	229.52	1	229.52	5.38	0.024
Error	2346.35	55	42.66		
Four Frequencies					
Age	11.67	1	11.67	0.25	0.618
Sex	26.88	1	26.88	0.58	0.450
Age × Sex	90.94	1	90.94	1.95	0.168
Error	2558.49	55	46.52		

The results indicated that eliminating peripheral ear differences led to the elimination of differences on the SSW at the L ear for both three and four frequency covariate conditions and for the four frequency covariate condition at the R ear.

For the three frequency covariate condition at the R ear, the main effect of age and the age × sex interaction were reduced but still significant. Older males made more errors than any other group for dichotic listening when hearing sensitivity was controlled. However, the major finding was that controlling for differences in hearing sensitivity led to the elimination and/or reduction of differences in SSW performances. Therefore the pathological, biological, environmental problems, etc. that influence hearing sensitivity as measured by pure tones will influence performance on the SSW.

The results also indicated that a degree of ear asymmetry was present for the three frequency covariate condition where significant differences were noted at the R but not at the L ear. One possible explanation is that this study did not have any medical verification of CANS pathology. Another possibility for the asymmetry between ears for SSW performance may be hemispheric dominance for the interpretation of speech. Studies by Dirks (1964) and Kimura (1963) have shown a L hemispheric dominance for dichotic listening tasks and a R hemispheric dominance for tonal properties. Therefore, it is possible that the L hemisphere may be more sensitive to changes in the auditory pathway from the R ear even when the peripheral ear is statistically controlled.

Summary

Two age groups (mns = 23 and 66 yrs; 15 M and 15 F per group) were given the SSW Test to assess the effects of age in both sexes and the effects of the peripheral ear on dichotic listening for each ear as measured on the SSW. An ANOVA noted a significant different ($F<.05$) for the main effects of age, sex, and their interaction. Post-hoc analysis indicated that differences could be accounted for by the poorer performances by older males. The Analysis of Covariance revealed that statistically controlling the pure-tone sensitivity covariates eliminated differences for age and for sex on the SSW for the L ear and for the four frequencies (.5, 1, 2, 4 kc/s) covariate condition for the R ear. For the three frequencies (.5, 1, 2 kc/s) covariate condition, age and age × sex interaction were significant for the R ear. The results indicated that the peripheral ear does influence dichotic listening and that older Ss would perform comparably to younger Ss if the peripheral ear performances were equal. An asymmetry was noted, between ears, for the three-frequency condition. It was suggested that as well as peripheral ear influences, pathological and structural changes above the cochlea and L hemisphere sensitivity may be involved.

References

1. Balas, R. R. Results of the SSW Test with old age population. Unpubl. Master's thesis, Northern Illinois University, 1962.

2. Balas, R. R. and Simons, G.R. The articulation function of the Staggered Spondaic Word List for a normal hearing population. J. Aud. Res., 1965, 5, 285–289.

3. Berlin, C. I. and Low, S. S. Temporal and dichotic factors in central auditory testing. pp. 280–312 in: Katz, J. (Ed.) Handbook of Clinical Audiology. Baltimore: Williams & Wilkins, 1972.

4. Bocca, E., Calearo, C. and Cassinari, V. A new method for testing hearing in temporal lobe tumors. Acta Otolaryngol., 1954, 44, 219–221.

5. Bocca, E., Calearo, C. and Cassinari, V. Testing "cortical" hearing in temporal lobe tumors. Acta Otolaryngol., 1955, 45, 289–304.

6. Brunt, Michael A. The Staggered Spondaic Word Test. pp. 334–356 (see Ref. 3).

7. Bunch, C. C. Age variations in auditory acuity. Arch. Otolaryngol., 1929, 9, 625–636.

8. Calearo, C. and Lazzaroni, A. Speech intelligibility in relation to the speed of the message. Laryngoscope, 1960, 67, 410–419.

9. Corso, J. Age and sex differences in pure tone thresholds. Arch. Otolaryngol., 1963, 77, 385–405.

10. Dirks, D. Perception of dichotic and monaural verbal material and cerebral dominance for speech. Acta Otolaryngol., 1964, 58, 73–80.

11. Glorig, A. and Nixon, J. Hearing loss as a function of age. Laryngoscope, 1962, 72, 1596-1609.

12. Hinchcliffe, R. The thresholds of hearing as a function of age. Acustica, 1959, 9, 303–308.

13. Katz, J. The use of staggered spondaic words for assessing the integrity of the central auditory nervous system. J. Aud. Res., 1962, 2, 327–337.

14. Katz, J., Basel, R. A. and Smith, J. M. A Staggered Spondaic Word Test for detecting central auditory lesions. Ann. Otol., Rhinol., Laryngol., 1963, 72, 908–918.

15. Kimura, D. Cerebral dominance and the perception of verbal stimuli. Canad. J. Psychol., 1961, 15, 116–171.

16. Kirikae, I., Sato, T. and Shitara, T. A study of hearing in advanced age. Laryngoscope, 1964, 74, 205–220.

17. Konigsmark, B. W. Aging of cells and structures. Internat'l. Audiol., 1969, 0, 191–195.

18. Kromptic-Nemanic, J. Presbycusis, presystosis, and presbosomia as consequences of the analogous biological process. Acta Otolaryngol., 1969, 67, 217–223.

19. Kromptic-Nemanic, J. Presbycisus and retrocochlear structures. Internat'l. Audiol., 1969, 8, 211–220.

20. Sataloff, J. and Menduke, H. Presbycusis. Arch. Otolaryngol., 1957, 66, 271–274.

21. Turner, L. A. A normative study on the SSW Test for various age groups. Unpubl. Master's thesis, University of Kansas, 1966.

Abstract

Procedural Aspects of the SSW Test With a Geriatric Population

Lynn Price-McDonald, M.A.

The performance of a geriatric population was evaluated using the Staggered Spondaic Word Test presented at both the standard level and at a PB-max-based level. The purpose of the present study was to determine if the reliability of the SSW Test could be improved when used to assess central auditory system integrity of geriatric subjects.

The subjects were 20 individuals (11 male; 9 female) ranging in age from 60–81 years. The mean age for the group was 66.9 years. The subjects had no known history of CANS disorders or evidence of middle ear pathology, as measured by impedance audiometry. Pure-tone air conduction thresholds, speech reception thresholds, and performance intensity function for phonetically balanced words (PI–PB) were obtained for both ears of each subject. Mean hearing loss for the age groups 60–69, 70–79, and 80 and above is shown in Table 1. It should be noted that the 3-frequency pure-tone average does not reflect the high frequency hearing loss in most subjects.

The SSW Test was presented at the standard level of 50 dB-SL (re: 3-frequency PTA) and at the PB-max, as determined by the PI–PB function for each ear. R-SSW and C-SSW results were compared for both presentation levels (see Table 2 and 3).

Master's thesis, California State University, Fresno, 1979.

TABLE 1

Decade	N	3 Freq PTA (Range) RE	LE
6th	14	15.3 (0.40)	16.0 (0.35)
7th	5	25.0 (5.35)	28.0 (15.35)
8th	1	40.0	35.0

TABLE 2

Mean R-SSW Scores as Function of Age and Sex

	Standard			PB-max		
	M	**F**	**Both**	**M**	**F**	**Both**
60–64	9.67	2.30	4.78	15.30	3.30	7.33
65–69	27.30	2.00	17.20	25.30	3.00	16.40
70 and over	17.40	48.00	22.50	15.00	32.00	17.80
Total	18.00	7.33	13.20	17.90	6.44	12.70

The results of this study revealed that manipulation of the presentation level of the SSW Test did not significantly affect R-SSW scores. The use of a PB-max presentation level with a peripheral correction factor obtained from a PB-max word discrimination score did reduce variability of the C-SSW scores between subjects and possibly provided for a more consistent measure of the central auditory function of geriatric subjects.

In addition, the following observations were made:

1) Response bias was reduced at the PB-max level, perhaps due to the different presentation levels for each ear. Many times PB-max occurred at a different SL for each ear.
2) C-SSW scores increased as peripheral hearing loss increased despite the peripheral correction factor.
3) An ear laterality effect was found favoring the right ear. It was assumed that this effect was the result of the dominance of the contralateral pathway to the left hemisphere.
4) Female subjects performed consistently better than male subjects.

TABLE 3

Mean C-SSW Scores as Function of Age and Sex

	Standard Procedure			PB-max Procedure		
	M	**F**	**Both**	**M**	**F**	**Both**
60–64	−3.67	−1.17	−2.00	10.67	1.67	4.67
65–69	22.00	0	13.20	24.70	3.00	16.00
70 and over	6.60	38.00	11.83	8.00	24.00	10.67
Total	7.91	3.44	5.95	13.27	4.44	9.30

5) Performance appeared to be better on the second presentation of the test. (Presentation levels were counterbalanced.)

6) A slight tendency for performance to decrease with increasing age was noted. This relationship was not as marked as expected.

While interpretation of the results obtained on the SSW Test with geriatric subjects will provide an estimate of the subject's overall central auditory function, defining a geriatric "normal" range possibly using the PB-max procedure, may enable the clinician to differentiate central impairment due to normal aging processes from pathologic, nonpresbycuisic central disorders. It appears that the SSW Test has the potential to become an important tool in the evaluation of normal and non-normal central function in a geriatric population with further research.

The Staggered Spondaic Word Test: A Normative Investigation of Older Adults

James D. Amerman and Martha M. Parnell

The use of the Staggered Spondaic Word Test (SSW) J. Katz et al., J. Speech Hear. Disord. 33, 132–146, for measurement of central auditory ability in adults beyond the age of 60 years is presently limited by the lack of an adequate normtive data base by which to differentiate typical and atypical response patterns obtained from elderly subjects. To provide a description of SSW performances for older age groups, the SSW was administered to 41 subjects, ranging in age from 60 to 79 years. Average word discrimination scores for the experimental population were within normal limits. The subjects evidenced a decrease in response accuracy and an increase in response variability relative to previously reported SSW results obtained from younger subjects. Nonsignificant correlations between age and SSW scores suggest minimal change in those central auditory functions assessed by the SSW test for subjects between the ages of 60 and 79 years. The need for stricter control over cognitive awareness and capability in the design of experiments that involve elderly subjects is discussed.

Ear and Hearing, 1, 42–45, 1980.

According to a recent survey of clinical testing procedures (22), the Staggered Spondaic Word Test (SSW) (16) is one of the most frequently used tests of central auditory function and is used now by almost 40% more clinicians than in 1971. The SSW utilizes a competing message technique which is sufficiently demanding to detect the presence of central auditory dysfunction. The test is composed of 40 pairs of 2 spondaic words each recorded and presented contralaterally in overlapped fashion. Specifically, the second syllable of the first spondee is overlapped with the first syllable of the second spondee, resulting in the following 4 conditions: right noncompeting, right competing (R-C), left competing (L-C), and left noncompeting. The diagnostic value of the SSW test has been supported by numerous investigators (5, 15, 20).

To determine the validity and reliability of diagnostic evaluations using the SSW, a strong normative base is mandatory. Reliable performance data derived from all age groups would best ensure the accurate application of the SSW to the study of subtle auditory problems that may exist at the central level. The SSW test has been standardized on a substantial number of relatively young and middle aged (11 to 60) normal and pathological individuals. However, adequate normative data is not available for older adults. The only documented information regarding the performance of subjects beyond the age of 60 years was contributed by Balas (1) who found significantly higher raw SSW scores for his twenty 60- to 79-year-old subjects as compared to young subjects. Balas' work did not incorporate the correction factor that was subsequently developed to minimize the influence of peripheral hearing loss on SSW performance. Therefore, clinical application of his results is not advised.

Recent research has emphasized the role of central factors as significant determinants of the changes in language decoding behavior associated with the aging process (7, 12, and others). Alterations in the structural and functional integrity of the central nervous system have been well documented for the elderly population. For example, an increase in reaction time and brain wave pattern fluctuation (2, 7, 23), decrease in brain mass (4), a 20% blood supply reduction, and neuron depreciation (3) have been observed in elderly individuals. More specifically, degeneration of the auditory pathways and auditory cortex have been documented by Kirikae et al. (19). Additionally, diminution of auditory skills (9) and speech decoding deficits disproportionately greater than would be predicted from pure-tone configurations have been frequently observed (14). All of these anatomical and physiological changes may have an effect on central auditory interpretation.

Due to the increasingly frequent clinical use of the SSW test of central auditory ability, the lack of normative information concerning performance of individuals over 60 years of age on the SSW and the reported central neurological depreciation that derives as a result of the aging process prompted this investigation of individuals between 60 and 79 years of age.

Method

Subjects

The experimental population consisted of 41 subjects, ranging in age from 60 to 79 years. Twelve male and 10 female subjects comprised the 60- to 69-year-old group; 11 males and 8 females were included in the 70- to 79-year-old group. The subjects were selected on the basis of cognitive awareness; medical, speech, language, and hearing history; and native English language background. Their ability to maintain independent lifestyles did not suggest that the performance of these individuals on the experimental battery would reflect characteristics of mental confusion or senility. However, inclusion of older adults into an experimental design introduces the possibility of these additional confounding variables. To eliminate participation of subjects whose performance might reflect behavioral features of senile dementia or mental confusion, a 32-point questionnaire was designed as a screening instrument. This questionnaire was based on a previously reported mental test devised by Hodkinson (13). Questionnaire items required accurate description of time, place, occupational history, names or current and former U.S. presidents, recitation of the months of the year and numbers from 1 to 20 backwards and forwards, and similar responses. Scores of 30 correct or better were achieved by all subjects, a criterion which is more stringent than the minimum 25 of 34 score established by Hodkinson to differentiate senile dementia and mental confusion from normal cognitive behavior. No subjects were rejected on the basis of their mental test scores. Each subject demonstrated further evidence of mental and physical competence by transporting himself/herself to the experimental setting at the proper time and date. Subjects reported negative histories in regard to previous neurological disorders, hearing loss, ear disease, or speech and language therapy. None were receiving tranquilizing or depressing medication that might have altered their responses to the experimental tests.

Procedures

To obtain a more complete description of threshold sensitivity, pulse-tone, sweep frequency Bekesy audiometry rather than traditional methods of evaluation of pure-tone thresholds was used. The Bekesy tracings provided a means of detecting abrupt changes in threshold values occurring in the intervals between octave frequencies. None of the subjects in this investigation evidenced such changes. Broad-band masking (86 dB SPL) was applied to the nontest ear as a precautionary measure to increase economy of testing time in the event that these elderly subjects demonstrated a high incidence of sizable interaural sensitivity difference. Threshold measurements were obtained from the midpoint of the tracings. The pure-tone averages (PTA's) displayed in Table 1 are believed to suggest a degree of sensitivity poorer than thresholds yielded by traditional audiometric procedures. According to Martin (21), threshold decrements of as much as 10 dB may occur as a function of a central masking effect resulting from the 86 dB SPL masking applied to the nontest ear during Bekesy examination. Subsequent intrasubject comparisons using both Bekesy and traditional pure-tone audiometry for 10 of the subjects supported this contention.

Monitored live-voice presentations were utilized to determine Speech Reception Thresholds (SRT's) and word discrimination scores (W-22 lists; 40 dB above SRT) from right and left ears separately (refer to Table 1). This method of presentation was utilized to avoid potential difficulties posed by elderly subjects who might experience difficulty in responding to the relatively rapid pace of available recorded materials (8, 11). Subsequently, all subjects responded to the binaural competing and noncompeting verbal stimuli included in the the 40-item SSW, List EC. Subject instructions, presentation procedures, and method of analysis have been previously reported by Katz (16). In this investigation, subjects were randomly tested with regard to age and sex. Test instructions were presented by the same examiner.

Equipment and Setting

Pure-tone air condition thresholds were derived from Bekesy audiometry (Grason-Stadler model E800). A Maico model MA-24 dual-channel research and diagnostic audiometer was used to establish SRT's, word discrimation values, and subsequently for presentation of the SSW. A Sony model TC-660 dual-channel reel-to-reel tape recorder was used in conjunction with Telephonics stereophonic headphones (TDH-39; 10 ohm) for stimulus presentation in a sound-treated audiometric suite.

Results

Table 1 displays the mean PTA's, the SRT's, and word discrimination scores for right and left ears for each of the 4 subject groups. Minimal differences in SRT's were observed for the subject groups. Average

TABLE 1.

Age, right ear and left ear pure-tone averages [PTA (500, 1k, 2k Hz)], speech reception thresholds (SRT), and discrimination (percentage correct) values for male and female subjects for both decades [HL (1)].

Subjects	Age (yr) Mean	Age (yr) Range	SRT (RE)[a] (dB)	SRT (LE) (dB)	D(RE) (%)	D(LE) (%)	PTA (RE) (dB)	PTA (LE) (dB)
M (n = 12)	66.66	62–69	24	20	95	95.33	29	28
M (n = 11)	74.64	70–79	21	21	96	91.1	25	25
F (n = 10)	65.40	61–69	23	21	98	98.6	27	26
F (n = 8)	73.25	70–78	22	20	98	98	28	25

[a]RE, right ear; LE, left ear; D, discrimination.

group discrimination scores were within normal limits (8). However, percentages for both female groups were superior to those achieved by the male groups.

Raw and Corrected SSW Scores

Raw SSW scores are shown in Table 2. The only significant difference ($t = 2.253$; $p < 0.05$) in mean total raw error scores was found between males and females (age decades pooled). RC and LC condition values and ear score differences accounted for this significant sex effect. After the application of the correction factor (minus percentage of error for word discrimination) to the raw scores, the male-female differences for the competing and noncompeting conditions and for mean ear scores were reduced as revealed in Table 3. An ultimate nonsignificant difference in total corrected staggered spondaic word test (C-SSW) scores between sexes was obtained. The greater difficulty involved in responding to the overlapped quasisimultaneous words was reflected in the increase in error responses elicited by the competing conditions. This response behavior is consistent with previous findings for younger populations.

As shown in Table 4, 10 subjects (24%) and 4 subjects (10%), respectively, evidenced mildly and moderately abnormal scores, as interpreted with reference to the upper and lower limit standard for normal SSW performances given by Brunt (6). No subjects were categorized as severely abnormal based on overall performance. However, 2 subjects' scores (5%) for the left competing condition fell within the severely abnormal range. The 60- to 79-year-old subjects of this investigation showed a decrease in response accuracy and an increase in response variability when compared with the results of previous research involving subjects ranging in age from 14 to 61 years. The

TABLE 2. ▬▬
Male and female group mean error scores for total raw SSW, right ear, left ear, right noncompeting, RC, LC, and left noncompeting conditions

	Mean Error Scores for Raw SSW						
	Total SSW	**RE**[a]	**LE**	**RNC**	**RC**	**LC**	**LNC**
Male 60–69	11.10	13.23	9.06	5.83	20.63	14.38	3.75
Male 70–79	14.43	11.71	17.16	6.82	16.59	27.27	7.05
Female 60–69	5.38	6.00	4.75	4.25	7.75	7.75	1.75
Female 70–79	6.88	5.78	7.97	3.44	8.13	12.50	3.44
Males (age pooled)	12.79	12.47	13.11	6.33	18.61	20.82	5.40
Females (age pooled)	6.13	5.89	6.36	3.84	7.94	10.13	2.59
All subjects	9.45	9.18	9.74	5.09	13.27	15.48	4.00

[a]RE, right ear; LE, left ear; RNC, right noncompeting; LNC, left noncompeting.

studies cited by Brunt (6) (5, 10, 17, 18) show a range of total raw SSW percentage correct from 97.1 to 98.8%. The 90.6% mean raw correct value for this study fell approximately 7 percentage points below the lower limits of this range. Mean error C-SSW scores reported from

TABLE 3. ▬▬
Male and female group mean error scores for total corrected SSW, right ear, left ear, right noncompeting, RC, LC, and left noncompeting conditions

	Mean Error Score for Corrected SSW						
	Total SSW	**RE**[a]	**LE**	**RNC**	**RC**	**LC**	**LNC**
Males 60–69	6.35	8.33	4.38	1.04	15.63	9.25	−0.92
Male 70–79	7.97	7.71	7.84	2.82	12.59	18.36	−1.96
Female 60–69	3.68	3.64	3.35	2.25	5.75	6.35	0.35
Female 70–79	5.03	3.94	5.13	1.75	6.13	10.50	−1.75
Males (age pooled)	7.16	8.02	6.12	1.93	14.12	13.81	−1.44
Females (age pooled)	4.35	3.79	4.24	2.00	5.94	8.43	1.05
All subjects	5.76	5.90	5.17	1.97	10.02	11.12	−0.19

[a]RE, right ear; LE, left ear; RNC, right noncompeting; LNC, left noncompeting.

TABLE 4.

Number and percentage of subjects ($n = 41$) showing normal to severely abnormal test values on the C-SSW relative to the upper and lower limit standard scores given by Brunt (6).

Score	Normal	Mildly Abnormal	Moderately Abnormal	Severely Abnormal
Total	27 (66)[a]	10 (24)	4 (10)	0
RE[b]	33 (81)	5 (12)	2 (5)	1 (2)
LE	34 (83)	3 (7)	4 (10)	0
RNC	41 (100)	0	0	0
RC	31 (76)	7 (17)	2 (5)	1 (2)
LC	33 (81)	3 (7)	3 (7)	2 (5)
LNC	41 (100)	0	0	0

[a]Numbers in parentheses, percentage of subjects.

[b]RE, right ear; LE, left ear; R-NC, right noncompeting; LC, left noncompeting.

previous research ranged from −4.6 to 3.0 errors. A higher mean error score of 5.8 was found for C-SSW scores in this investigation. Also, a standard deviation of 6.03 observed for the older adults indicated greater response variability for this 60- to 79-year-old group than for the experimental populations previously mentioned by Brunt (6) (range of SD—1.5 to 4.97). The discrepancy between our data and those presented by Brunt was primarily a reflection of the high degree of variability exhibited by the male subjects, who evidenced standard deviations of 10.2 and 9.12 for the 60 to 69 and 70 to 79 age groups, respectively.

Correlations were computed to compare age and the following SSW performance values: total C-SSW score; corrected right and left ear scores; and RC and LC condition scores. The resulting coefficients indicated no significant relationship with increasing age and response accuracy. Our observations of a 60- to 79-year-old population suggest that the central auditory abilities assessed by the SSW competing message procedure may undergo relatively minimal change for this age bracket.

Discussion

The aging process must be clinically acknowledged when evaluating C-SSW values derived from older individuals. Characteristics of the SSW performances of these subjects may be determined not only by age-related changes in primary auditory areas, but may also reflect individual levels of cognitive awareness or mental confusion.

Depreciated levels of cognitive awareness and orientation related to neurological degenerative processes operative in older individuals must be carefully scrutinized. With further research effort, a correction factor for level of mental awareness might be realized and incorporated into the scoring procedure to differentiate this factor from auditory perceptual dysfunction.

The subjects in this investigation reported no undue difficulties in understanding speech in everyday situations. They generally evidenced no difficulty in understanding the examiner's questions, conversation, or test instructions. Their history and performance during the testing procedures indicated that these individuals were essentially "normal" communicators. However, the decreased accuracy and increased variability observed in their SSW scores relative to younger subjects strengthens the suggestion of Brunt (6) that ". . . although the SSW may prove useful in studying CANS changes with age . . . the question remains whether the SSW test would be able to differentiate CANS age changes from a centrally located lesion (pp.273–274)." At present, the authors concur with Brunt's admonition that abnormal SSW results for young children below 11 years of age or individuals over 60 years be interpreted cautiously.

The desirability of developing useful clinical procedures for the assessment of central auditory processing in the aged encourages attempts to compile a more extensive data base from elderly subjects drawn from a wider age range and from a variety of occupational and educational backgrounds. Information relative to test–retest reliability of the SSW for a comprehensive age range is desirable to establish more precisely the magnitude and signficance of SSW performance differences related to maturational and aging processes. Furthermore, description of performances of subjects who evidence varying degrees of cognitive awareness and varying types of CNS lesions would aid the primary goal of determination of an index for differentiation of normal from pathological central auditory conditions exhibited by persons in older age groups.

References

1. Balsa, R. R. 1962. Results of the staggered spondaic word test with an old age population. Unpublished masters thesis, Northern Illinois University.

2. Bauer, H. G. 1965. Measurements of brain wave period and auditory reaction time as related to advancing age. Electroenceph. Clin. Neurophysiol. 19, 318.

3. Bergman, M, 1977. Aging speech perception. Short course presented at the Annual Meeting of the American Speech and Hearing Association. Chicago, Illinois.

4. Bondareff, W. 1959. Morphology of the aging nervous systsem. in J. E. Birren, ed. Handbook of Aging and the Individual: Psychological and Biological Aspects. University of Chicago Press, Chicago.

5. Brunt, M. 1969. Auditory sequelae of diabetes. Doctoral dissertation, University of Kansas.

6. Brunt, M. A. 1978. The Staggered Spondaic Word Test. in J. Katz, ed. *Handbook of Clinical Audiology*. The Williams & Wilkins Co., Baltimore.

7. Feldman, R. M., and S. N. Reger. 1967. Relations among hearing, reaction time, and age. J. Speech Hear. Res. 10, 479–495.

8. Goetzinger, C. P. 1978. Word discrimination testing. in J. Katz, ed. *Handbook of Clinical Aduiology*. The Williams & Wilkins Co., Baltimore.

9. Goldman, R., M. M. Fristoe, and R. W. Woodcock. 1976. *The Goldman-Fristoe-Woodcock Auditory Skills Test Battery*. American Guidance Service, Inc., Circle Pines, MN.

10. Goldman, S., and J. Katz. 1965. A comparison of the performance of normal hearing subjects on the Staggered Spondaic Word Test given under four conditions: dichotic, diotic, monaural (dominant ear), and monaural (nondominant ear). Paper presented at the Annual Meeting of the American Speech and Hearing Association, Chicago.

11. Harris, J. D. 1965. Speech audiometry. in A. Glorig, ed. *Audiometry: Principles and Practices*. The Williams & Wilkins Co., Baltimore.

12. Hinchcliffe, R. 1962. The anatomical locus of presbycusis. J. Speech Hear. Disord. 27, 301–310.

13. Hodkinson, H. M. 1973. Mental impairment in the elderly. J. Roy. Coll. Phys. (Lond.) 7, 305–317.

14. Jerger, J. 1973. Audiological findings in aging. Adv. Oto-Rhino-Laryngol. 20, 115–124.

15. Jerger, J., and S. Jerger. 1976. Clinical validity of central auditory tests. J. Scand. Audiol. 4, 147–163.

16. Katz, J. 1968. The SSW test: an interim report. J. Speech Hear. Disord. 33, 132–146.

17. Katz, J., R. A. Basil, and J. M. Smith. 1963. A staggered spondaic word test for detecting central auditory lesions. Ann. Otol. 72, 908–917.

18. Katz, J., and P. Fishman. 1964. The use of the staggered spondaic word test as a means of detecting differences between age groups. Unpublished study.

19. Kirikae, I., T. Sato, and T. Shitara. 1964. A study of hearing in advanced age. Laryngoscope 74, 205–220.

20. Lynn, G., and J. Gilroy. 1972. Neuro-audiological abnormalities in patients with temporal lobe tumors. J. Neurol. Sci. 17, 167–184.

21. Martin, F. N. 1977. Clinical masking. in L. J. Bradford, ed. *An Audio Journal for Continuing Education*. Vol. 2, p. 7. Grune and Stratton, Inc., New York.

22. Martin, F. N., and N. K. Forbis. 1978. The present status of audiometric practice: a follow up study. Asha 20, 531–541.

23. Surwillo, W. W. 1963. The relation of simple response time to brain wave frequency and the effects of age. Electroenceph. Clin. Neurophysiol. 15, 105–114.

Acknowledgement

The authors wish to recognize the helpful consultation offered by J. Brad Allard, M.C.D., clinical audiologist, and Donald G. Williamson, associate professor, Area of Speech Pathology-Audiology, University of Missouri-Columbia.

Author's Note

Table 2 has been expanded to include the standard deviations for this data.

TABLE 2a.
Mean Error Scores for R-SSW

	Total-SSW	RE	LE	RNC	RC	LC	LNC
Male 60–69	11.10 (12.91)*	13.23 (17.77)	9.06 (8.74)	5.83 (11.35)	20.63 (27.70)	14.38 (14.35)	3.75 (4.00)
Male 70–79	14.43 (11.67)	11.71 (8.45)	17.16 (16.38)	6.83 (6.43)	16.59 (12.46)	27.27 (28.54)	7.05 (5.90)
Female 60–69	5.38 (4.17)	6.00 (4.52)	4.75 (4.07)	4.25 (3.14)	7.75 (7.21)	7.75 (6.82)	1.75 (2.37)
Female 70–79	6.88 (3.19)	5.78 (3.95)	7.97 (3.95	3.44 (2.97)	8.13 (5.47)	12.50 (6.12)	3.44 (2.65)
Males (age pooled)	12.79 (13.03)	12.47 (13.82)	13.11 (13.32)	6.33 (8.94)	18.61 (21.41)	20.82 (22.73)	5.40 (5.25)
Females (age pooled)	6.13 (3.74)	5.89 (4.15)	6.36 (4.23)	3.84 (3.20)	7.94 (6.32)	10.13 (6.78)	2.59 (2.57)
All Subjects	9.45	9.18	9.74	5.09	13.27	15.48	4.00

* Standard deviations
From: "The Staggered Spondaic Word Test: A Normative Investigation of Older Adults"

Performance of Older Adults on the SSW Test

Dennis James Arnst, Ph.D.

(Note: This paper was presented immediately following "SSW Test Results with Peripheral Hearing Loss" p. 287. Consequently, a separate introduction was not included.)

The SSW Test has been standardized on individuals between the ages of 10 and 60 years. Because a "central aging" effect has been shown with individuals over 60, the influence of age on a test for central function is of interest.

One hundred and fifty-six subjects were included in the present study and grouped by decade, as shown in Figure 1. The mean pure-tone audiogram for each decade is presented in Figure 2 and compared with the mean audiogram of the YNG bilateral cochlear hearing loss group described in the previous paper. (The data obtained from the YNG cochlears have been included for comparison purposes throughout this discussion.)

FIGURE 1.
Distribution of Subjects: Age

Decade	(N)	Mean Age (S.D.)
6th	67	64.0 (2.6)
7th	54	73.0 (2.5)
8th	35	83.9 (2.4)

Presented at the American Speech-Language-Hearing Association Convention, November 21–24, 1980

FIGURE 2.

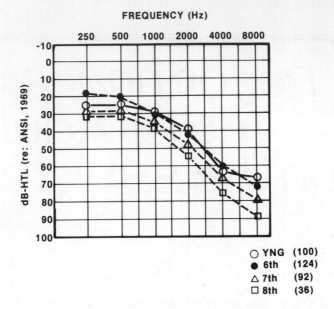

FREQUENCY (Hz)

○ YNG (100)
● 6th (124)
△ 7th (92)
□ 8th (36)

Mean audiometric data (Figure 3) clearly show the effects of age in this population. Note the increased 3- and 5-frequency averages. Also, note the similarities between the HL in YNG cochlears and the 60-year-old group. The difference between the 3- and 5-frequency average is similar across all decades, suggesting consistency in the slope of the threshold curve despite increased amount of HL occurring as age increases. Finally, note the increased errors which occur on the WDS as subjects get older. In short, the expected effects of presbycusis appear to be reflected in the audiometric data for the groups in this study.

The SSW Test was administered according to standard procedures and the results are shown in the comparative SSW-gram in Figure 4. Note that the R-SSW scores (represented by filled circles) increase, as do the C-SSW scores (represented by empty circles). Also note the increased separation between these scores as age increases. Remember that this separation is characteristic of cochlear type problems and the C-SSW reflects the status of central auditory function.

As for the response bias results, note that the ear effects REF versus LEF errors) were not significant in a majority of cases at all age levels. But, when it was significant, more errors were made when the word sequence was begun LEF. (See Figure 5.)

FIGURE 3.

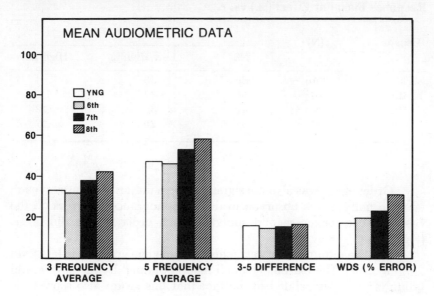

MEAN AUDIOMETRIC DATA

☐ YNG
▨ 6th
■ 7th
▨ 8th

3 FREQUENCY AVERAGE
5 FREQUENCY AVERAGE
3-5 DIFFERENCE
WDS (% ERROR)

FIGURE 4.

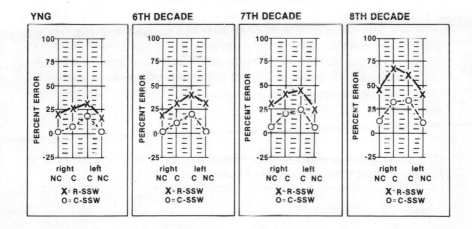

YNG | 6TH DECADE | 7TH DECADE | 8TH DECADE

PERCENT ERROR

right left
NC C C NC

X = R-SSW
O = C-SSW

FIGURE 5. ══════════════════════════════════════

Response Bias: Ear Effect (%) vs. Age

Decade	(N)	REF vs LEF		
		NS	Low/High	High/Low
YNG	(50)	58	38	4
6th	(67)	56	37	7
7th	(54)	49	39	12
8th	(35)	57	26	17

Order effect was also not significant in a majority of cases at each age. No pattern was observed in the preponderance of errors on the first spondee versus second spondee when order effects did occur (Figure 6).

The mean number of reversals for each age group was less than 2.0 (Figure 7). The extremely small mean obtained by the 80-year-old group is probably related to the fact that this group also scored the greatest number of errors and, consequently, reduced the probability of reversals occurring.

The percentage of each age group making more than four reversals is shown in Figure 8. In general, individuals changing the word sequence on more than four items has been shown by Katz and Pack (1975) to be associated with confirmed cortical dysfunction not involving Heschl's gyrus (i.e., NAR problems). It can be assumed that since reversals never occurred more than 10% in any age group, the type of cortical dysfunction suggested by reversals was not prevalent in the cochlear HL population. A more detailed analysis of response bias in older adults needs to be made, but will not be considered here. The question to be addressed then is, does the SSW Test reflect a central aging effect?

FIGURE 6. ══════════════════════════════════════

Response Bias: Order Effect (%) vs. Age

Decade	(N)	1st vs. 2nd Spondee		
		NS	Low/High	High/Low
YNG	(50)	62	12	26
6th	(67)	51	28	21
7th	(54)	43	33	24
8th	(35)	66	17	17

FIGURE 7.
Response Bias: Reversals (%) vs. Age

		Number of Reversals					
Decade	(N)	0	1	2-6	7-12	≥13	Mean
YNG	(50)	64	10	16	4	6	1.8
6th	(67)	63	19	13	3	2	1.1
7th	(54)	60	15	21	2	2	1.4
8th	(35)	94	6	0	0	0	0.2

In comparing raw and corrected SSW scores across age groups, it is apparent that both increase systematically with age (Figure 9). The Pearson product–moment correlation coefficient between the R-SSW and WDS error decreased with age. This change may have been due to the greater amount of HL in the older groups. Yet, a low correlation between C-SSW and WDS was maintained across all age groups. Therefore, the WDS-correction factor appears to be consistent at all age groups despite WDS-level.

The percentage of each age group obtaining a particular SSW category is shown in Figure 10. Note the increase in the *Moderate* and *Severe* categories as age increases. These categories are typically associated with higher level CANS dysfunction. A Chi-square analysis suggested a significant relationship exists between age and SSW category.

Because the C-SSW score reflects the status of the central auditory system and SSW category has been shown to increase with age, it is necessary to evaluate the concurrent influence of age and HL on the C-SSW score.

FIGURE 8.
Percentage of Subjects With More Than 4-Reversals

Group	(N)	%
Normal Hearing	(86)	2
Young Cochlears	(50)	10
6th Decade	(67)	7
7th Decade	(54)	6
8th Decade	(35)	0
* * *		
NAR (Katz & Pack, 1975	(17)	76

FIGURE 9.

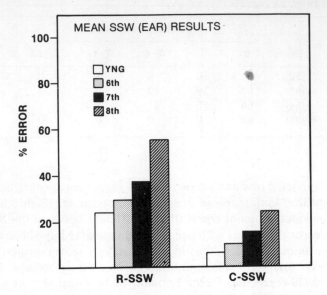

A two-way ANOVA and Duncan post-hoc test revealed the following: (1) C-SSW scores increased as a function of age; however, the YNG cochlears performed similarly to the 60-year-old group; (2) C-SSW scores in subjects with more than 40 dB HL were significantly greater at all ages than C-SSW scores in subjects with HL less than 40 dB; (3) interaction effects between age and HL were not significant.

The general implications of these results are shown in Figure 11. Note the slight upward slope of the curves between the YNG and 8th Decade data. Also, note the clustering of the curves above and below 40 dB HL.

FIGURE 10.
SSW Category (combined) vs. Age (%)

Group	(N)	SSW Category	
		N–O–Mi	Mo–S
Normal Hearing	(86)	100	0
Young Cochlears	(50)	76	24
6th Decade	(67)	72	28
7th Decade	(54)	50	50
8th Decade	(35)	26	74

FIGURE 11.

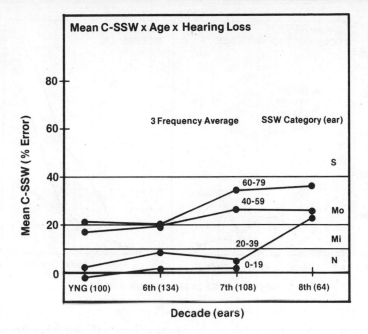

Decade (ears)

Both graphs in Figure 12 reflect the differences between the YNG cochlears and each of the older age groups as HL increases. The graph on the left plots the individual differences for each decade; the one on the right plots the cumulative effects of HL and age and the impact on C-SSW. Both demonstrate that

1. C-SSW differences for the 70-year-olds and 60-year-olds are similar up to 40–50 dB HL

2. Above 40–50 dB HL, the 70-year-olds behave more like the 80-year-olds

3. 80-year-olds are very different from all other data, no matter how much HL is involved.

In conclusion, it appears that the C-SSW score is influenced by age and may reflect a "central aging" effect that differs by decade. Sixty-year-olds appear to perform like YNG bilateral cochlears at all levels of HL. Therefore, the ceiling of the SSW might be raised to include all 60-year-olds. Secondly, 70-year-olds with HL up to 40 dB appear to show no difference from the 60-year-old group and may also be included in the upward extension of the age limit. However, C-SSW results for 70-year-olds with more than 40 dB HL need to be carefully

FIGURE 12. ═══════════════════════════════

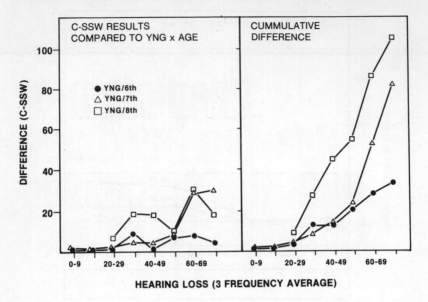

HEARING LOSS (3 FREQUENCY AVERAGE)

evaluated so that the influence of hearing loss will not be misrepresented. And finally, since 80-year-olds represent the oldest population studied and showed more hearing loss and the most desperate scores, interpretation of SSW results with this population is at best guarded.

Ultimately, the application of these results would be realized in a "central aging" correction that could be applied to C-SSW so that differential diagnostic use of the SSW would not be limited.

Prediction of Hearing Handicap With the Staggered Spondaic Word Test

Michael Brunt

Introduction and Review of the Literature

Fairbanks' Hearing Handicap Scale [HHS] (High, Fairbanks, and Glorig, 1964) has been used in many studies as a measure of self-assessment of communication problems arising from hearing loss (Speaks, Jerger, and Trammel, 1979; Schow and Tannahill, 1977; Mc-Cartney, Maurer, and Sorensen, 1976; Berkowitz and Hochberg, 1971; Blumenfeld, Bergman, and Milner, 1969). The results have been similar in all. Correlations have been larger for measures of sensitivity—speech reception threshold and pure-tone average—and smaller for measures of communication ability—speech discrimination. These findings suggested that a suprathreshold test sampling a greater proportion of the auditory system might be a better predictor of communication skills than speech discrimination.

A second consideration that initiated this study is the increasing proportion of the population who are elderly. Presently, there are 23 million individuals aged 65 years and older (U.S. Census, 1977).

ASHA Convention, Atlanta, Georgia, 1979.

Prevalence of hearing loss in the elderly is estimated at 231 per 1000 for ages 65 to 74, increasing to 399 per 1000 for the age group 75 and over (Metropolitan Life Insurance Company, 1976).

Presbycusis, or hearing loss in the elderly, has been described as a high-frequency, sensory-neural loss implying dysfunction at the cochlea and/or VIIIth nerve. However, research has shown that hearing problems in the elderly do *not* stop at the auditory nerve. Schuknecht (1955, 1967) and others have found changes in the auditory system from the cochlea to the auditory cortex (Brody, 1955; Hansen and Reske-Neilsen, 1965; Harbert, Young and Menduke, 1966; Kirikae, Sato, and Shitara, 1974). Behavioral tests of site of lesion have suggested auditory dysfunction of both the peripheral and central auditory systems (Konkle, Beasley, and Bess, 1977; Gang, 1976; Jerger and Jerger, 1975; Traynor, 1975; Proud, Dirks, and Embrey, 1961; Jerger, 1960, 1973; Jerger, Shedd, and Harford, 1959). Finally, additional factors related to auditory changes would be *nosoacusis* (disease) *socioacusis* (noise/everyday life) and noise-induced hearing loss. One implication of the above review is that the elderly are not a homogeneous group with respect to hearing and, perhaps, communication problems.

Katz' Staggered Spondaic Word (SSW) Test (Katz, 1968, 1977) was designed and has been found useful in detecting central auditory problems (Katz, 1962, 1968, 1977; Jerger and Jerger, 1975; Katz and Pack, 1975; Balas, 1971). In addition, this test is sensitive to problems in the cochlea and VIIIth nerve. Correlations with the CID W-22's of .86 and higher have been shown in individuals with peripheral loss (Katz, 1968, 1977; Katz and Pack, 1977). Therefore, the SSW is corrected for discrimination errors purported to be related to peripheral loss. Any remaining error is assumed to reflect central auditory nervous system dysfunction.

Since the SSW samples a greater proportion of the auditory system than routine speech discrimination tests, it might be a better predictor of communication skills in the elderly. The purpose of this study was to examine performance on the SSW as it relates to hearing handicap judged on the Hearing Handicap Scale. Results for pure-tone average, speech reception threshold, and speech discrimination were compared to the HHS as well.

Method

Subjects

Thirty subjects, 57–90 years of age, with a mean age of 71.8 years were evaluated. There were 14 males and 16 females. Individuals with a known history of central nervous system disorder were excluded as were those with a conductive loss.

Test Equipment and Materials

All hearing tests were done in an IAC sound booth meeting ANSI 1969 standards. Either a Grason-Stadler Model 1701 or a Maico 24B audiometer coupled with a Sony TC-366 tape recorder was used for test administration. Output was routed through TDH-49 earphones mounted in standard (MX-41/AR) cushions. All speech tests were given via tape recorded lists.

CID W-1 word lists were used for speech reception thresholds (SRT). CID W-22's served for measuring speech discrimination (WDS). The SSW Test, List EC, was used. The HHS was used to assess self-reported hearing handicap.

Procedure

Subjects initially were given the HHS. Following this, the pure tone, SRT, WDS, and SSW tests were administered, in that order.

Pure-tone air and bone conduction thresholds were obtained for 500 through 4000 Hz (Carhart and Jerger, 1959). SRT's were established using the Chaiklin-Ventry procedure (1964). WDS was assessed at 40 dB SL per ear re: SRT. The SSW Test was given at 50 dB SL per ear re: SRT (Katz, 1968, 1977).

Standard scoring was used for the pure tones, the SRT, and WDS. A PTA was computed also. The HHS was scored in percent (High, Fairbanks, and Glorig, 1964). The greater the percentage, the greater the perceived handicap.

The SSW allows for seven raw scores (R-SSW), each given in percent incorrect (Brunt, 1978). The seven scores were for the right noncompeting (R-NC) and competing (RC) words, left noncompeting (L-NC) and competing (LC) conditions, for the right ear (RE), left ear (LE), and for total raw score (Total). In this study the SSW Test was given to evaluate a large proportion of the auditory system. Therefore, no correction for speech discrimination errors was made.

Results and Discussion

The subjects did not evidence much hearing loss by pure tones. There was decreasing sensitivity toward the high frequencies. Any loss was sensory-neural in nature.

Table 1 presents ranges, means, and standard deviations for each ear for the PTA, SRT, and WDS. As expected, results for the PTA and SRT were quite similar.

TABLE 1.
Means and standard deviations for pure-tone average (PTA), speech reception threshold (SRT), and speech discrimination (WDS) for right and left ears

		dB HL PTA	dB HL SRT	% Correct WDS
Right	Mean	30.5	27.5	82.9
Ear	SD	11.7	11.7	16.3
Left	Mean	29.9	26.7	87.5
Ear	SD	12.7	13.4	12.2

TABLE 2.
Mean, standard deviation, and range for the Fairbanks Hearing Handicap Scale (HHS)

Mean	SD	Range
31.1	18.7	0–64

Scores on the HHS, as seen in Table 2, ranged from 0 to 64%, with a mean of approximately 31%. These results were compared to Schow and Tannahill's (1977) classification of hearing handicap on the HHS. The mean—31.1%—placed the group in the *slight handicap* category. Of the 30 subjects, 10 fell in the *no handicap* category (0–20%) and 10 in the *slight handicap* range (21–40%). The remaining 10 fell in the *mild-moderate* category (41–70%). In short, 20 of the 30 subjects demonstrated some handicap, at least as measured by the HHS.

TABLE 3.
Means and standard deviations for the R-SSW

	Right Noncompeting	Right Competing	Left Competing	Left Noncompeting
Mean	14.3	24.8	26.4	15.6
SD	13.8	16.9	19.4	16.6
	Right Ear	Total	Left Ear	
Mean	19.7	20.5	21.1	
SD	14.8	15.4	17.5	

TABLE 4. ━━━━━━━━━━━━━━━━━━━━━━━━━━━
Means and standard deviations for the better and poorer ear for the PTA, SRT, WDS, and SSW

		dB PTA	dB SRT	% WDS	% SSW
Better	Mean	27.4	23.3	88.9	16.6
Ear	SD	12.0	11.0	11.1	14.6
Poorer	Mean	33.1	30.8	81.1	24.3
Ear	SD	11.4	12.9	16.4	17.1

Table 3 presents the ranges, means and standard deviations on the seven raw percent error scores on the SSW Test. There were more errors on the competing (RC, LC) than on the noncompeting (R-NC, L-NC) words, a common pattern on the SSW.

In published studies HHS performance is usually related to the better ear. Table 4 shows results in that light for the PTA, SRT, WDS, and SSW.

Pearson product-moment correlations were computed between the HHS and PTA, SRT, WDS, and SSW for the better as well as the poorer ear. The sample comprised a relatively small N. Therefore, a significance level of .01 (28 df) was chosen to reduce the chances of making a Type I error; that is, assuming a significant correlation when there is none. Significant correlations can be noted from Table 5 for the SSW as well as the PTA and SRT for the better and poorer ears.

TABLE 5. ━━━━━━━━━━━━━━━━━━━━━━━━━━━
Correlations of the Hearing Handicap Scale (HHS) with PTA, SRT, WDS, and SSW for the better and poorer ears.

	dB HL PTA	dB HL SRT	% WDS	% SSW
Better Ear	.70[1]	.57[1]	−.46	.61[1]
Poorer Ear	.72[1]	.49[1]	−.40	.66[1]

[1]Significant at .01 (28 df)

TABLE 6. ▬▬▬▬▬▬▬▬▬▬▬▬▬▬▬▬▬▬▬
Correlations of the Hearing Handicap Scale with the R-SSW

Right Noncompeting	Right Competing	Left Competing	Left Noncompeting
.59[1]	.56[1]	.59[1]	.63[1]

Right Ear	Total	Left Ear
.62[1]	.66[1]	.63[1]

[1]Significant at .01 (28 df)

As noted previously, the SSW Test consists of seven possible raw error scores. All of these were correlated with the HHS. All correlations were significant (see Table 6).

These preliminary results on 30 subjects suggest that the SSW Test may be a viable predictor of hearing handicap in the elderly. Correlational data suggest that all seven raw SSW scores are approximately equivalent in their relationship to HHS.

Table 7 lists results of this study and others with correlations comparing the HHS to PTA and WDS relative to the better ear. Correlations generally are larger for the PTA and are similar to the correlation of .61 for the better ear relative to the SSW. Correlations with WDS are smaller. The present findings suggest that the SSW assesses the complexity of the auditory system in a more complete fashion than routine

TABLE 7. ▬▬▬▬▬▬▬▬▬▬▬▬▬▬▬▬▬▬▬
Correlations between the HHS, PTA, and WDS for various studies. (Results for the better ear.)

Study	Mean Age	PTA	WDS
High et al. (1964)	49.0	.65	−.15
Blumenfeld et al. (1969)	60–82	−	−.58
Speaks et al. (1970)	59.0	.72	−.29
Berkowitz and Hochberg (1971)	70.3	.57	−.30
McCartney et al. (1976)	74.0	.40	−.44
Schow and Tannahill (1977)	45.8	.73	−.20
Brunt (1979)	71.8	.70	−.46

tests of communication ability such as speech discrimination. Previously, this had been shown in the elderly by McCoy, Butler and Broekhoff (1977), Balas (1962), and Katz (1961). Furthermore, in this study there were significant correlations of the SSW with the HHS, while there was no correlation of either of these with WDS.

Summary

Preliminary findings suggest that the raw SSW test scores may be viable predictors of communication handicap in the elderly. Of the various SSW measures, perhaps the total raw score should be the score of choice as it represents the client's response to signals to both ears. Administration of the SSW may be a useful addition to a basic audiologic evaluation. It would serve as a measure of communication skill while having the advantage of providing information on the auditory system as well.

References

Balas, R. Staggered spondaic word test: Support. Annals of Otol. Rhino Laryngol., 80, 134–139 (1971)

Berkowitz, A. and Hochberg, I. Self-assessment of hearing handicap in the aged. Arch. Otolaryngol., 93: 25–28 (1971).

Blumenfeld et al. Speech discrimination in an aging population. J. Speech Hearing Res., 12: 210–217 (1969).

Brody, H. Organization of cerebral cortex: III. A study of aging in the human auditory cortex. J. Compar. Neurol., 102: 511–556 (1955).

Brunt, M. The staggered spondaic word test. In J. Katz (ed.) Handbook of Clinical Audiology, Baltimore: Williams and Wilkins (1978).

Carhart, R. and Jerger, J. F. Preferred method for clinical determination of pure-tone thresholds. J. Speech Hearing Dis., 24: 330–345 (1959).

Chaiklin, J. B. and Ventry, I. M. Spondee threshold measurement; a comparison of 2- and 5-dB methods. J. Speech Hearing Dis., 29: 47–59 (1964).

Goetzinger, C. et al. A study of hearing in advanced age. Arch. Otolaryngol., 72: 662–674 (1961).

Gang, R. The effects of age on the diagnostic utility of the rollover phenomenon. J. Speech Hearing Dis., 41: 63–69 (1976).

Harbert, F. et al. Audiologic findings in presbycusis. J. Aud. Res., 6: 297–312 (1966).

Hansen, C. and Reske-Nielsen, E. Pathological studies in presbycusis. Arch. Otolaryngol., 82: 115–132 (1965).

High, W. S. et al. Scale for self-assessment of hearing handicap. J. Speech Hearing Dis., 29: 215–230 (1964).

Jerger, J. Audiological findings in aging. Adv. Otorhinolaryngol., 20: 115–124 (1973).

Jerger, J. Bekesy audiometry in analysis of auditory disorders. J. Speech Hearing Res., 3: 275–287 (1960).

Jerger, J. and Jerger, S. Clinical validity of central auditory tests. Scand. Audiol. J., 4: 147–163 (1975).

Jerger, J., Shedd, J., and Harford, E. On the detection of extremely small changes of sound intensity. Arch. Otolaryngol., 69: 200–211 (1959).

Katz, J. The SSW test: An interim report. *J. Speech Hearing Dis.*, 33: 132–146 (1968).

Katz, J. The staggered spondaic word test. In R. Keith (ed.), *Central Auditory Dysfunction.* New York: Grune and Stratton (1977).

Katz, J. and Pack, T. New developments in differential diagnosis using the SSW test. In M. Sullivan (ed.), *Central Auditory Processing Disorders.* Lincoln: University of Nebraska Press (1975).

Kirikae, I., Sato, T., and Shitara, T. Study of hearing in advanced age. *Laryngoscope,* 74: 205–221 (1964).

Konkle *et al.* Intelligibility of time-altered speech in relation to chronological aging. *J. Speech Hearing Res.,* 20: 108–115 (1977).

McCartney *et al.* A comparison of the Hearing Handicap Scale and the Hearing Measurement Scale with standard audiometric measures on a geriatric population. *J. Aud. Res.,* 16: 51–58 (1976).

McCoy, C., Butler, M., and Broekhoff, J. Effects of age and sex in dichotic listening: The SSW Test. *J. Aud. Res.* 17: 263–268 (1977).

Metropolitan Life Insurance Company. Hearing Impairments in the United States. *Metropolitan Life Insurance Statistics,* 57: 7–9 (1976).

Schow, R. L. and Tannahill, J. C. Hearing handicap scores and categories for subjects with normal and impaired hearing sensitivity. *J. Amer. Aud. Soc.,* 3: 134–139 (1977).

Schuknecht, H. Presbycusis. *Laryngoscope,* 65: 402–419 (1955).

Schukneckt, H. Further observations on the pathology of presbycusis. *Arch. Otolaryngol.,* 80: 369–382 (1964).

Speaks, C. *et al.* Measurement of hearing handicap. *J. Speech Hearing Res.,* 13: 768–776 (1970).

Traynor, R. A method of audiological assessment for the non-ambulatory geriatric patient. Unpublished dissertation, University of Northern Colorado, Greeley, Colorado (1975).

U.S. Bureau of Census. Current Population Reports, Series P-25, No. 704. Projections of the population of the U.S.: 1977–2050. Washington, D.C.: U.S. Government Printing Office, July 1977.

A Study of Central Auditory Functioning in Adult Aphasics

Dorothy Haberkamp Air, Ph.D.

The purposes of this study were to determine whether adult aphasics perform differently than normals on a central auditory test battery comprised of both verbal and non-verbal stimuli, and whether aphasic performance on the central auditory test battery correlates with specific language functions as tested on an aphasia test.

Two groups of subjects, ten aphasics and ten normals, were selected for the study. The test battery administered to each subject consisted of the Staggered Spondaic Word Test (SSW), Competing Environmental Sounds Test (CES), and Assessment of Aphasia and Related Disorders.

The results of a t-test analysis indicated that aphasics performed significantly poorer than normals on the SSW Total score, all four SSW conditions, order effect bias, ear effect bias, and reversals. A significant difference was found between groups for mean CES performance and right ear performance. Further analysis of the data showed that four aphasics showed a left ear advantage on both the SSW and CES while two aphasics showed a right ear advantage on both tests. The remaining subjects showed a mixed advantage or no ear advantage. Normal subjects demonstrated no ear advantage or minimal differences between ears on the SSW and CES. Interpretation of the ear advantages demonstrated by the aphasics on both verbal and non-verbal stimuli lends support to the lesion effect theory which has been proposed in the literature, i.e. a degrading of the signal occurs regardless of whether the stimuli is verbal or non-verbal.

Pearson correlation results showed a number of significant relationships between central auditory processing performance of the aphasics and performance on the aphasia subtests. SSW right ear scores showed a significant correlation only with repetition of words, while left ear scores showed a number of correlations in the areas of naming ability, auditory comprehension, paraphasias, reading skills, and writing skills. Ear effect correlated with repetition tasks and verbal paraphasias. First word order effects showed a significant correlation

---

Reprinted from *Dissertation Abstracts International*, Volume 40, Number 7, 1980.

with repetition tasks, paraphasias and writing skills while second word order effects correlated only with repetition tasks. Reversal responses on the SSW correlated with general speech characteristics and auditory comprehension of complex materials. Pearson correlation results between CES performance and the aphasia subtests indicated a significant relationship between poor right ear performance and overall severity of aphasia, naming, oral reading, and paraphasias. Poor left ear performance correlated with auditory comprehension, paraphasias, reading, and writing. While a number of significant correlations were found between central auditory processing performance and specific language skills, caution should be exercised in interpreting these results because of the small number of subjects upon which it is based.

Localizing Lesions and Treatment Measurements of Aphasics by the SSW

Richard K. Peach and Glen M. Baquet

Introduction

The neuropsychological correlation between language performance and the circumscribed cortical centers which subserve language comprehension and production has long been integral to the study of aphasia. Beginning with the early localizationists, the determination of specific aphasic syndromes resultant from lesions to selected sites of the cortex has contributed significantly to a better understanding of the neurological processes underlying language. While language is contemporarily viewed as the product of several integrated functional systems, it is currently accepted that some language processes are more dependent than others on functions performed by particular cortical areas, and that aphasic symptoms are the result of selective impairment to one or another of these areas (Luria, 1966). Consequently, diagnosis of specific forms of aphasia has focused on this differential variation in language disturbance due to lesions in separate regions of the cortex.

While the nature of aphasic deficits has primarily been described in terms of linguistic parameters, the diagnostic categorization of aphasic subgroups has been diverse depending upon the testing instrument utilized. Emphasizing the relationship between cortical pathology

Presented to the American Speech-Language-Hearing Association Annual Convention, Atlanta, Georgia, 1979.

of selected areas and resultant language disturbance, the Boston Diagnostic Aphasia Examination (Goodglass and Kaplan, 1972) classifies aphasic syndromes according to site of cerebral lesion based upon characteristic patterns of performance on a variety of both linguistic and nonlinguistic tasks. Reexamination of response profiles on other testing instruments has recently been undertaken to further provide evidence for the localization of lesions (Porch, 1978). The clinical necessity for obtaining information concerning site of lesion and resultant types of aphasia is manifest in that it provides prognostic information for recovery of speech and language function (Kertesz and McCabe, 1977; Eisenson, 1964).

Specifying the site of lesion in aphasic patients is therefore an important aspect of treatment and it behooves the clinician to use localizing data from a variety of sources (Darley, 1972). In addition to the diagnostic instruments already discussed, valid means of securing localization information are often available in the patients' medical records. However, obtaining these records may sometimes be difficult, especially in clinics outside a medical environment, or they may not contain information concerning specific localizing procedures at all. It is also common that the patients' medical records are unavailable at the time of the speech and language evaluation. To alleviate this problem, it is suggested that significant information concerning determination of site of lesion can be contributed through use of the Staggered Spondaic Word (SSW) Test (Katz, 1962, 1968).

The SSW is a dichotic listening task which has been used and refined as a central auditory processing diagnostic tool. Considerations in the development of the SSW Test have included the effect of peripheral hearing loss, test–retest reliability, sensation level, intelligence, and simplicity (Brunt, 1978). The test was devised not only to detect central auditory disorders, but also to be free of contamination due to peripheral hearing loss. In addition, it requires little sophistication or training on the part of the person being tested and is applicable to a wide range of patients regardless of age, intelligence, or education.

Katz, Basil, and Smith (1963) and Katz and Pack (1975) have indicated that the SSW is most useful in detecting cortical auditory disorders, especially those of primary auditory reception. Interpretation of test results provide patterns of response which may be indicative of patients having central nervous system lesions affecting the areas of the sensory and mortor cortices around the Rolandic fissure or perhaps the anterior temporal lobe. The correlation between audiological tests, including the SSW, and hemispheric lesions has previously been demonstrated (Lynn, Benitez, Eisenbrey, Gilroy, and Wilner, 1972). Valid SSW test results have been reported when studying an aphasic population (Johnson and Katz, 1971).

The potential applicability of dichotic listening tasks in clinical management of aphasia, especially as a measurement of observable recovery, has also been proposed (Johnson, Sommers, and Weidner, 1977). Inasmuch as the SSW provides an index of central auditory processing skills, utilization of the test as an instrument to measure improvement in the auditory comprehension of aphasic patients following treatment appears to be a worthwhile application. Results of such measurements may contribute information to the intactness of the central auditory processing system of the aphasic patient or to the compensatory functions which the brain adopts in response to deficits in that system. Currently, instruments primarily designed to test auditory comprehension are limited, with the Token Test (DeRenzi and Vignolo, 1962), Supplementary PICA Testing (Berry, 1976), and the Revised Token Test (McNeil and Prescott, 1978) as the most prominent examples.

The purpose of the present study, therefore, was twofold: (1) to compare the SSW Test with the Boston Diagnostic Aphasia Examination to determine the applicability of the former test in supplying localizing data for cerebral site of lesion, and (2) to investigate the relationship between the measurement of auditory processing skills in an aphasic population by the SSW and the Boston Diagnostic Aphasia Examination.

Subject Selection

Ten adults, seven males and three females, with a mean age of 43.0 years (SD = 15.22 years), were included in this study. All subjects presented had a history of cerebral pathology due to one of the following etiologies: (1) cerebral vascular accident, either of thrombo-embolic or hemorrhagic origin, (2) arteriovenous malformation, (3) cerebral trauma, or (4) infectious disease. The mean months post onset for the group was 14.3 (SD = 18.46 months). Medical records were obtained either concurrent with or subsequent to testing of all subjects. All subjects were right handed previous to the cerebral insult and were monolingual, native speakers of English. All subjects had normal hearing sensitivity within 25 dB HTL and speech discrimination scores of no less than 30% in each ear.

From this group of subjects, a subgroup of five adults, consisting of five males, with a mean age of 46.6 years (SD = 14.26 years) was selected. All subjects in this group were receiving treatment for aphasia in the Speech and Hearing Center clinic and met all selection criteria as defined in the overall subject group. The mean months post onset for this group was 10 (SD = 10.53 months) at the initiation of therapy.

Procedure

All subjects received pure-tone audiometry (500 1K, 2K, and 4K Hz). Conductive involvement was ruled out either by pure-tone thresholds or impedance audiometry. Speech reception threshold and speech discrimination tests were obtained using monitored live voice. Following this procedure, the SSW was administered using the recommended clinical guidelines. The responses were scored and related to the established patterns of dysfunction for selected cerebral areas as described by Katz (1973). These seven areas represent general loci of cortical pathology within the frontal and temporal lobes and are not exact to the specific gyri or fasciculi within those major components. The correspondence between these areas as defined by the SSW and the specific cerebral sites involved in those regions are approximately as follows: 1 and 2—posterior aspect of superior temporal gyrus (primary and secondary auditory cortex), 3—posterior aspects of midregion from medial to superior frontal gyri (primary motor cortex), 4—posterior aspects of midregion from medial to inferior frontal gyri (primary motor cortex), 5—anterior aspects of superior and medial temporal gyri (tertiary cortex), 6—extensive region, including posterior inferior frontal gyrus (primary motor cortex), inferior portions of supplementary motor cortex, premotor area (secondary motor cortex) and complete overlap of area 5, and 7—entire frontal lobe with temporal area included in area 5 (see Appendix).

All subjects were also administered the Boston Diagnostic Aphasia Examination (Goodglass and Kaplan, 1972). Z-score profiles for aphasia subscores and rating scale profiles for speech characteristics were charted to determine the location of the causative site of lesion.

A dichotomous system of classification was used to compare the group results of the two testing instruments for determination of site of lesion due to the dissimilar distribution of areas for identification. All but one of the diagnostic categories of the Boston Diagnostic Aphasia Examination are characterized by lesions which are posterior to the Rolandic fissure, while the opposite is true for the SSW (emphasis on anterior lesions). Two common sites of identification between the instruments involve Broca's and Wernicke's areas. Therefore, the results were generally classified on an anterior–posterior basis to study the agreement between the tests along this dimension. Intraindividual results were subsequently compared to each other and to the medical records to evaluate agreement among the measures and to specify any instances where the agreement along the anterior–posterior dimension was not supported by the relative categorical areas indicated by the two tests.

In order to examine the feasibility of the SSW as an instrument to measure recovery in auditory processing skills, each patient who was selected for the subgroup of the study and enrolled in treatment received an administration of the test concurrent with other therapy measures previous to and following the treatment period. The results of the SSW administration were then paired with the patients' performance on the auditory comprehension subtests of the Boston Examination to obtain a measure of association between the two.

Results and Discussion

The localization data were organized in a fourfold table to test for significance of changes between anterior–posterior identification of lesions as indicated by the Boston and SSW tests. Due to the small expected frequencies, the probability for the observed frequencies at $\alpha =$ .05 was determined by binomial expansion. With $p < 2.5$, it was concluded that the two measures demonstrated no difference between them in the probability for identification of anterior versus posterior lesions.

Analysis of intraindividual results indicated consistency in identification of site of lesion for 80% of the cases studied. The greatest agreement between the two tests was found for lesions involving Wernicke's area of the temporal lobe, in which there was complete correspondence. This evidence is support for the premise that the SSW is ideally sensitive to disorders of central auditory processing. There was also good agreement for lesions involving Broca's area, in which a bimodal profile of SSW results were observed based upon severity of involvement. For those patients who showed mild aphasic symptoms (overall PICA $\geq$ 80%), identification of solely motor involvement was demonstrated. Patients who presented moderate aphasic symptoms (overall PICA $\leq$ 60%) were identified as having a lesion of the motor area as well as involvement of the auditory reception area. This effect was apparently due to either the patient's inability to phonemically encode the required response, which had been correctly comprehended auditorily, or to the more general involvement of auditory processing skills, which is concomitant with cerebral infarcts that are more massive than the circumscribed area of the inferior frontal convolution and extend posteriorly to involve additional areas.

The two cases of disagreement between the SSW and Boston Examination involved posterior lesions not including the auditory reception area. One patient presented primarily word finding and reading comprehension difficulties and was identified as having an anterior lesion of SSW area 7. While not corresponding to the lesion seemingly responsible for the presenting symptoms at the time of testing, it is suggested that such information be used as a basis for further investigating the patient's case history to determine if a previous cerebral insult had occurred and which, in some cases, may effect the diagnosis of the present characteristics. The second case exhibited a conduction aphasia as determined by the Boston Examination and was identified as having a lesion of SSW area 4. Inasmuch as repetition is a primary diagnostic characteristic of this type of aphasia, the identification of a lesion in the motor cortex with intact auditory comprehension is consistent with the presenting symptoms of conduction aphasia on an imitative task. Consideration of other phenomena—for example, literal and verbal paraphasia, which the SSW does not take into account—seem necessary in these cases to correctly identify the site of lesion.

The corrected scores from the administrations of the SSW and the raw scores of the Boston Diagnostic Aphasia Examination were converted to standard scores for the purpose of comparing the results of the two tests in terms of auditory processing skills (Table 1). The difference scores between the standardized measures following pre- and post-therapy testing were correlated to derive an estimation of the association between the two tests in demonstrating auditory processing recovery following treatment. The SSW was found to demonstrate a moderate correlation ($r_s = -.50$) with the auditory comprehension scores from the Boston Diagnostic Aphasia Examination. Perhaps one reason why a stronger correlation was not observed is that the SSW is not a measure of true language comprehension as is the Boston, requiring only the ability to perceive and make the phonetic associations inherent in the incoming stimuli before producing an auditory–verbal response. The small sample size was likely a contributing factor also in that a larger sample would more adequately represent the distribution

TABLE 1.
Comparison of standardized scores derived from Boston Diagnostic Aphasia Examination auditory comprehension scores and SSW corrected scores.

Subject	Type of Aphasia	Boston		SSW	
		Pre	Post	Pre	Post
1	Broca's	+0.75	+0.74	−0.41	−1.00
2	Anomic	+0.97	+1.00	−0.33	−0.06
3	Wernicke's	−1.36	+1.52	+0.27	+1.10
4	Conduction	+0.50	+0.71	+1.10	−0.97
5	Mixed	−0.08	+0.32	+1.56	+0.94

of scores which can be derived from the two tests and provide a better estimate of their association. However, it appears that the SSW may be sensitive to changes due to recovery in some aspects of communication which are not observed in receptive language testing due to their subtle nature. This was especially found to be the case in our patients who presented mildly to moderately involved comprehension abilities with Boston scores that demonstrated relatively little pre/post changes, but whose SSW scores reflected differences of a proportionately greater magnitude. As such, it appears that the SSW may contribute to the aphasiologists' diagnostic battery in further describing the nature of the aphasic patient's auditory deficits, that is, whether they are primarily perceptual or associative. Further research with the SSW in the aphasic population will be necessary in order to address these issues.

Certain limitations on the use of the SSW with an aphasic population were observed during the course of this study. Because of the expressive requirements of the response task, only patients who demonstrated an ability to repeat the spondaic words on several practice items could be included in the experiment. Development of a picture-pointing task to indicate the patient's responses could help to alleviate the difficulty imposed in the expressive response mode, but would negate those response errors which occur due to a phonological substitution in the imitative production of the auditory presented stimulus. Then again, phonological and semantic substitutions (literal and verbal paraphasias) are characteristic of certain types of aphsia and certainly confound the response profile obtained for these particular patients by SSW testing. Utilization is not recommended for testing with all aphasic patients, especially the severely involved (PICA < 30%) or easily frustrated, in which the appearance of a catastrophic response is probable.

Additional research appears warranted to study the relationship between the results of SSW testing and those obtained utilizing comprehension testing instruments of similar or different formats than that of the Boston Examination. When used in this way, a supplemental source for lesion localization or recovery of auditory processing skill measurement may be gained. With continued application, interpretation of test profiles may yield significant information to aid in diagnosis of aphasic patients.

References

Berry, Wm. Testing auditory comprehension in aphasia: Clinical alternatives to the Token Test. In Brookshire, R. H. (ed.). *Clinical Aphasiology: Proceedings of the Conference*, 1976. Minneapolis: BRK Publishers (1976).

Brunt, M. The Staggered Spondaic Word Test, in Katz, J. (2nd edition), *Handbook of Clinical Audiology*. Baltimore: Williams & Wilkins (1978).

Darley, F. The efficiacy of language rehabilitation in aphasia. *JSHD*, 37, 3–21, 1972.

DeRenzi, E. and Vignolo, L. A. The token test: a sensitive test to detect receptive disturbances in aphasia. *Brain*, 85, 665–678, 1962.

Eisenson, J. Aphasia: A point of view as to the nature of the disorder and factors that determine prognosis for recovery. *Int. J. Neurol.*, 4, 287–295, 1964.

Goodglass, H. and Kaplan, E. *The Assessment of Aphasia and Related Disorders*. Philadelphia: Lea and Febiger (1972).

Johnson, M. and Katz, J. Relationship between dichotic listening and language abilities of aphasic subjects. Paper presented at First Annual Conference on Clinical Aphasiology, Albuquerque, NM, 1971.

Johnson, J., Sommers, R., and Weidner, W. Dichotic ear preference in aphasia. *JHSR*, 20, 116–129, 1977.

Katz, J. The use of Staggered Spondaic Words for assessing the integrity of the central auditory nervous system. *J. Aud. Res.*, 2, 327–337, 1962.

Katz, J., Basil, R. A., and Smith, J. M. A staggered spondaic word test for detecting central auditory lesions. *Anals of Otol. Rhinol. Laryngol.*, 72, 908–918, 1963.

Katz, J. The SSW Test—An interim report. *J. Speech Hear. Disorders.*, 33, 132–146, 1968.

Katz, J. *The SSW Test Manual*. Auditec of St. Louis, Brentwood, MO, 1973.

Katz, J. and Pack, G. New developments in differential diagnosis using the SSW test. In Sullivan, M. (ed.), *Central Auditory Processing Disorders*. Omaha: University of Nebraska Press (1975).

Kertesz, A. and McCabe, P. Recovery patterns and prognosis in aphasia. *Brain*, 100, 1–18, 1977.

McNeil, M. and Prescott, T. *Revised Token Test*. Baltimore: University Park Press (1978).

Luria, A. R. *Higher Cortical Functions in Man*. New York: Basic Books (1966).

Lynn, G., Benitez, J., Eisenbrey, A., Gilroy, J., and Wilner, H. Neuro-audiological Correlates in Cerebral Hemisphere Lesions. *Audiology*, 11, 115–134, 1972.

Porch, B. E. *The Porch Index of Communicative Ability*. Palo Alto: Consulting Psychological Press (1967).

Porch, B. Profiles of aphasia: test interpretation regarding the localization of lesions. In R. H. Brookshire (ed.), *Clinical Aphasiology: Proceedings of the Conference, 1978*. Minneapolis: BRK Publishers (1978).

Appendix

SSW Response Bias

(adapted from Katz and Pack, 1975)

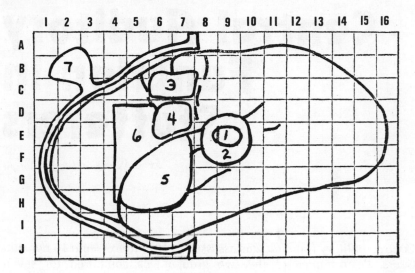

Central Auditory Function in Stutterers

James W. Hall and James Jerger

Central auditory function was assessed in 10 stutterers and 10 nonstutterers. Performance of the two groups was compared for seven
audiometric procedures including acoustic reflex threshold, acoustic
reflex amplitude function, performance intensity function for
monosyllabic phonetically balanced (PB) words, performance intensity
function for Synthetic Sentence Identification, Synthetic Sentence
Identification with Ipsilateral Competing Message, Synthetic Sentence
Identification with Contralateral Competing Message, and the Staggered Spondaic Word test. Relative to the control group, the performance of the stuttering group was depressed on three procedures—the
acoustic reflex amplitude function, Synthetic Identification with Ipsilateral Competing Message, and Staggered Spondaic Word test. As a
group, the stutterers presented evidence of a central auditory deficiency. The pattern of test results suggests a disorder at the brainstem
level. The subtlety of the deficiency is emphasized.

Perhaps as a result of advances in the sophistication of auditory
test procedures, central auditory function in stuttering has received
renewed attention during the past two decades. Rousey, Goetzinger,
and Dirks (1959) investigated sound localization abilities in 20 normal,
seven hemiplegic, 20 emotionally disturbed, and 20 stuttering children.

Journal of Speech and Hearing Research, 106, 224–29, 1980.

The stutterers, as a group, demonstrated a relatively poorer sound-localizing ability. Sound localization impairment may be a characteristic of temporal lobe auditory disorder (Sanchez Longo, Forster, and Auth, 1957; Jerger et al., 1969), although not invariably (Jerger, Lovering, and Wertz, 1972). Gregory (1964) administered tests of binaural loudness balance, median plane localization, and intelligibility of unaltered and distorted speech to a group of 30 stutterers and 10 nonstutterers. The groups performed comparably on the binaural loudness balance and median plane localization tests. A difference between groups on the speech intelligibility tests was not significant. Gregory concluded that his findings provided no evidence of a central auditory disorder in stutterers.

A major new approach to the old question of hemispheric dominance for speech in stutterers has been the use of dichotic listening tests. Curry and Gregory (1969) and Sommers, Brady, and Moore (1975), using meaningful words as stimuli, have reported that a significantly greater proportion of stutterers failed to demonstrate the expected right ear advantage (REA) in dichotic listening tasks than did nonstuttering control subjects. They conclude that stuttering may be related to the early Orton-Travis theory hypothesizing incomplete dominance for speech in stutterers (Orton, 1927; Travis, 1931). By contrast, Slorach and Noehr (1973), testing children with digits as stimuli, and Sussman and MacNeilage (1975), testing adults with consonant-vowel syllables, demonstrated that stutterers fell within the normal range for lateralization for speech, as indicated by the dichotic listening test. Results reported by Quinn (1972) assume an intermediate position on the issue of laterality for speech. Of Quinn's 60 stutterers, 20% demonstrated reverse dominance, that is, a left ear advantage. However, as a group, the stutterers were comparable to the control group in ear differences on the dichotic tests. Sommers, Brady, and Moore (1975), Moore (1976), and Moore and Lang (1977) offer some possible explanations for the disagreement in findings on dichotic listening tests. Moore (1976) points out that the amount of right ear advantage demonstrated is related to the nature of the dichotic verbal material (for example, syllables, digits, words). In those studies showing a reduced right ear advantage, or a left ear advantage (Curry and Gregory, 1969; Sommers, Brady and Moore, 1975; Quinn, 1972), meaningful linguistic stimuli were used. In addition, divergent results may, in part, be caused by a lack of homogeneity among stutterers (Sussman and MacNeilage, 1975). Although a group of stutterers may demonstrate relatively similar speech behavior, the bases for stuttering may, in fact, vary among them.

In addition to the dichotic studies, auditory processing abilities have also been recently assessed monotically (Manning and Rienche,

1976). Performance on auditory assembly tasks involving meaningful and nonmeaningful consonant-vowel-consonant syllables were found to be comparable for 30 stuttering and 30 nonstuttering children.

Finally, Toscher and Rupp (1975) administered portions of the central auditory test battery developed by Jerger (1973; 1975) to 14 stutterers and 14 nonstutterers. They reported statistically significant differences between groups on the Synthetic Sentence Identification Ipsilateral Competing Message (SSI–ICM) test. No ear differences, however, were noted among the stutterers.[1] Toscher and Rupp suggest that their findings might be "attributed to differences in neural function, neurophysiological organization, or the overall central auditory functions which are necessary to normal auditory processing and perception" (Toscher and Rupp, 1975).

Previous studies of central auditory function in stuttering have typically relied on a single type of test. The conclusions drawn from the dichotic-listening studies, for example, were based on the results of essentially one test paradigm. Recently, however, the value of administering a battery of audiologic tests has been stressed (Jerger, 1973; Jerger and Jerger, 1975a). The results of a single test measure may show considerable variability. Generally, positive results on a test will be obtained on a small proportion of patients having normal auditory function. Conversely, some patients with a definite auditory disorder may remain undetected even when assessed by a test sensitive to the disorder. This problem of false-alarms and false-negative findings weakens the power of single auditory tests. A battery of tests, however, permits comparison of the performance on several measures of auditory function.

This study assesses central auditory function in stutterers using a battery of clinically valid tests. The primary objective was to compare the relative pattern of test performance in stutterers to that of a control group of nonstutterers. A second objective was to compare the groups on the isolated results of each test measure.

Method

Subjects

The experimental group consisted of 10 stutterers. Nine were male, one was female. Their age range was 10 to 35 years, with a mean age of 23 years and four months. All stutterers wrote with their right hand. Degree of stuttering was distributed as follows: mild, one; mild to moderate, one; moderate, three; moderate to severe, two; and severe,

---

[1]M. M. Toscher, personal communication (1977).

three. The stutterers were diagnosed and classified by severity, independently by two speech-language pathologists. All stutterers had normal hearing based on (1) hearing threshold levels of 20 dB (re ANSI, 1969) or better at octave frequencies 250 Hz through 8000 Hz, and (2) normal findings on impedance audiometry. In no stutterer did the difference in hearing sensitivity between ears exceed 5 dB, as determined by pure-tone thresholds, thresholds for PB words, and thresholds for Synthetic Sentences.

The control group consisted of 10 persons with no apparent speech disorder, as determined by history and informal observations by a speech-language pathologist. Ten were male, one was female. The age range was 10 to 35 years, with a mean age of 23 years and six months. All wrote with their right hand. The control group was comparable to the stuttering group in educational background. All control subjects had normal hearing based on (1) hearing threshold levels of 25 dB or better at octave frequencies 250 Hz through 8000 Hz, and (2) normal findings on impedance audiometry. In no control did the difference in hearing sensitivity between ears exceed 10 dB, as determined by pure-tone thresholds and thresholds for PB words and Synthetic Sentences.

Test Battery

Seven audiometric test procedures were administered to all subjects. All of the procedures, with the exception of one, the amplitude function for the acoustic reflex, have been previously described in detail elsewhere (Katz, 1962; Jerger, 1973, 1974; Jerger and Jerger, 1975a, b).

Acoustic Reflex Threshold　　Contralaterally stimulated acoustic reflex thresholds were measured for broadband noise (BBN) and for pure tones at octave frequencies from 250 Hz through 4000 Hz. Ipsilaterally stimulated acoustic reflexes were measured for 1000 and 2000 Hz stimuli. Threshold levels were defined at the lowest hearing level (HL) in dB that produced reliable deflections of the balance meter.

In the contralateral mode, threshold levels were obtained when sound was presented to the ear opposite the ear containing the impedance bridge probe. In the ipsilateral mode, sound was presented and the acoustic reflex threshold measured in the ear containing the impedance bridge probe. The maximum intensity used to elicit reflex contractions in the contralateral and ipsilateral modes was 110-dB HL.

Acoustic Reflex Amplitude Function　　Using a 2000-Hz signal, the acoustic reflex threshold again was measured. Then, the signal intensity was increased in successive 5-dB increments to a maximum intensity of 110-dB HL. The signal duration was not fixed. Instead, the signal was presented for a time sufficient to allow the reflex to reach maximum amplitude. That is, an amplitude plateau was obtained for the reflex measurement at threshold and at each 5-dB increment greater than threshold. The reflex amplitudes at each intensity level were recorded on a strip chart for later analysis.

PI-PB Functions   Performance-intensity functions for monosyllabic (PB) word lists (PI–PB) were obtained by presenting blocks of 25 words at each of several suprathreshold levels. Generally, performance was defined from that intensity level yielding 0–20% correct up to a maximum speech intensity of 100-dB sound pressure level (SPL). White-noise masking was presented to the nontest ear whenever the speech level was sufficiently intense to cross over and be heard in the nontest ear.

PI-SSI Functions   Performance-intensity functions for Synthetic Sentences (PI-SSI) (Jerger, Speaks, and Trammell, 1968) were constructed by presenting lists of 10 sentences at each of several suprathreshold levels. As with the PI-PB functions, performance was defined from that intensity level yielding 0–20% correct up to a maximum speech intensity of 100-dB SPL. The SSI task was made more difficult by a competing speech message. Masking noise, again, was presented to the nontest ear whenever the speech level was sufficiently intense to cross over and be heard in the nontest ear.

SSI-ICM and SSI–CCM   Sentences were presented at an intensity level of 30-dB HL. Performance was measured at several message-to-competition ratios (MCRs) for both an ipsilateral competing message (ICM) and a contralateral competing message (CCM).

Staggered Spondaic Word (SSW) Test   The SSW test (Katz, 1962) was composed of 40 pairs of partially overlapping spondaic words. The presentation level was always 40-dB HL. The percentage of correct scores for the leading, competing, and lagging conditions was obtained. The average percentage of correct scores for each ear in the competing condition was compared.

Instrumentation and Test Materials

Pure-tone and speech audiometry were carried out on a specially constructed audiometer. During pure-tone and speech testing, the subjects were seated in a double-walled, sound-treated booth. Impedance audiometry was carried out with a clinical impedance audiometer. Acoustic reflex measurements used in the amplitude function analysis were written out on a single-channel strip-chart recorder.

Procedure

All subjects were tested in a single session of one to one-and-a-half hours' duration. The entire test battery was administered to each subject in the following order: impedance audiometry, including reflex thresholds and amplitude functions, pure-tone audiometry, PI–PB functions, SSW test, PI–SSI functions, SSI–CCM, and SSI–ICM. Equipment was calibrated biologically before testing. Earphones were reversed on alternate subjects to counterbalance any possible channel effects.

Results

Pure-Tone Sensitivity

Relatively normal peripheral auditory sensitivity is an essential prerequisite for the valid administration of the central test battery (Jerger and Jerger, 1975a). The presence of a slight asymmetry between ears, or a decrease in pure-tone sensitivity on both ears, however, has been described as a possible component of brainstem auditory disorders. Gravendeel (1958) noted a low-frequency loss in patients with brainstem disorder. He was unable to account for the loss on the basis of a peripheral auditory disorder. Jerger and Jerger (1974) reported mild high-frequency hearing impairment in eight out of 16 patients with intraaxial brainstem disorders. However, generally there was no sensitivity difference between ears. When an asymmetry was present, it was not reliably related to the lateral site of the brainstem disorder (Jerger and Jerger, 1974).

All subjects in the present study had, by criteria for inclusion in the study, hearing threshold levels equal to or better than 25 dB at octave intervals from 250 Hz through 8000 Hz. There was no difference in pure-tone sensitivity between groups for either ear. Also, the averaged pure-tone audiograms for the two ears were symmetrical for both groups.

Acoustic Reflex Thresholds

Acoustic reflex threshold abnormalities have been reported in patients with brainstem disorders (Griesen and Rasmussen, 1970; Jerger, 1973; Liden and Korsan-Bengsten, 1973; Jerger and Jerger, 1975a, b, c). When the acoustic reflex pathways are affected, acoustic reflexes are elevated or absent to contralateral stimulation, but present at normal levels to ipsilateral stimulation (Griesen and Rasmussen, 1970; Jerger, 1975; Jerger, Neely, and Jerger, 1975).

In this study, both contralateral and ipsilateral acoustic reflexes were present at normal levels in all stutterers and nonstutterers. The average SPARs (Sensitivity Prediction by Acoustic Reflex) (Jerger and Jerger, 1974) for the right and left ears for both groups were comparable.

Acoustic Reflex Amplitude Functions

Acoustic reflex amplitude curves, relating the change in acoustic reflex amplitude to a uniform increase in the intensity of the stimulus, have been studied by several investigators. Djupesland, Flottorp, and Winther (1967), Beedle (1970), Peterson and Liden (1972), and Jerger, Maudlin, and Lewis (1977) have all reported a progressively greater magnitude of reflex responses with an increase in contralateral acoustic stimulation with pure tones. Beedle (1970) and Peterson and Liden (1972) found a flattened reflex growth pattern in sensorineural ears when compared to normal ears. Peterson and Liden (1972) also noted a substantially flattened amplitude function for a patient with a corpus callosum lesion. In this patient, the reflex amplitudes did not equal those of the normal or sensorineural ears at any sensation level tested. The authors point out the possible diagnostic value of amplitude functions in patients with neurological disorders.

Acoustic reflex amplitudes in patients with brainstem disorder have been studied by Bosatra, Russolo, and Poli (1976). Using a 1000-Hz signal, these investigators found that acoustic reflex amplitudes were reduced in patients with pathologic lesions affecting the acoustic reflex arc. Their results also confirmed Borg's (1973) finding that the acoustic reflex threshold is often normal in brainstem dysfunction. In animal studies, considerably flattened amplitude functions have resulted from disruptions in the central acoustic reflex pathways at the brainstem level (Borg, 1973).

Figure 1 shows contralateral acoustic reflex amplitude functions for both ears of each group. The sensation level of the 2000-Hz signal increases above the acoustic reflex threshold in 5-dB steps to a maximum signal intensity of 110-dB HL. The amplitude of the acoustic reflex is shown as a percentage of the amplitude obtained for the control group at the maximum intensity level. The slope of the amplitude function is consistently more gradual for the stuttering group. At every sensation level above acoustic reflex, the amplitude for the stuttering group is smaller than that for the control group.

FIGURE 1.

Comparison of contralateral acoustic reflex amplitude functions for stuttering and control groups. The amplitude at each sensation level above acoustic reflex threshold is plotted as a percentage of the maximum amplitude for the control group. Key: **the open symbols are the control group, the black symbols represent the stutterers. Circles denote right ear; squares denote left ear.**

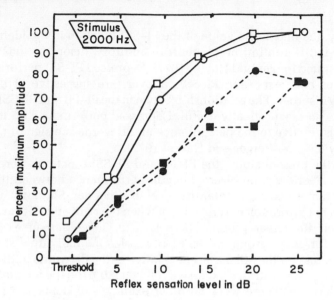

PI-PB

Depressed maximum speech intelligibility for PB words (PB max) is characteristic of some patients with brainstem disorders (Jerger, 1973; Jerger and Jerger, 1974; 1975a, b, c). According to these researchers, the interear comparison of full PI–PB functions is of more diagnostic value than a comparison of the PB scores obtained at a single intensity level. A mild loss in both ears, but greater in the ear contralateral to the site of the disorder, is considered a positive central auditory finding. Excessive PI–PB rollover is a common finding in patients with central auditory disorder (Jerger, 1973; Jerger and Jerger, 1974; 1975 a, b, c). Rollover is excessive if the performance decreases by greater than 20% at intensity levels above the level of maximum intelligibility.

In both the stuttering and control groups in this study, the percentage of correct scores readily increased to the 80%–90% range as the intensity reached 20-dB HL. An accurate level of performance (92%–100%) was then maintained from 40-dB HL to the maximum intensity level, 80-dB HL, for both groups. There was no ear difference in the performance of either group. Similarly, there was no evidence of the rollover phenomenon. When considered individually, none of the stutterers demonstrated a consistent ear difference on PI–PB functions; nor was there any individual case of excessive rollover.

PI-SSI

Recently, the diagnostic value of the PI–SSI function in the identification and differentiation of central auditory disorders has been demonstrated (Jerger and Hayes, 1977). Depressed PI–SSI performance in one or both ears, and PI–SSI rollover, are suggestive of central auditory disorder. The relationship between the PI–PB and PI–SSI functions is also diagnostically useful. Depressed performance on the SSI materials relative to the performance on PB words is a sign of central auditory disorder (Jerger and Hayes, 1977).

In the present study, the PI–PB and PI–SSI functions were comparable. There was no discrepancy in performance between the PBs and SSI materials at any intensity level in either ear. Similarly, no differences in performance were evident when the right and left ears were compared for either group. There was no suggestion of excessive rollover for either group on the PI–SSI task. One individual stutterer showed a loss on the SSI materials relative to the PB words in the right ear. He also demonstrated excessive rollover (30%) on the SSI materials for the left ear. There were no other examples of depressed performance on the SSI materials among members of the stuttering group.

SSI-ICM

Decreased performance on the Synthetic Sentence Identification with an Ipsilateral Competing Message (SSI-ICM) is characteristic of central auditory disorders (Jerger, 1973; Jerger and Jerger, 1974, 1975a, b, c). Usually the loss is in the ear contralateral to the site of disorder. When both ears show a deficit, the loss is usually greater in the contralateral ear.

Results for SSI-ICM in the present subjects are graphed in Figure 2. Percentage of correct sentence identification is plotted as a function of the message-to-competition ratio (MCR). Three MCRs were tested for each ear. At 0 MCR, the easiest listening situation, the message (sentences) and competition (continuous discourse) are at equal intensity levels. At −10 MCR, an intermediate level of difficulty, the competition is at an intensity level 10 dB greater than the message. and at −20 MCR, the most difficult listening condition used in this study, the competition is 20 dB more intense than the message.

Two findings were apparent from an analysis of the SSI-ICM data of this study. First, in both groups a higher average correct score was obtained for the right ear than for the left. The ear difference was greatest at the most difficult listening condition, −20 MCR. Second, the average percentage of correct scores for the stutterers was poorer than that for the control group at each MCR. The difference in performance between groups was seen for both ears. The average SSI-ICM scores for the three MCRs were computed. Relative to the control group, the stutterers show an 8% loss in the right ear and a 9% loss in the left ear. In terms of the criteria used in clinical interpretation of ear differences in performance on the SSI-ICM, however, this difference between groups is slight.

SSI-CCM

The SSI materials used with a contralateral competing message (CCM) are sensitive to temporal lobe auditory disorders (Jerger, 1973; Jerger and Jerger, 1974, 1975a, b, c). Of most importance in differentiating

FIGURE 2. ▬▬▬▬▬▬▬▬▬▬▬▬▬▬▬▬▬▬▬▬▬▬▬▬▬
Comparison of performance for stuttering and control groups for the Synthetic Sentence Identification test with Ipsilateral Competing Message (SSI-ICM). The percentage of correct scores for both groups are shown for each of the three message-to-competition ratios (MCRs) tested: Key: The open symbols are the control group, the black symbols represent the stutterers. Circles denote right ear, squares denote left ear.

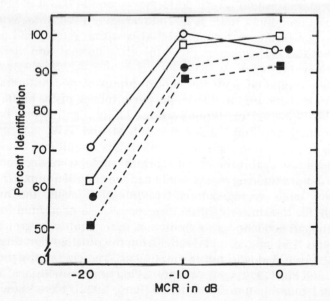

brainstem from temporal lobe auditory disorders is the performance on the SSI-CCM relative to the SSI-ICM. A greater loss on the ICM suggests a brainstem site. A greater performance deficit on the CCM suggests a temporal lobe site (Jerger, 1973; Jerger and Jerger, 1974, 1975a, b, c). In this study, the average performance for the SSI-CCM for both groups was 100%.

SSW Test

The SSW (Staggered Spondaic Word) Test is sensitive to auditory impairment primarily at the temporal lobe level (Katz, 1962, 1968; Jerger and Jerger, 1975a, b). A positive sign of a temporal lobe auditory disorder is a performance difference between ears for the simultaneous dichotic condition of the test (Katz, 1968; Jerger and Jerger, 1975a, b).

The percentage of correct scores for the leading, lagging, and competing conditions of the SSW test were compared between groups for each ear. In the competing condition, the control group demonstrated a 2% right ear advantage (REA), based on these percentages of correct scores. The stuttering group, however, demonstrated no right ear advantage (REA). The two groups were comparable in the leading and lagging noncompeting conditions.

Discussion

The overall pattern of central auditory test findings for the group of stutterers, when evaluated in terms of normal expectations, fails to suggest substantial central auditory disorders. Acoustic reflexes are present at normal threshold levels, performance on PI-PB and PI-SSI functions shows no deficit, there is no rollover on either PBs or Synthetic Sentences, performance on the SSI-ICM is within established normal limits, SSI-CCM performance is unequivocally normal, and there is no dramatic ear difference on SSW.

When compared with the control group of nonstutterers comparable in age and sex, however, the performance of the stutterers is somewhat depressed on three portions of the central test battery; acoustic reflex amplitude functions, SSI-ICM, and SSW.

The average contralateral acoustic reflex amplitudes at each intensity level tested, threshold and suprathreshold, were decreased for each ear in the stuttering group, relative to the control group. When the amplitudes were averaged over five intensity levels, the average amplitude for the stuttering group was 60%–65% of normal for both ears. Although acoustic reflex thresholds in the stuttering group were normal, this finding does not detract from the possible significance of their decreased acoustic reflex amplitudes. The findings of Bosatra, Russolo, and Poli (1977) with patients having brainstem lesions, and experimental investigations in animals (Borg, 1973), have shown that disruption in the central acoustic reflex arc may severely affect the suprathreshold amplitude while reflex threshold remains essentially normal.

Deficits on the SSI-ICM, when not in combination with an SSI-CCM loss, have been clinically documented as characteristic of disorders affecting the auditory brainstem pathways (Jerger, 1973; Jerger and Jerger, 1974, 1975a, b, c). Compared to the control group, the performance of the stuttering group on the SSI-ICM was depressed bilaterally. Yet the stutterers' high level of performance on the PI-PB and PI-SSI functions and the absence of rollover on either of these tests contradict the SSI-ICM results. A long-recognized problem in designing tests of central auditory function has been the need to stress the auditory system sufficiently to bring about a deterioration in performance (Antonelli, Calearo, and Demitri, 1963; Bocca and Calearo, 1963; Parker, Decker, and Richards, 1968). In terms of their demands on the auditory system, the speech tests used in this study are varied. Repeating PB words presented in quiet constitutes a relatively easy listening task. Identifying the Synthetic Sentences in competition at 0 MCR is more difficult, but still not sufficiently demanding to detect some central auditory disorders. By presenting either the PB words or the SSI materials at high-intensity levels, additional stress is put on the central auditory system. Thus, a greater proportion of central auditory disorders generally are detected.

A unique advantage of the SSI-ICM is that the difficulty can be selectively controlled by varying the message-to-competition ratio (MCR). An MCR of -10, and especially -20, puts an unusual demand on the speech decoding capabilities of the central auditory system. Thus, the difficult conditions of the SSI-ICM are sensitive to even subtle central auditory disorders, primarily at the brainstem level. Such disorders may remain undetected with less demanding speech tests. It was at these difficult listening conditions on the SSI-ICM that a difference in performance emerged between the stuttering group and the control group. This result is in agreement with the findings of Toscher and Rupp (1975), who also showed a difference between stutterers and nonstutterers at an MCR of -20 dB on SSI-ICM.

The present stutterers all performed with 100% accuracy on the SSI-CCM. This test, however, is less sensitive to temporal lobe disorders than SSW (Jerger and Jerger, 1975b). The SSW test has proved to be a highly sensitive measure of cerebral auditory function (Katz, 1968; Jerger and Jerger, 1975b). Therefore, central auditory signs, usually reflecting an auditory impairment at the temporal lobe level, may appear on SSW but not on SSI-CCM. The stutterers' normal performance on the SSI-CCM, and depressed performance on the SSW test, is not, therefore, contradictory. Rather, the combination of findings points up the subtlety of any possible impairment in central auditory function in stutterers. The present SSW test results are in close agreement with those previous dichotic listening studies with stutterers that have used meaningful linguistic stimuli (Curry and Gregory, 1969; Sommers, Brady, and Moore, 1975). The results from the present study and these two previous studies are compared in Table 1. The proportion of nonstutterers demonstrating the REA is consistently 70%–75%, while only 40%–45% of the stutterers show the REA.

Isolated test results obtained on the stuttering group are characterized by inconsistencies. This finding corroborates the observation made by Toscher and Rupp.[2] Members of their stuttering group showed a greater degree of variability than did the members of the control group. It is also in agreement with reports of clinical experience with the same tests of central auditory function (Jerger and Jerger, 1975b). The inconsistencies in test performance seriously restrict the conclusions that may be drawn from studies employing a single central auditory test.

With this limitation in mind, it is reasonable to conclude that, as a group, the stutterers did present evidence of a central auditory deficiency. More specifically, the pattern of test results suggests a disorder at the brainstem level.

The acoustic reflex amplitude functions and SSI-ICM are sensitive to brainstem level auditory disorders (Bosatra, Russolo, and Poli, 1977; Jerger, 1973; Jerger and Jerger, 1974, 1975a, b, c). The SSW has typically been considered a test of temporal lobe function (Katz, 1962, 1968). However, Jerger and Jerger (1975b) have suggested that, while substantial SSW deficits were consistently obtained on patients with

---

[2]M. M. Toscher, personal communication (1977).

TABLE 1. ━━━━━━━━━━━━━━━━━━━━━━━━━━━━━
Comparison of the percentage of stutterers and nonstutterers showing a right ear advantage (REA) for the Staggered Spondaic Word (SSW) test in the present study, and for the dichotic listening test in studies reported by Curry and Gregory (1969) and Sommers, Brady, and Moore (1975).

	Percentage of Subjects Showing REA		
Subjects	Curry & Gregory (1969)	Sommers et al. (1975	Present Study
Control Group	75%	72%	70%
Stuttering Group	45%	41%	40%

temporal lobe disorders, SSW deficits were also obtained on some patients with brainstem disorders. Performance on the SSI-ICM provided the distinction between the groups. Those patients with brainstem disorders showing an SSW deficit also consistently showed a loss on the SSI-ICM. In view of these observations, the performance of the stutterers as a group is consistent with a brainstem level auditory disorder.

The subtlety of the deficiency must be emphasized. Even the stuttering group data are not dramatically characteristic of central auditory disorder, as described in the literature. The depressed performance of the stuttering group becomes apparent only when compared with a carefully matched control group. Still, there is considerable potential value in investigating auditory function in stuttering with the clinical central auditory test battery. Subgroups of stutterers may be distinguished based on unique patterns of test performance. In addition, specific suspicious findings, such as the acoustic reflex amplitude function discrepancies, may be followed up with intensive study in selected stutterers. Clearly, more investigation of central auditory function in stuttering is warranted.

Acknowledgement

Sally McKee and Thelma Zirkelbach graciously assisted in providing subjects. Requests for reprints should be addressed to James W. Hall, Audiology Service, Mail Station NA 200, The Neurosensory Center, Texas Medical Center, Houston, Texas 77030.

References

American National Standards Bureau, *Specification for Audiometers*. ANSI S3.6-1969. New York: American National Standards Bureau (1969).

Antonelli, A., Calearo, C., and De Mitri, T., On the auditory function in brainstem diseases. *Int. Audiol.*, 2: 55–61 (1963).

Beedle, R. K. An investigation of the relationship between the acoustic reflex growth and loudness growth in normal and pathologic ears. Doctoral dissertation, Northwestern Univ. (1970).

Bocca, E., and Calearo, C., Central hearing processes. In J. Jerger (Ed.), *Modern Developments in Audiology*. New York: Academic, 337–370 (1963).

Borg, E., On the neuronal organization of the acoustic middle ear reflex. A physiological and anatomical study. *Brain Res.*, 49, 101–123 (1973).

Bosatra, A., Russolo, M., and Poli, P., Oscilloscope analysis of the stapedius muscle reflex in brain stem lesions. *Archs Otolar.*, 102, 284–285 (1976).

Curry, F., and Gregory, H., The performance of stutterers on dichotic listening tasks thought to reflect cerebral dominance. *J. Speech Hearing Res.*, 12, 78–82 (1969).

Djupesland, G., Flottorp, G., and Winther, F., Size and duration of acoustically elicited impedance changes in man. *Acta oto-lar. Suppl.*, 224, 220–228 (1967).

Gravendeel, D. W., *Perceptive Bass₁ Deafness*. Utrecht: H. J. Smits (1958).

Gregory, H., Stuttering and auditory central nervous system disorder. *J. Speech Hearing Res.*, 7, 335–341 (1964).

Greisen, O., and Rasmussen, P., Stapedius muscle reflexes and otoneurological examination in brain stem tumors. *Acta oto-lar.*, 70, 366–370 (1970).

Jerger, J., Diagnostic audiometry. In J. Jerger (Ed.), *Modern Developments in Audiology.* (2nd ed.) New York: Academic, 75–115 (1973).

Jerger, J., Diagnostic use of impedance measures. In J. Jerger (Ed.) *Manual of Impedance Audiometry,* New York: American Electromedics (1975).

Jerger, J., and Hayes, D., Diagnostic speech audiometry. *Archs Otolar.*, 103, 216–222 (1977).

Jerger, J., and Jerger, S., Auditory findings in brain stem disorders. *Archs Otolar.*, 99, 342–350 (1974).

Jerger, J., and Jerger, S., Diagnostic audiology. In Donald Tower (Ed.), *The Nervous System: Human Communications and its Disorders.* (Vol. 3) New York: Raven Press, 199–205 (1975a).

Jerger, J., and Jerger, S., Clinical validity of central auditory tests. *Scand. Audiol.*, 4, 147–163 (1975b).

Jerger, S., and Jerger, J., Extra- and intra-axial, brain stem auditory disorders. *Audiology,* 14, 93–117 (1975c).

Jerger, J., Lovering, L., and Wertz, M., Auditory disorder following bilateral temporal lobe insult: Report of a case. *J. Speech Hearing Dis.*, 37, 523–535 (1972).

Jerger, J., Mauldin, L., and Lewis, N., Temporal summation of the acoustic reflex. *Audiology,* 16, 177–200 (1977).

Jerger, S., Neely, G., and Jerger, J., Recovery of crossed acoustic reflexes in brain stem auditory disorder. *Archs Otolar.*, 101, 329–332 (1975).

Jerger, J., Speaks, C., and Trammell, J., A new approach to speech audiometry. *J. Speech Hearing Dis.*, 33, 318–328 (1968).

Jerger, J., Weikers, N., Sharbrough, F., and Jerger, S., Bilateral lesions of the temporal lobe: A case study. *Acta oto-lar. Suppl.*, 258 (1969).

Katz, J., The use of staggered spondaic words for assessing the integrity of the central auditory nervous system. *J. aud. Res.*, 2, 327–337 (1962).

Katz, J., The SSW test: An interim report. *J. Speech Hearing Res.*, 33, 132–146 (1968).

Liden, G., and Korsan-Bengtsen, M., Audiometric manifestations of retrocochlear lesions. *Scand. Audiol.*, 2, 29–40 (1973).

Manning, W. H. and Riensche, L., Auditory assembly abilities of stuttering and nonstuttering children. *J. Speech Hearing Res.*, 19, 777–783 (1976).

Moore, W. H., Bilateral tachistoscopic word perception of stutterers and normal subjects. *Brain & Lang.*, 3, 434–442 (1976).

Moore, W. H., and Lang, M. K., Alpha asymmetry over the right and left hemispheres of stutterers and control subjects preceding massed oral readings: A preliminary investigation. *Percept. & Mot. Skills,* 44, 223–230 (1977).

Orton, S. T., Studies in stuttering. *Arch. Neurol. Psychiat., Chicago,* 18, 671–672 (1927).

Parker, W., Decker, R., and Richards, N., Auditory function and lesions of the pons. *Archs Otolar.*, 87, 228–240 (1968).

Peterson, J. L., and Liden, G., Some static characteristics of the stapedial muscle reflex. *Audiology,* 11, 97–114 (1972).

Quinn, P. T., Stuttering: Cerebral dominance and the dichotic word test. *Med. J. Aust.,* 2, 639–643 (1972).

Rousey, C. L., Goetzinger, C. P., and Dirks, D., sound localization ability of normal, stuttering, neurotic, and hemiplegic subjects. *Arch. gen. Psychiat.,* 1, 640–645 (1959).

Sanchez Longo, L. P., Forester, F. M., and Auth, T. L., A clinical test for sound localization and its applications. *Neurology,* 7, 655–663 (1957).

Slorach, N., and Noehr, B., Dichotic listening in stuttering and dislalic children. *Cortex,* 9, 295–300 (1973).

Sommers, R. K., Brady, W.A., and Moore, W.H., Dichotic ear preferences of stuttering children and adults. *Percept. Mot. Skills,* 41, 931–938 (1975).

Sussman, H. M., and MacNeilage, P. F., Hemispheric specialization for speech production and perception in stutterers. *Neuropsychologia,* 13, 19–26 (1975).

Toscher, M. M., and Rupp, R. R., A study of the central auditory processes in stutterers using the Synthetic Sentence Identification (SSI) test battery. [*J. Speech Hearing Res.,* in press] (1978) Poster Session, Annual meeting of the American Speech and Hearing Association. Washington, D.C. (1975).

Travis, L. E., *Speech Pathology.* New York: Appleton-Century-Crofts (1931).

Central Auditory Dysfunction Among Chronic Alcoholics

Jaclyn B. Spitzer, PhD, and Ira M. Ventry, PhD

The relationship between chronic alcoholism and auditory processing problems was examined using a central auditory test battery. Fifteen carefully selected alcoholic subjects and 15 age-matched nonalcoholic control subjects were evaluated using pure-tone thresholds, spondee thresholds, speech discrimination, acoustic reflex thresholds, performance-intensity function, Staggered Spondaic Word (SSW) test, Synthetic Sentence Identification (SSI), and temporal summation. Significant differences between the groups were obtained for acoustic reflex measurement, SSW, and SSI. A significant subject-related interaction was obtained for temporal summation measurement. Approximately half of the alcoholics yielded results consistent with brainstem pathologic features.

Alcohol has long been considered an ototoxic drug.[1] Clinical reports of the occurrence of hearing loss,[5,6] tinnitus, and auditory hallucinations have served as the basis of the classification as ototoxic. However, findings of histopathologic examination and studies of pure-tone thresholds[9,10] have failed to document conclusively the effect on peripheral auditory structures.

Wolff and Gross[8] reported the results of the examination of 16 temporal bones of alcoholic patients. The investigation was prompted by clinical observations of loss of equilibrium, complaints of fullness of

Reprinted from the Archives of Otolaryngology, April 1980, Volume 106 the ears, auditory hallucinations, high incidence of tinnitus, and reversible sensorineural hearing loss. The findings indicated multiple fractures of the ampullae among the specimens, but in view of the possible contamination by head trauma, the results were deemed comparable with findings on routine examinations.

Studies of pure-tone thresholds have produced contradictory conclusions. Nordahl[9] studied the incidence of hearing loss among 83 institutionalized alcoholics. Fourteen (17%) of the patients demonstrated sensorineural loss. Nordahl concluded that the observed hearing loss was not alcoholism-related, but reflected the noise exposure commonly experienced by alcoholics in their work environment. In contrast, Montauti and Paterni[10] reported detecting sensorineural hearing loss of various degrees and configurations in 15 of the 16 alcoholics in their sample. The latter authors stated that "bilateral, symmetrical, perceptive" hearing loss is almost always present among alcoholics. Clearly, the conflicting findings of Nordahl and Montauti and Paterni leave uncertain the relationship between alcoholism and peripheral degeneration.

Alcohol's effect on central auditory function has been examined, primarily through studies employing experimental administration of the drug to nonalcoholic subjects. The central depressant effect has been documented, as revealed by elevated acoustic reflex thresholds with magnitude of reflex contraction decreased and latency increased,[11,12] and prolonged components of auditory evoked responses.[13] Central processing effects among alcoholics have received less attention. A single study by Chandler et al[14] failed to find significant temporal lobe dysfunction among non-brain-injured chronic alcoholics using a dichotic listening paradigm.

In view of the inconclusive evidence relating alcoholism to peripheral auditory pathologic features and the superficial examination of the effect on levels beyond the cochlea, the present study was undertaken to investigate the central auditory effects of chronic alcoholism. The technique selected was twofold, using (1) an intensive diagnostic battery, as described by Jerger and Jerger,[15,16] for the determination of the site of lesion: and (2) for the temporally manipulated signals, for the determination of change in perceptual abilities as a function of change in duration or percent compression.

Method

Subjects

Two subject groups composed of 15 alcoholics and 15 control subjects were selected. The alcoholic subjects were veterans undergoing a four-week detoxification program in an alcohol rehabilitation unit. Individuals admitted to the program were classified as gamma-stage[17] alcoholics, in whom loss of self-control and social function are characteristic. Participants in the study were selected on the basis of chart review and personal interview by the first investigator. Subjects were included who met the following criteria: hearing within the normal range for their age; negative history of ear infection, noise exposure, head injury, use of ototoxic drugs, and addiction to drugs other than alcohol; and negative otologic and neurologic examination results. Some individuals were included whose neurologic examination demonstrated alcoholic neuropathy or who reported a history of delirium tremens. All subjects spoke English as their native language and were able to read simple sentences. The purpose of the study was explained to qualified individuals. After signing an informed consent, volunteers underwent an EEG and approximately six hours of auditory testing. Individuals whose EEG was consistent with focal pathologic features were excluded from the sample.

The mean age of the alcoholic group was 42.7 years (SD = 8.99); they ranged in age from 26 to 55 years. The alcoholic subjects were heterogeneous regarding duration of alcoholism and preferred beverage. All subjects in the alcoholic group reported excessive drinking for more than ten years.

An age-matched nonalcoholic control group was selected from general medical wards. They met the same selection criteria as the alcoholics. The mean age of the control subjects was 42.1 years (SD = 8.81); the age range was 26 to 53 years old.

Procedures

All subjects underwent a basic audiologic evaluation and two diagnostic sessions. The basic test battery included pure-tone air and bone conduction thresholds, and speech discrimination using taped Central Institute for the Deaf (CID) W-22 words. Site-of-lesion testing of the alcoholics included Short Increment Sensitivity Index (SISI),[18] tone decay testing,[19] tympanometry and acoustic reflex measurement, and sweep frequency Bekesy threshold measurement. During the two diagnostic sessions, the subjects underwent an intensive central auditory battery[15] that included performance intensity function for phonetically balanced words (PI-PB functions); Staggered Spondaic Word (SSW) test; Synthetic Sentence Identification with ipsilateral competing message (SSI-ICM) and with contralateral competing message (SSI-CCM); and listening to temporally altered signals. The subjects traced temporal summation thresholds for taped trains of brief tones with equivalent durations[20] of 640, 320, 160, 80, 40, 20, and 10 ms at the stimulus frequencies of 500, 1,000, 2,000 and 4,000 Hz. Four lists of Everyday Sentences[21] at compression ratios of 0% (uncompressed), 20%, 40%, and 60% were presented monaurally to a subsample of alcoholics and control subjects.

The testing was performed at the Brooklyn Veterans Administration Hospital. The subjects were seated inside a double-walled audiometric booth. Stimuli from the pure-tone and speech circuits of a 1½ channel audiometer were delivered into a TDH-49 earphone mounted in an MX-41/AR cushion. Taped CID W-22 word lists were played on a high-quality cassette tape recorder fed into the audiometer's speech circuit; other taped stimuli were played on a high-quality reel-to-reel tape deck. Sweep frequency Bekesy tracings and responses to brief-tone stimuli were obtained using the automatic circuit of the audiometer and recorded on the associated X-Y plotter. Measurement of the admittance changes accompanying acoustic reflex contraction were made with an otoadmittance meter using a 220-Hz probe tone. All equipment was calibrated in conformance with the American National Standards Institute 1969 standards. A more detailed description of procedures has been provided elsewhere.[22]

Results

The results of individual components of the basic and diagnostic batteries will be reported. The battery results will be examined to determine if there is a pattern suggestive of site-of-lesion that characterized the alcoholic sample.

Basic Battery

Table 1 illustrates mean pure-tone thresholds and standard deviations for the alcoholic and control groups. The subject selection criterion of normal hearing for their age is reflected in the higher thresholds and increased variability above 2,000 Hz. The alcoholics' mean threshold at 4,000 and 8,000 Hz were 7 to 13 dB higher than those of the control subjects, although standard deviations indicate overlap between the groups. All subjects had an acceptable pure-tone average-spondee threshold correspondence. Speech discrimination scores at 40 dB sensation level (SL) were comparable for both ears as determined by Student's t tests for correlated samples ($P > .05$, two-tailed; insignificant findings for both right and left ears). Pure-tone configurations, spondee thresholds, and speech discrimination scores are indicative of hearing within normal limits and subject group comparability for these measures. Therefore, measures of central auditory function were not influenced by pure-tone hearing loss or discrimination loss.

TABLE 1.
Mean Pure-Tone Thresholds in Alcoholic and Control Groups*

Group	Frequency, Hz					
	250	500	1,000	2,000	4,000	8,000
Alcoholics						
Right ear	14.00	12.33	9.33	11.0	25.66	30.33
SD	(5.07)	(5.62)	(8.63)	(9.85)	(16.99)	(27.08)
Left ear	13.33	13.00	9.66	13.66	28.66	30.33
SD	(3.61)	(7.74)	(7.66)	(11.72)	(20.13)	(20.21)
Control subjects						
Right ear	14.28	7.66	7.33	7.00	17.66	17.33
SD	(6.75)	(7.28)	(6.51)	(5.60)	(15.79)	(17.91)
Left ear	11.00	8.66	6.66	8.66	21.66	16.66
SD	(5.07)	(6.67)	(4.49)	(7.18)	(13.58)	(14.59)

*Thresholds in decibels hearing level; alcoholics, $N = 15$; control subjects, $N = 15$.

The results of the peripheral test battery are summarized in Table 2. Results of tone decay testing were negative for the entire sample. Positive SISI scores (80% or higher) were obtained unilaterally in four subjects and bilaterally in one subject; positive findings were limited to 4,000 Hz, where pure-tone thresholds indicated sensorineural loss in the high frequencies only. Bekesy thresholds were typed according to a widely accepted classification system.[23] Twelve subjects had type I thresholds for either ear; 11 (73% of the sample) had type I tracings bilaterally. Type II thresholds were traced by one individual unilaterally and two bilaterally. A single subject had a type IV threshold unilaterally. The findings described may be summarized as consistent with cochlear site-of-lesion affecting the high frequencies. No evidence of neural involvement was detected among the alcoholic subjects on these measures.

Diagnostic Battery

The components of the battery were acoustic reflex measurement, generation of PI-PB functions, SSW, and SSI. Mean acoustic reflex thresholds (in decibels SL) and their standard deviations appear in Table 3. Reflexes were elicited at mean SLs, which ranged from 69.6 to 84.6 dB. There is a trend for the SL of reflex threshold to decrease and for variability to increase with increased frequency. Some of the cell means in Table 3 are based on a reduced number, since reflex contraction may not have been elicited at that frequency. The observation of absent acoustic reflexes is of diagnostic importance.[15,16] The number of absent reflexes at each frequency is displayed in Table 4. The total number of absent reflexes was significantly greater among the alcoholic subjects than the control subjects ($\chi^2 = 13.7$; $P < .001$, two-tailed).

Based on discrimination scores obtained during PI-PB measurement, a rollover index[23] was calculated for each subject using the formula $(PB_{max} - PB_{min})/PB_{max}$. The mean rollover indices and standard

TABLE 2.

Findings on Modified Carhart Tone Decay Test, SISI, and Bekesy Thresholds Categories Among Alcoholic Subjects*

| | No. of Observations | | | | | |
Ear	Positive Tone Decay	Positive SISI	I	II	Bekesy Type III	IV
Right	0	3†	12	3	0	0
Left	0	3†	12	2	0	1

*N = 15; SISI indicates Short Increment Sensitivity Index.
†At 4 kHz only.

TABLE 3.

Mean Acoustic Reflex Thresholds and Standard Deviations*

| | Frequency, Hz | | | |
Group	500	1,000	2,000	4,000
Alcoholics (N=15)				
Right ear	80.41	82.50	80.76	72.00
SD	(9.15)	(12.04)	(16.05)	(17.19)
Left ear	78.75	79.58	70.45	72.00
SD	(11.10)	(11.37)	(14.39)	(22.38)
Control subjects (N=15)				
Right ear	84.00	82.66	83.00	75.38
SD	(12.56)	(10.49)	(7.51)	(17.84)
Left ear	81.78	84.64	80.71	69.61
SD	(11.02)	(9.08)	(8.95)	(18.08)

*Thresholds in decibels sensation level.

TABLE 4.
Number of Observations of Absent Acoustic Reflexes at Each Frequency

Group	Frequency, Hz			
	500	1,000	2,000	4,000
Alcoholics (N=15)				
Right ear	3	2	2	5
Left ear	3	3	4	5
Control subjects (N=15)				
Right ear	0	0	0	2
Left ear	1	1	1	2

deviation appear in Table 5. Student's t tests for correlated samples failed to differentiate between the groups for either ear ($P > .05$, two-tailed).

Mean total corrected SSW scores (alcoholics, $\bar{x}. = -2.73$; control subjects, $\bar{x}. = -0.13$) fell within the normal range.[24] Nine alcoholics' total scores were classed as normal, while all 15 control subject scores fell into the normal category. The six abnormal scores by alcoholics were all in the overcorrected category; according to Jack Katz, Ph.D. (October 1977), the latter classification is consistent with either sensorineural[25] or brainstem pathologic features. The performance of the alcoholic subjects was compared with that of their age-matched control subjects using a Wilcoxon Matched Pairs Signed Rank Test, which indicated a significant difference between the groups ($P < .05$, two-tailed) for the corrected total score.

TABLE 5.
Mean Rollover Index Findings

Group	Ear	
	Right	Left
Alcoholics (N = 15)	.28	.27
SD	(.15)	(.13)
Control subjects (N = 15)	.18	.20
SD	(.09)	(.12)

TABLE 6.

Mean Scores on Synthetic Identification-Ipsilateral Competing Message Test

Group	Message-to-Competition Rule				
	+10	0	−10	−20	−30
Alcoholic (N = 15)					
Right ear	98.66	88.00	67.33	39.33	10.00
SD	(5.16)	(13.73)	(16.24)	(21.86)	(12.53)
Left ear	100.00	70.66	78.00	42.66	11.33
SD	(0.00)	(15.79)	(16.98)	(21.53)	(16.41)
Control subjects (N = 15)					
Right ear	100.00	96.66	84.66	55.33	14.66
SD	(0.00)	(4.87)	(15.05)	(18.07)	(13.02)
Left ear	100.00	98.66	86.00	54.00	20.00
SD	(0.00)	(3.51)	(14.04)	(16.81)	(16.47)

Mean scores on the SSI with an ipsilateral competing message (SSI-ICM) and standard deviations are displayed in Table 6. As expected, both groups tended to make more errors as the message-to-competition ratio (MCR) was increased. Another noteworthy trend in Table 6 is for mean scores at each MCR to be lower for the alcoholics than for the control subjects. In order to examine the individual alcoholic's results, the results for each ear were plotted with percent correct responses as a function of MCR (Fig 1 and 2). The mean data obtained from using the control subjects were plotted using ±1 SD as the normal range. This was done since the heterogeneity of the alcoholic and control samples with respect to age may have introduced variation in scores absent in the Jergers' norms. The number beside the X in Fig 1 and 2 reveals that fewer abnormal responses were obtained during left ear ICM trials than during right ear trials.

Nine alcoholics scored below the normal range in right ear trials, as compared with two control subjects. During left ear trials, seven alcoholics performed poorly, whereas only one control subject did. The differences in ICM performance reached statistical significance for both right ($\chi^2 = 7.1$; $P < .01$, two-tailed) and left ($\chi^2 = 6.1$; $P < .05$, two-tailed) ears. Four alcoholics scored abnormally bilaterally during ICM conditions. Scores on the SSI-CCM were high; the lowest score obtained was 80% for an alcoholic at 1 MCR. Poor performance; then, on ICM trials was obtained in the presence of good scores on CCM conditions.

FIGURE 1.
Right ear performances on Synthetic Identification-ipsilateral competing message as function of message-to-competition ratio. Shaded area represents control group's mean ± 1 SD; X represents alcoholic subjects who fell outside of range; numbers indicate frequency of observations that fell outside of range.

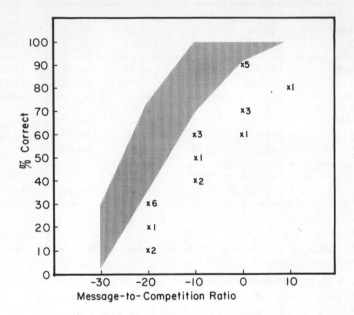

Temporally Manipulated Signals

The two procedures in the temporal battery were temporal summation at threshold and compressed speech. Thresholds were obtained at the four stimulus frequencies for seven durations. The thresholds were converted from decibels hearing level to decibels relative to the threshold for the shortest duration at that frequency. The converted thresholds underwent a four-way analysis of variance (frequency × duration × subject × group × ear, replicated within subjects 15 times). Significant main effects were obtained for frequency ($F = 9.76$, $df = 3$) and duration ($F = 493.30$, $df = 6$). Significant interaction effects were obtained for subject × ear ($F = 4.36$, $df = 1$), ear × duration ($F = 2.64$, $df = 6$), and subject × ear × duration ($F = 3.02$, $df = 6$). The obtained significant duration main effect was expected, since it reflects the well-recognized time and intensity trading characteristic of the auditory system.[26] The observed significant frequency main effect may be attributed to high-frequency threshold loss noted earlier. Aberrant temporal summation functions have been observed in individuals

FIGURE 2.
Left ear performance on Synthetic Sentence Identification-ipsilateral competing message as function of message-to-competition ratio. Shaded area represents control group's mean ± 1 SD; X represents alcoholic subjects who fell outside of range; numbers indicate frequency of observations that fell outside of range.

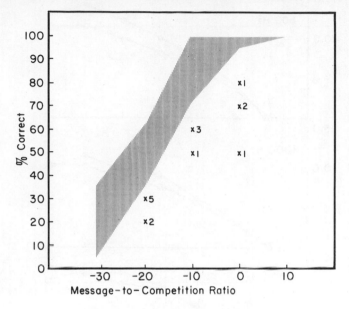

with cochlear site-of-lesions.[27] The failure to obtain a significant subject main effect indicates that temporal summation differences between the groups attributable solely to alcoholism cannot be documented.

However, a signficant subject × ear interaction was calculated. Figures 3 and 4 illustrate the interaction. During right ear trials (Fig 3), on the average, alcoholics required 1 to 3 dB greater intensity to reach threshold than the control subjects. Figure 4, illustrating mean left ear responses, reflects the comparability of the groups' responses in the interweaving of functions.

A subsample of seven alcoholics and their matched controls listened to compressed CID Everyday Sentences at 20 dB SL. Table 7 summarizes the mean performance and ranges on the compressed speech task. The spread of scores is essentially comparable for the two groups. When scores of 70% or below were examined, the most markedly reduced scores were obtained for six alcoholics under left ear stimulation and five control subjects under right ear stimulation.

FIGURE 3. ▬▬▬▬▬▬▬▬▬▬▬▬▬▬▬▬▬▬▬▬▬▬▬▬▬▬▬
Mean temporal summation functions obtained from right ear of alcoholic (open circle) and control (closed circle) groups (N = 15 in each group).

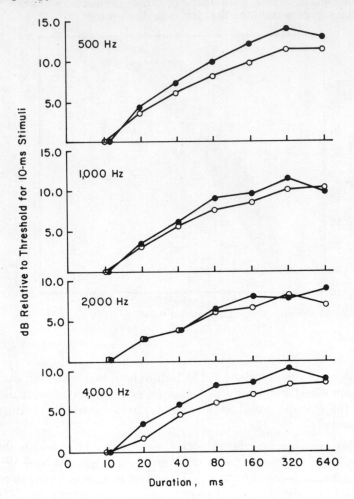

Constellation of Findings

The diagnostic decision regarding site-of-lesion is based on inspection of the indvidual alcoholics' findings on the battery. Tables 8 and 9 display the positive results for each member of the alcoholic sample. As indicated in Table 9, the cooccurrence of positive findings on two or more measures was limited to seven subjects. Two subjects had absent

FIGURE 4.

Mean temporal summation functions obtained from left ear of alcoholic (open rectangle) and control (closed rectangle) groups (*N* = 15 in each group).

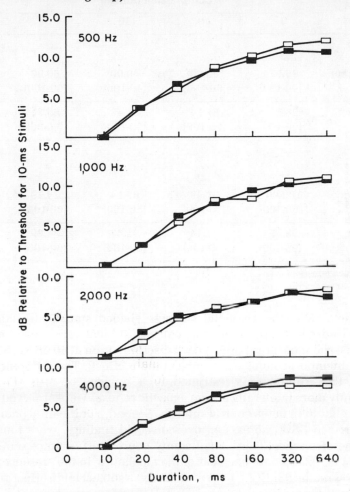

acoustic reflexes and poor SSI-ICM performance. Four alcoholics performed poorly on the SSI-ICM and SSW tests. Two subjects demonstrated high rollover indices (0.45 or higher) and poor SSI-ICM scores. Two alcoholic subjects had high rollover scores and overcorrected SSW scores. Subject 13 was the only individual to have abnormal performance on acoustic reflex, SSI, and rollover index. Subject 8 was the sole alcoholic subject to perform normally (yield negative results) on all the measures.

TABLE 7.
Mean Scores and Ranges for Compressed Speech Conditions*

Group	% Compression (Range)			
	0	20	40	60
Alcoholic (N = 7)				
Right ear	98.57	80.00	80.00	80.00
SD	(90-100)	(30-100)	(40-100)	(60-100)
Left ear	98.57	87.14	81.43	65.71
SD	(90-100)	(70-100)	(50-100)	(60-80)
Control subjects (N = 7)				
Right ear	100.00	91.43	87.14	74.29
SD	(100-100)	(70-100)	(50-100)	(60-100)
Left ear	98.57	87.14	91.43	84.29
SD	(90-100)	(50-100)	(80-100)	(60-100)

*Presented at 20 dB sensation level.

In summary, the alcoholic subjects yielded statistically comparable findings to those of the control subjects for pure-tone thresholds, spondee thresholds, speech discrimination at 40 dB SL, SSI-CCM, and temporal summation (subject main effect). The differences between the groups were restricted to a nucleus of tests. First, significantly more bilaterally absent acoustic reflexes were observed in the alcoholics than in the control subjects. Second, significantly poorer total corrected SSW scores, i.e., overcorrected findings, were found among the alcoholics. Third, signficantly poorer performance on the SSI-ICM was obtained for each ear of the alcoholics, in the presence of good scores on the SSI-CCM. Fourth, although a subject main effect was not obtained for temporal summation measurement, a signficant subject × ear interaction effect indicated that the alcoholics required 1 to 3 dB more intensity during right ear trials than did the control subjects. Finally, the deleterious effect of compression on speech discrimination was greatest in the alcoholics' left ear, although noted bilaterally.

Comment

It is apparent that no single pattern of abnormal findings characterized the alcoholic sample. Positive results were scattered throughout the diagnostic and temporal batteries. Although the present data are not

TABLE 8.
Constellation of Alcoholic Subjects' Test Results: Basic Evaluation

Subject Code No.	Pure-Tone Threshold		Speech Reception		Discrim. at 40-dB SL†		Bekesy Type‡		Tone Decay		SISI§	
	R	L	R	L	R	L	R	L	R	L	R	L
3												
4												
5												
6	+	+										
8							II					
9	+	+						IV				
11												
12	+	+					II	II			+	+
13	+	+									+	+
14												
15												
16	+	+					II	II			·|	+
18												
19	+	+									+	+
20	+											+

*Threshold loss for frequencies above 2 kHz only.
†SL indicates sensation level. Only scores poorer than 80% noted.
‡Type I tracings not included.
§SISI indicates Short Increment Sensitivity Index. Positive findings limited to 4 kHz only.

conclusive due to small sample size and heterogeneity of the groups regarding age and alcoholic abuse, auditory processing dysfunction is nevertheless suggested.

Absent acoustic reflexes (at frequencies at which there was no threshold loss), poor performance on the SSI-ICM (in the presence of good performance on the SSI-CCM), and over-corrected SSW scores (in the presence of very good speech discrimination scores) are considered consistent with brainstem site-of-lesion. In addition, high rollover scores (higher than 0.45) have been observed in individuals with brainstem pathologic features, as well as in eighth nerve lesions.[24]

TABLE 9.
Constellation of Alcoholic Subjects' Test Results: Diagnostic Battery and Compressed Speech

Subject Code No.	Acoustic Reflex*		Roll-Over		SSW‡	SSI-ICM§		SSI-CCMII		Compressed ☆	
	R	L	R	L		R	L	R	L	R	L
3	+(4)	+(4)					+				
4	+(2)										
5	+(4)	+(4)									
6					+						
8											
9					+	+	+				
11					+	+	+				
12			+				+				
13		+(4)	+		+	+	+				+
14				+	+						+
15			+		+	+				+	+
16			+	+						+	
18					+	+					+
19								+		+	+
20		+(2)				+				+	

*Only individuals who had absent reflexes at two or more frequencies are included. Numbers in parentheses indicate number of freqencies where reflexes were absent.
†Only scores higher than 0.45 noted.
‡SSW indicates Staggered Spondaic Word test. All scores were overcorrected.
§SSI-ICM indicates Synthetic Sentence Identification with ipsilateral competing message. Only scores falling below normal range noted.
IISSI-CCM indicates Synthetic Sentence Identification with contralateral competing message. Only scores of 80% or poorer noted.
☆Only scores of 70% or poorer noted.

Therefore, the results of the diagnostic battery may be interpreted as strongly suggestive of brainstem dysfunction affecting approximately half the sample.

The compressed speech findings, poor performance on which is regarded as consistent with cortical degeneration,[28,29] need not be regarded as in conflict with the brainstem findings. The coexistence of multiple lesions within the CNS, including sites within the central auditory nervous system, has been reported.[30] Therefore, the present findings should be regarded as indicative of coexistent brainstem and cortical degeneration reflective of the diffuse degenerative process of alcoholism.

The present study must be considered a preliminary exploration of the effects of chronic alcoholism on sites beyond the cochlea. Further research is required to clarify trends in the present data. When aberrant responses are obtained in central auditory evaluation, alcoholism should be considered as a possible etiologic, or minimally contributory, factor.

References

1. Bleuler E: *Textbook of Psychiatry.* New York, Dover Publishers, 1951, p 306.

2. Heller M F: *Functional Otology.* New York, Springer Publishers, 1955, pp 100–109.

3. Morrison W W: *Diseases of the Ear, Nose and Throat,* ed 2. London, Staples Press, Ltd, 1956, p 204.

4. Quick C: Chemical and drug effects on inner ear, in Paparella M M, Shumrick D A (eds): *Otolaryngology.* Philadelphia, W B Saunders Co, 1973, vol 2, p 392.

5. Duchon V J, Bauer M: Hypakusis nach akuter Alkoholvergiftung. *Pract Otorhinolaryngol* 22:94–98, 1960.

6. Courbon P, Chapolaud J: Halluncinations visuelles et unilateralment auditives chez un alcoolique otopathe. *Ann Med Psychol* 95:764–767, 1937.

7. Gross M M, Halpert E, Sabot L, et al: Hearing disturbances and auditory hallucinations in the acute alcoholic psychoses: I. Tinnitus: incidence and significance. *J Nerv Ment Dis* 137:445–465, 1963.

8. Wolff D, Gross M M: Temporal bone findings in alcoholics. *Arch Otolaryngol* 87:350–358, 1968.

9. Nordahl T: Examination of hearing in alcoholics. *Acta Otolaryngol;* suppl 188, 1964, pp 362–370.

10. Montauti G, Paterni F: Rilievi audiometrici negli alcolisti cronici. *Boll Mal Orecchio* 83:500–504, 1965.

11. Cohill E N, Greenberg H J: Effect of ethyl alcohol on the acoustic reflex threshold. *J Am Audiol Soc* 2:121–123, 1977.

12. Robinette M A, Brey R H: Influence of alcohol on the acoustic reflex and temporary threshold shift. *Arch Otolaryngol* 104:31–37, 1978.

13. Gross M M, Begleiter H, Tobin M, et al: Changes in auditory evoked response induced by alcohol. *J Nerv Ment Dis* 143:152–156, 1966.

14. Chandler B C, Vega A, Parsons O A: Dichotic listening in alcoholics with and without a history of possible brain injury. *Q J Stud Alc* 34:1099–1109, 1973.

15. Jerger J, Jerger S: Clinical validity of central auditory tests. *Scand. Audiol* 4:147–163, 1975.

16. Jerger S, Jerger J: Extra- and intra-axial brain stem auditory disorders. *Audiology* 14:93–117, 1975.

17. Jellinek E M: *The Disease Concept of Alcoholism.* New Haven, Conn, Hillhouse Press, 1968.

18. Jerger J, Shedd J, Harford E: On detection of extremely small changes in sound intensity. *Arch Otolaryngol* 69:200–211, 1959.

19. Olsen W O, Noffsinger D: Comparison of one new and three old tests of auditory adaptation. *Arch Otolaryngol* 99:94–99, 1974.

20. Dallos P J, Olsen W O: Integration of energy at threshold with gradual rise-fall tone pips. *J Acoust Soc Am* 36:743–751, 1964.

21. Davis H, Silverman S R: *Hearing and Deafness*, New York, Holt, Rinehart and Winston, 1970, p 493.

22. Spitzer J: *The Auditory Processing Abilities of Chronic Alcoholics*, doctoral dissertation. Teachers College, Columbia University, New York, 1978.

23. Jerger J: Bekesy audiometry in analysis of auditory disorders. *J Speech Hear Res* 3:275–287, 1960.

24. Jerger J, Jerger S: Diagnostic significance of PB word functions. *Arch Otolaryngol* 93:573–580, 1971.

25. Katz J: *The SSW Manual*. St. Louis, Audiotec of St Lous, 1973.

26. Watson C S, Gengel R: Signal duration and signal frequency in relation to auditory sensitivity. *J Acoust Soc Am* 64:989–997, 1969.

27. Wright H N: Clinical measurement of temporal auditory summation. *J Speech Hear Res* 11:109–127, 1968.

28. DeQuiros J B: Accelerated speech audiometry, an examination of test results. *Trans Belton Inst Hear Res*, 1964, No. 17, pp 5–47.

29. Kurdziel S, Noffsinger D, Olsen W: Performance by cortical lesion patients on 40 and 60% time-compressed materials. *J Am Audiol Soc* 2:3#7, 1976.

30. Victor M, Adams R, Collins G: *The Wernicke-Korsakoff Syndrome*. Philadelphia, F A Davis, 1971.

Abstract

Central Auditory Dysfunction in Multiple Sclerosis

David Hicks, M.A.

The use of the SSW Test and performance-intensity functions for phonetically balanced word lists and the Synthetic Sentence Index (SSI) was evaluated for detecting central auditory impairment in a group of 18 individuals with clinically identified multiple sclerosis (MS). Results revealed that 33.3% of the cases studied were identified as having some central auditory involvement. The P–I functions appeared to show the possibility of central auditory dysfunction in 6 of the 18 cases. The SSW Test was consistent with cortical involvement in 2 of the 18 cases. In those cases, the SSW was highly accurate in identifying the area of dysfunction as defined by neurologic reports. The shortcomings of the basic audiometric test battery were remarkably evident in that no central involvement was suggested by the pure-tone audiogram and/or word discrimination scores.

Master's Thesis, California State University, Fresno, 1979

F. Jarman 2-10-84

Abstract

Evaluation of Central Auditory Dysfunction in Temporal Lobe Epilepsy

Martha J. Todebush, M.A.

Ten subjects with clinically confirmed temporal lobe epilepsy were evaluated using the SSW and CES tests. Most of the subjects has experienced grand mal seizures in addition to temporal lobe seizures. All of the subjectswere currently taking Dilantin, usually in combination with another drug, for control of seizure activity. Overall performance revealed the absence of significant abnormal responses suggesting central auditory dysfunction, although 60% of the cases revealed abnormal response patterns, which indicated the presence of nonauditory reception area (NAR) involvement. Of the six subjects revealing abnormal results: (1) two had mildly depressed C-SSW scores; (2) five demonstrated from 2–14 reversals; (3) one showed difficulty on the CES Test; and (4) four showed positive SSW/CES indicators. Four of these subjects indicated well-defined neurological test (e.g., EEG, EMI scan) results. Among the four, three subjects displayed central performance that was highly consistent in the identification of existing localized (nonauditory) lesions. The subjects with the least specific neurological findings, and possibly more diffuse abnormalities, tended to perform normally.

California State University, Fresno, 1979.